Birth Politics

Birth Politics

Colonial Power, Medical Pluralism, and Maternity in Nigeria

Ogechukwu Ezekwem Williams

JOHNS HOPKINS UNIVERSITY PRESS   BALTIMORE

Johns Hopkins University Press
2715 North Charles Street
Baltimore, Maryland 21218
www.press.jhu.edu

Library of Congress Cataloging-in-Publication Data
Names: Williams, Ogechukwu E., author.
Title: Birth politics : colonial power, medical pluralism, and maternity in Nigeria / Ogechukwu E. Williams.
Other titles: Global studies in medicine, science, race, and colonialism.
Description: Baltimore : Johns Hopkins University Press, 2025. | Series: Global studies in medicine, science, race, and colonialism | Includes bibliographical references and index. | Summary: "This book examines the political, religious, and cultural dynamics of childbirth in Nigeria, focusing on how traditional midwives, biomedical maternities, faith-based birthing homes, and international organizations shaped its reproductive landscape"—Provided by publisher.
Identifiers: LCCN 2025001358 (print) | LCCN 2025001359 (ebook) | ISBN 9781421452760 (paperback ; alk. paper) | ISBN 9781421452777 (ebook)
Subjects: MESH: Maternal Health Services—history | Parturition | Birthing Centers—history | Midwifery | Medicine, African Traditional—history | Colonialism—history | History, 20th Century | Nigeria
Classification: LCC RG963.N53 W55 2025 (print) | LCC RG963.N53 (ebook) | NLM WA 11 HN5 | DDC 362.198209669—dc23/eng/20250408
LC record available at https://lccn.loc.gov/2025001358
LC ebook record available at https://lccn.loc.gov/2025001359

A catalog record for this book is available from the British Library.

Special discounts are available for bulk purchases of this book. For more information, please contact Special Sales at specialsales@jh.edu.

EU GPSR Authorized Representative
LOGOS EUROPE, 9 rue Nicolas Poussin, 17000, La Rochelle, France
E-mail: Contact@logoseurope.eu

To Adam, Zikora, Amara, and Ezimma
for all of your sacrifices

Contents

Figures

Acknowledgments

The popular African saying, "It takes a village," applies very much to this project. Research for this book began in 2013, first as a dissertation and then as a book, and involved several summers of archival and ethnographic work. During the extended life of the project, I have encountered the kindness and generosity of many. I am grateful to my family in Nigeria and the United States, as well as countless colleagues, friends, archivists, and research assistants who have contributed in various capacities to this project's success.

My utmost gratitude goes to my husband and biggest cheerleader, Adam Williams, without whose constant support and prodding the timely completion of this project, as a wife and mother, would have been impossible. Many times, he assumed sole care of our babies and encouraged me to get on that airplane to Nigeria or the United Kingdom and complete my archival research and oral histories. For an extended time during the COVID-19 shutdown, when we were both working full-time at home with a toddler and an infant, Adam ensured that I had dedicated hours of protected writing time, during which he assumed full responsibility of the kids while I focused on nothing else but writing. I completed two chapters in that manner in the first two months. I will always remain grateful for all of his kindness and support.

In this book's first life as a dissertation, I received generous guidance from Toyin Falola, Abena Osseo-Asare, Philippa Levine, Gloria Chuku, and Juliet Walker, whom I consider my dream team. Each scholar provided a unique kind of perspective and guidance to my work. Abena's ever generous counsel ensured that I interwove my field experiences into my narratives and analysis, an approach that continues to influence my writing. Juliet Walker made certain that I always thought about my work in terms of the diaspora and how the global may have shaped the local. Philippa Levine kept my work grounded in a gender and empire lens and pointed me toward some key collections in the United Kingdom that I had been unaware of. Gloria Chuku's analytical insight always pushed me to explore boundaries otherwise untouched. Toyin Falola was everything all at once, and I remain grateful for all of the countless hours that he invested in my scholarship.

A number of friends, colleagues, scholars, and intellectual community at UT Austin and Creighton University made an impact on this work. My special thanks to Abimbola Adelakun, Shery Chanis, Dotun Ayobade, Cacee Hoyer, Elizabeth O'Brien, Henry W. Brands, Judith Coffin, and others at UT whose generosity shaped this project at various points during its early stages. I am particularly grateful to UT's Gender Symposium and the history department's Dissertation Colloquium, where several aspects of the dissertation were workshopped. At Creighton University, colleagues Andy Hogan, Surbhi Malik, Adam Sundberg, Lydia Cooper, and Matthew Reznicek provided feedback on various chapters. Elizabeth Elliot-Meisel and Chiwengo Ngwarsungu ensured that my academic work remained on track as I juggled research, teaching, and African studies leadership. Research assistants Thomas Haggstrom and Ethan Meuret helped organize my data at various stages of my research.

Beyond Creighton, I am especially grateful to Saheed Aderinto, Deirdre Cooper Owens, and Jacqueline-Bethel Mougoue, who readily provided layers of support, counsel, and feedback over the course of my research. Barbara Cooper and Lynn Thomas's reading of my chapter on birth control was instrumental in reframing that aspect of my work, and I am grateful for their insights. To all of the scholars at the African Studies Association, American Association for the History of Medicine, Lagos Studies Association, UT Africa Conference, and other academic organizations whose critical insights shaped the ideas for this book at multiple stages, I remain grateful.

In Nigeria, several people made my fieldwork as smooth as possible. I give profound thanks to Chukwuma Opata, Ijeoma Ezenwuba, Emmanuel Chukwuneke, and Esther Ezekwem, who connected me with many interviewees and accompanied me to multiple interviews in oft inaccessible locations, especially in Enugu State. Emmanuel Ogungbemi made my research experience at Ibadan and Lagos seamless by serving as my research assistant and occasional interpreter and helping me navigate the faith-healing community in Ibadan. His connections to Christ Apostolic Church proved priceless over the course of several years. Mama Sewa and Mama Dami, introduced to me by my friend Abimbola Adelakun, organized some of my interviews and accompanied me to several locations in Ibadan during my first visit to that city. Despite the fuel scarcity at Ibadan during that trip, Mama Sewa queued for gas, secured the elusive commodity, and came rushing over to my hotel room to ensure that I attended several interviews on time. Dr. Adebowale Ayobade connected me with many useful contacts at Ibadan who made my experiences in the city even more rewarding.

I want to especially acknowledge the group of scholars at the University of Nigeria whose stewardship shaped my scholarship in multiple ways. My sincere gratitude to Egodi Uchendu, whose mentorship and commitment to women's history at the University of Nigeria solidified my path to studying women. I thank Uchenna Anyanwu, Onwuka Njoku, Chukwuma Opata, Jones Ahazuem, Paul Obi-Ani, Apex Apeh, and Chidi Amaechi for their contributions to the scholarly journey that yielded this project.

Part of this research was completed during the COVID-19 pandemic, setting my work back and making it impossible to travel to my research sites for two years. My research assistants in Nigeria—Emmanuel Ogungbemi, Adeola Adeyemi, Sikiru Yusuff, and Adaobi Ezekwem—kept my work alive and made it possible for me to ultimately get the data that I needed.

My research project would have been impossible to complete without the confidence of the communities who entrusted me with their oral histories and granted me access to their spaces. I am grateful to the midwives and members of the Christ Apostolic Church whose trust has enabled me to tell an important aspect of Nigeria's childbirth story about CAC faith delivery homes that is largely untold. To the countless midwives, nurses, and community elders that trusted me with their oral histories, you have my gratitude.

I am grateful to my family in Nigeria for the numerous times that one or multiple siblings paused their own schedule to accompany me across the country as I completed my work, making sure that I had some assistance, especially when I traveled with kids. My youngest sibling, Onyeka, often doubled as my unofficial research assistant during several visits to the archives in Enugu.

To Heather Fryer, thank you for the careful close reading of my final draft and for the detailed suggestions that enriched the final version of this manuscript. Your generosity as a colleague and a coach will not be forgotten. To the book's peer reviewers and readers, and to my series editor at Johns Hopkins, Ahmed Ragab, I am grateful for all of the time that you invested in this project.

Research for this book was funded in part by multiple grants from the University of Texas at Austin; CURAS, Creighton University; The Kingfisher Institute; and the Rockefeller Archives Center. Publication funding was provided jointly by the University at Buffalo's Humanities Institute (HI) and the Office of the Vice President for Research and Economic Development (OVPRED). I remain grateful for the support of these institutions in bringing this research to fruition.

This is no exhaustive vote of thanks. I appreciate every individual or group that has contributed to this project in any way. *Anyukoo mamiri onu, ogbaa ufufu* (when we join together to accomplish a thing, it is more productive). *Daalu nu . . .* thank you.

On the Politics of Childbirth in Nigeria

An Introduction

This peaceful penetration through the motherhood of the country must do much at least to ensure . . . training of the rising generation.

W. H. S. Curryer, "Mothercraft in Southern Nigeria," *The Nigerian Daily Times*, 1927

The Key Actors

In 2013, I sat outside an old building made of mud and cement as a retired traditional midwife, Mary Ugwuanyi, reminisced about her experiences as a midwife. Mary had originally refused to grant me an audience unless I paid a stipulated sum of money for what she believed to be a training session. She could not understand that I was a researcher attempting to conduct an oral history interview with her on childbirth in Nigeria. To Mary, I was just another midwifery student in one of these "big schools" trying to harness knowledge of local methods. Apparently, Mary, who comes from a line of traditional midwives with a wealth of herbal and therapeutic knowledge that was ancestral, not academic, had received many inquirers from midwifery schools in the city. These students sought to learn traditional techniques for managing pregnancy. Ultimately, Mary began to charge fees for her instructional sessions with the students, marking this kind of engagement not as a mere transfer of knowledge but as a transaction.

Mary's unwavering belief that our oral history interview was instruction in midwifery was not unique to her. In 2016, I met Onyeugwu nwa Ogwo, a retired midwife who was 102 years old at the time and the oldest woman in her community. Like Mary, Onyeugwu could not understand that I was merely a researcher and was convinced that I was training to be a midwife. Nothing I said shifted her perception or how she would engage with me, so I accepted this view and settled into my interview session. Throughout the interview, Onyeugwu punctuated her stories with admonitions of being "selfless and strong-hearted," as this was the greatest quality needed in a midwife.[1] She emphatically stated in the middle of our session, "You have to be courageous and not fidget because at times a woman in labor could be screaming, which could unnerve the midwife, but you don't need to get nervous."[2] I nodded in acknowledgment, without attempting to explain further that I was no midwife. These encounters with Mary, Onyeugwu, and a few other older traditional midwives began to reshape what had begun as an inquiry into traditional birthing practices to an interest in the elaborate landscape of childbirth in Nigeria and the intersections that had become apparent between biomedical maternities and non-Western birthing institutions.

When I left Onyeugwu in Lejja and returned to Nsukka town, I met Chizoba, a traditional midwife who was a household name in the community and the health centers. Chizoba's story of her midwifery practice completely solidified the decision to examine the dominant modes of childbirth in Nigeria and their intertwined relationships. Chizoba, who, like Mary, was from a lineage of traditional midwives, recounted how she had been invited by medical personnel at a major hospital in Enugu to demonstrate her renowned skills as a midwife. This hospital often invited and partnered with well-known traditional midwives in their maternity wards. Here, doctors, nurse-midwives, and matrons watched their traditional counterparts manage complex cases such as breech pregnancies or cord entanglements under close supervision. For several years until 2014, Chizoba, whose skill as a midwife was well proven in this hospital, spent time intermittently in the facility and attended deliveries. She only ended this collaboration because she feared that biomedical personnel might exploit or frame her as she could neither read nor write and relied on people's interpretations of documents and their written renditions of her words. As she put it, "Those who felt threatened and intimidated by my skill might cause me harm."[3]

These sorts of relationships between Chizoba and the hospital in Enugu or Mary and the midwifery students indicated the importance of the contests and intersections that have shaped the relationships between biomedical hospitals and their non-biomedical counterparts. These intersections framed the broader questions that have shaped this project: What was the nature of the connections, intersections, and co-constitutions between traditional midwives and their biomedical counterparts? What did these various modes of childbirth look like on their own, and under what circumstances had it become possible for nurse-midwives to seek out traditional practitioners for training in the traditional ways of managing childbirth? What cultural, religious, and political dynamics in the history of childbirth made these intersections and interconnections possible?

During my research in 2015, a new indigenous maternal health care actor featured in my narrative of Nigeria's political and sociocultural landscape of birth—Aladura (prayer people) faith homes. These were a product of a religious movement, the Aladura movement, that began in the late 1920s largely as a response to racial hierarchies in European missionary churches, the economic depression that followed World War I and the 1918 influenza pandemic, and the failure of Western medicine to provide respite from recurring disease outbreaks and other public health challenges due partly to poor infrastructure and underdeveloped biomedical technology.[4] On the recommendation of a colleague, I visited Lagos and Ibadan in 2015 in search of faith homes where women delivered their babies according to a set principle of faith healing. It became apparent in these cities that the faith homes of an early Aladura denomination, Christ Apostolic Church (CAC), were widespread and organized, and they had a well-established midwifery training school and headquarters in Ede, a city in southwestern Nigeria. Although it was typical throughout the 1930s for Aladura churches to have prayer houses dedicated to tending the sick, what distinguished the CAC was that it was the only Aladura church that focused on the institutionalization of faith homes at a large scale beginning in the colonial era, replete with its own training institution, trained midwifery corps, a set of codified practices, and a national supervisory framework.

At Ede, the Faith Home Midwifery Training Center sported a certificate from the state Ministry of Health identifying it as a certified provider of maternal and infant welfare services. The training center itself had classrooms and a curriculum featuring an academic calendar whose subjects included courses in health education, homiletics, basic anatomy, and parts of speech. This raised the question of how a faith-based maternity center acquired a state-recognized midwifery school and recognition by the Ministry of Health as a legitimate provider of maternity services. As the contemporary narrative of this faith home headquarters unfolded, so did its historical origins as a product of a religious movement in western Nigeria identified by the colonial government as the Aladura movement.[5]

As my field research progressed, I learned that a biomedical nurse-midwife led the faith home in Ede. This was no accident. From 1959, when Joseph Babalola, one of the CAC's founders and its most prominent figure, collaborated with the women's wing of CAC to establish a midwifery school for the church's faith homes, he deliberately reached out to a CAC female evangelist and nurse, Mrs. D. O. Oladiran, to take charge of the training center and the network of CAC faith homes that would spread afterward under the mandates of the training center graduands. Since then, the Ede headquarters have maintained the practice of appointing professionally trained nurses as matrons.

For a church whose doctrine of faith healing eschewed traditional medicine and biomedicine and encoded in its 1946 constitution that CAC women must desist from using hospitals during childbirth, this practice of hiring biomedical nurses to lead its top institution of faith healing stood out.[6] As I explored this trajectory and the faith home's history, it became evident that Babalola made this decision at a time when the church's practice of faith healing was under attack by government officials, who argued that they lacked any structure and jeopardized public health. This move was, therefore, part of an attempt to create a birthing institution that was seen as legitimate and respectable in government and public circles while sustaining its core mission of faith healing. It marked the beginning of a sustained attempt by CAC faith homes to remain relevant in a changing world whose economic and political landscape heralded the need for change.

This book is, thus, a history of intersections, rivalries, negotiations, adaptations, and ultimately pluralism. It explores the politics of childbirth in Nigeria as a product of decades-old rivalry, coexistence, and evolutions that emanated with the onset of colonial rule and the introduction of a Western maternal health care framework in the country. It frames childbirth as a political, religious, and cultural battleground for individual agency and social control, and it demonstrates how various Western and African actors sought to acquire elements of each other's healing practices to build legitimacy in a changing socioeconomic and political landscape. It makes a novel contribution to the literature on childbirth in Africa by examining faith-based delivery homes in the context of colonial and postcolonial struggles to control reproduction. Its approach to co-constitutions and intersections between faith homes, traditional midwifery, and biomedical maternities moves existing narratives on medical pluralism beyond patients' combination of healing therapies to how health care professionals and institutions across various birthing traditions altered their techniques at institutional levels to incorporate or accommodate other healing traditions and, as such, satisfy the needs of the society. The book unravels the history behind Nigeria's contemporary maternal and reproductive landscape and the intersectional roles that indigenous, colonial, and international actors played in the shaping of this arena.

A Subject of Strategic Importance: Birth in Nigeria

Birth Politics is the first comprehensive history of childbirth in Nigeria that not only provides accounts of the predominant birthing traditions in the country but also demonstrates how traditional midwives, agents of biomedicine, and Aladura faith healers collectively shaped the culture of birth or what I describe as Nigeria's *birthscape*—the political, sociocultural, and economic environment that defined Nigeria's maternal health care scene. Scholars like Hibba Abugideiri and Meghan Vaughan have argued for the importance of studying indigenous and Western medical systems in comparison.[7] According to Vaughan, African participation in biomedicine was sometimes a path to constructing new identities.[8] I highlight these new paths by analyzing traditional, biomedical, and faith-based midwifery as distinct and yet intertwined institutions whose evolutions can only be completely understood in context with each other. Ralph Schram's now-classic history of Nigerian health services lays a good foundation for understanding medical missions and the colonial medical in Nigeria.[9] Other scholars provide specific insights into colonial and missionary interventions in childbirth as well as developments in indigenous birthing traditions.[10] However, historical studies of birth in Nigeria remain fragmented and focus largely on the independent examinations of indigenous birthing institutions and biomedical maternities in the colonial era. The historiography is also heavily epidemiological, emphasizing immediate trends that are equally important but lack the background for understanding the present.[11] The field remains short on historical studies of birth, an essential focus area, considering Nigeria's ranking by UNICEF as the second largest maternal and infant death contributor in the world during the early stages of this research in 2014.[12] *Birth Politics*, therefore, makes a vital contribution to current scholarship by evaluating the outcome of a century-long struggle for the control of childbirth, in which traditional midwives, faith healers, and doctors consistently (re)shaped each other's histories and coopted elements of their healing practices in the search for sustained legitimacy in a changing sociopolitical landscape. It lays the background for understanding the contemporary challenges of maternal health care in Nigeria.

Pushing beyond the focus on the traditional childbirth versus colonial maternity framework that dominates current literature, *Birth Politics* examines the persistent phenomenon of faith-based birthing homes, which have become an important component of maternal health in Nigeria and elsewhere in Africa. The book demonstrates how the limits of biomedicine in Nigeria during public health crises and disease outbreaks in the second and third decades of the twentieth century resulted in intervention by Aladura (praying people) churches, a set of independent African churches that arose in western Nigeria during the first quarter of the twentieth century. Aladura congregations established faith homes in the early 1930s that tended to women's reproductive concerns through the tenets of faith healing—based firmly on prayers and divine intervention. The inclusion of faith homes and their practice of maternal health care in this history challenges a plot that privileges colonial and missionary actors as the major protagonists in colonial reproductive politics and as the disruptors of traditional frameworks. This book, thus, has implications for how we can begin to study the history of childbirth in the colonial and postcolonial era, with attention to the roles that African churches continue to play in health-seeking.

Early studies of the Aladura by scholars such as J.D.Y. Peel and Harold Turner in the 1960s have established insights into the origins and organizational structures of various Aladura churches.[13] Other works followed in the 1980s that dwelt largely on the gender dynamics, leadership structure, and theology of the Aladura.[14] While these works have been important to our understanding of these independent African churches, they have mostly overlooked what contemporary members of the CAC, the Aladura church that is explored in this book, refer to as faith homes or faith delivery homes and the historical nature of the positions that they occupied in Nigeria's maternal health care setting. I demonstrate how the CAC, which was not aligned with traditional or biomedical conceptions of maternal care, maneuvered between and within these dominant systems and adopted elements from each realm to remain relevant and responsive in a changing colonial and postcolonial landscape. By advancing discourses of the Aladura beyond the realm of theology and into colonial and postcolonial medicine, *Birth Politics* brings the agency of African spiritual actors in the contests over the control of reproduction clearly into view.

Similarly, the urgency of incorporating the Aladura in this or any study of childbirth highlights the expanding role of spirituality and spiritual spaces in understanding the interpretations of health and well-being in African societies.[15] African traditional religions have, in general, reflected the important role of the supernatural in health care. This belief in the spiritual dimensions of certain health conditions plays a dominant role in women's decisions and that of their families to access care within a hospital network, in a faith home or other faith-based organization, or with a traditional medicine practitioner. A 2014 study by three Nigerian gynecologists concluded, for instance, that "our women desire spiritual care during pregnancy and childbirth. Its incorporation into maternal health services will improve hospital delivery rates," highlighting the importance of institutions like the Aladura in shaping health-seeking behaviors.[16] Also, the sustained inadequacies of biomedical maternities in Nigeria continue to play a role in the preponderance of faith-based medicine. Decades after they arrived on the scene, CAC faith homes' popularity remains fueled by the primary reason that brought them into existence: the shortcomings of biomedicine. Understanding the roles that CAC's faith homes have historically played in maternity care, as well as the services that make them attractive to the populace, offers glimpses into health-seeking behaviors and how they have shaped the choice of care.

Birth Politics is very much a history of medical pluralism—a term that researchers of African medicine have described as an intersection of therapies, patients, and medical frameworks, or the nonexclusive multiple layers of therapeutics that individuals and families embrace in the search for healing—as it is of childbirth.[17] Works on medical pluralism, such as Olsen and Sargent's *African Medical Pluralism*, Acobson-Widding and David Westerlund's *Culture Experience and Pluralism*, M. Dekker and Rijk van Dijk's *Markets of Wellbeing*, and Jonathan Roberts's *Sharing the Burden of Sickness*, focus on how patients in Africa combine therapies.[18] Olsen and Sargent begin their important volume with the following question: "How do individuals and communities make sense of disease in contemporary Africa? What medical options arise in the pursuit of medical care?"[19] These questions are reflective of the focus of scholarship on medical pluralism. *Birth*

Politics follows a different trajectory and focuses not only on the diverse healing modalities that communities draw from but also largely on how various medical professionals and institutions have altered their therapies and methods, notably at the institutional level, to harness opportunities and fulfill the demands that communities' health-seeking behaviors have created. In other words, it examines the ways in which institutions of healing have sought to adopt techniques within their own practice that bridge with the methodologies of other healing traditions.

As the book demonstrates, these professional and institutional-level pluralisms manifested in how traditional midwives, for instance, modified their trainings to include apprenticeships with nurses or sought certifications as a Traditional Birth Attendant (TBA), a term that the World Health Organization introduced in the 1980s to identify individuals who received informal training on safe delivery from biomedical staff.[20] These pluralisms also materialized in the ways that faith homes professionalized and created a midwifery school and referral systems that served the changing needs of the society, as well as in the changes that biomedical professionals permitted within the hospitals or enacted in their training policies to accommodate local attitudes.

Beyond the examination of medical pluralism as the institutional intersection of healing traditions, I also explain medical pluralism as a process created by intersections and power struggles in the political, economic, sociocultural, and religious realm, which in turn created the atmosphere for the existence of new or co-constituted medical traditions. *Birth Politics*, therefore, views the crossings of various birthing traditions in Nigeria within the broader lenses of political power struggles, socioeconomic survival, and fights for legitimacy. Narratives of medical pluralism in Africa also focus heavily on the changes and adaptations made by the less dominant or marginalized indigenous systems. *Birth Politics* addresses this area but also highlights the overlooked series of negotiations and changes that occurred within the biomedical realm itself, especially as a result of personnel shortages, competition from the Aladura, and low utilization of hospitals for birth throughout the colonial era.

Women's Reproduction: Contested Sites

Throughout history, women's reproduction has been a site of constant struggle for power, control, and nation-building. In Africa, this politics of reproduction received heightened attention during the colonial era as Western colonial powers grappled with and sought to reshape the colonial landscape based on their own perceptions of women, gender, and reproduction. In colonial Nigeria, gendered ideologies were reconfigured to reflect that of the British metropole and manifested themselves in sociocultural processes like marriage and education, new or redefined political and economic institutions, and gendered divisions of labor.[21] In Britain during the late nineteenth and early twentieth centuries, a high infant mortality rate and panic over a declining population resulted in a focus on mothers as the culprits for and solutions to this problem of an unhealthy nation. By the twentieth century, it became even more so "the duty and destiny of women to be 'mothers of the race.'"[22] Other roles that British women increasingly undertook, notably as workers outside the home, received condemnation as proof of incompetence and irresponsibility to mothercraft.[23] The latter term, *mothercraft*, had become defined by public health professionals and voluntary organizations in Britain in the early twentieth century as encompassing the proper approaches to mothering and childrearing. These nineteenth- and early twentieth-century ideologies of British women's positions in society became relied on by missionaries in Nigeria as a roadmap for Christianizing and "civilizing" the local population.

The importance of childbirth and reproduction in colonial and missionary constructions of empire is well established.[24] Scholars like Nancy Hunt, Walima Kalusa, Carol Summers, and Jean Allman have highlighted the new forms of social power that intervention in childbirth opened up to missionaries.[25] Lynn Thomas, Amy Kaler, and Beverly Chalmers similarly demonstrate the importance of birth and reproduction to local politics.[26] The fight to Christianize and civilize manifested in various ways, but (re)constructions of birth and motherhood soon became identified as the vulnerable event in women's lives through which missionaries and the colonial administration could gain access to families and change individual lives and social structures.[27] Missionary interventions in the reproductive lives of Nigerian women were matched by greater government involvement in maternal welfare services from the 1930s and the consequent professionalization of midwifery as a viable field of employment for Nigerian women based on the now-familiar belief that interventions in the home and in the upbringing of children would make for a healthier population. A healthier society was also believed to cast the colonial enterprise more favorably. Lord Frederick Lugard, the first governor-general of Nigeria, explained the rationale for future expansions of hospitals and dispensaries based on the logic that this would "popularize our rule, and to check the present mortality."[28]

The interventions that ensued in the realm of gender and reproduction altered the traditional balance of power in the indigenous society, which consequently had far-reaching effects in the professional field of midwifery. Ndubueze Mbah makes the point, for instance, that British colonial rule was a patriarchal assault that eroded parallel male–female political institutions and instead mass-produced "wage earning men and domesticated women."[29] In many cases, missionaries and colonial officials were ignorant of precolonial institutions that balanced power between male and female political and social institutions. As such, they established a male-dominated colonial machinery that was ignorant of or oblivious to female power and empowered men over women in the emerging colonial framework. Under these circumstances, access to Western education for women under the colonial regime in Nigeria took the back seat until conversations about securing the future labor supply of the colony through government interventions in birth and motherhood forced a review of female education and gave a boost to the expansion of nursing and midwifery facilities, including training institutions, as an avenue through which women could increasingly participate in the colonial machinery in the 1940s.

Nonetheless, the colonial establishment did not enact these goals of altering cultural trends in birth and motherhood without resistance. In the traditional politics of reproduction, motherhood was an important milestone for married women, and mothering was a communal affair. The rituals associated with birth also reinforced sociocultural ties and familial relations and propagated age-old views of gender and gendered spaces, such as the space of childbirth itself. Those who presided over birth were mostly older women from expecting parents' families or traditional midwives, all of whom served as custodians of the society's views of acceptable motherhood and legitimate births. The colonial encroachment into these spaces, therefore, threatened multiple cultural processes that various community figures sought to protect either through direct or subtle resistance or through their own reappropriation of the unfolding process of Westernization for their own purposes.

This local reappropriation of colonial processes manifested itself clearly in the case of twin infanticide, a culture-bound practice in parts of southern Nigeria that missionaries identified as one of the woes of local mothercraft.[30]

Under this practice, locals believed that the birth of twins or multiplets was a taboo outcome that could spell negative repercussions for the community. While missionaries threatened legal action and arrest of those found guilty of twin killings, local communities sought ways to exploit missionary actions for their own convenience. When missionaries expressed the desire to establish twinneries—accommodations for discarded twins—some local communities readily offered to build these homes in mission outposts with the goal of removing these twin children from the communities to mission outposts, the new "evil forest" in the community for discarding cursed or unwanted items. Others had more sinister goals of quietly eliminating one or both twins in these mission-run properties so that it was impossible for such deaths to be traced to them. In other cases, some communities in the 1920s and 1930s resorted to the neglect of one or both twin babies or the elimination of one at birth because such deaths could not be proven as murder in colonial courts due to the plethora of health challenges that ordinarily confronted twins.

In some cases, interventions in birth required government officials to forge alliances with the very female local authorities and institutions they sought to undermine. In Ondo Province, for instance, medical officers resorted to relying on female chiefs and other prominent women to supervise the activities of junior midwives in village clinics and local dispensaries and, therefore, use the women's authority to compel midwives' compliance with health officers' demands.[31] Medical officers hoped that "these women chiefs who had a good deal of influence" would also become instrumental in encouraging women in their communities to take part in activities hosted at the maternity homes.[32] Advances in colonial maternal and infant welfare projects sometimes depended on such collaborations. These locals participated likely because of the visibility, access, and recognition within the colonial service that such roles gave them.

In the new space of birth created by the Aladura, women's reproduction featured as a point of contention between the colonial government and the Aladura but also as a building block for CAC's popularity. The conceptions of reproduction as crucial to economic life and, for the locals, as important to a woman's security and reputation in her marital home compelled Yoruba women to seek solutions for infertility in the revival services of Joseph Babalola. Babalola himself did not set out to undertake issues of maternity care as the building block for his religious ministry, but the needs that women presented as well as the persistence of infertility, higher in western Nigeria according to colonial records than elsewhere in the country, gave him a reputation for undertaking "welfare work (pre-natal and post-natal) for the craving woman."[33]

Beyond the colonial era, the contest over women's reproduction featured in the international race, rooted in early twentieth-century eugenicist ideals, to save the world from domination by lesser elements—the nonwhite races—and ultimately from a population crisis that was anticipated to be triggered by the developing world. In Nigeria, this international politics of population control manifested on the bodies of women as canvasses for enacting social and political change. The suppression of women's reproduction, different from the colonial-era goal of encouraging it, led once again to a push to educate women. This time, this education was not in the service of maximizing reproduction, as in the colonial era, but its curtailment. Those who pushed for the expansion of women's education during this era viewed this as an avenue for delayed childbearing and, ultimately, fewer children. The pushback in Nigeria against what became known as the birth control movement and family planning led to an indigenization of this movement to reflect local values and highlight ties with local cultures of child spacing. Those who opposed birth control, predominantly men and religious authorities, argued that it erased society's ability to map the sins of immorality on the bodies of women who could evade the policing of their bodies through the use of birth control.

The Fields of Play: Scope

This contest over birth spans the twentieth century, beginning in the early 1900s and ending in the 1990s, and occurred in various phases as colonial, national, and global developments changed the fields of play and the outcomes that were sought. It manifested in attempts that began in the early twentieth century to relocate birth from the home and the control of traditional midwives to hospitals and government- or mission-trained personnel. It also featured a birth control politics in the postindependence era, driven by international population control activists who sought to curtail birth and reshape interpretations of women's reproduction. The Nigerian infant—the product of birth—was viewed differently by the various main actors—traditional midwives, medical missions, colonial maternities, Aladura faith healers, and international population control advocates—at varying points in this struggle. These various outlooks of birth and babies manifested in conflicts, intersections, and adaptations that have shaped Nigeria's colonial and postcolonial history of childbirth.

For traditional midwives and their local communities, babies represented the bonds that reinforced society's social networks and were, thus, subject to the care and protection of not only their parents but also their local communities. For Christian missionaries, they were souls to be saved from paganism: the desired embodiments of Western civilization. The colonial government viewed them from the late 1920s as future labor supply that guaranteed continued extraction of the colony's agricultural resources for the benefit of the metropole. Their survival through childhood was, therefore, important for the colonial machinery. As a Christian organization, Aladura faith healers viewed their work of faith healing as a godly service to their community and proof of God's healing power over traditional and biomedical remedies. Their intervention in childbirth became an avenue for evangelism but also the platform on which they could build political and sociocultural legitimacy. The international organizations that joined the fray in the late 1950s viewed women's reproduction differently from Britain's outlook of maximizing birth and minimizing wastages from infant deaths. Each potential birth in Nigeria was regarded by some in these organizations as tipping the balance of power between Black and white peoples across the world and triggering a population explosion.

Birth Politics opens with an examination of the traditional contexts of birth and motherhood as well as the birth rituals and sociopolitical networks that the local birthing traditions upheld. Using a case study of the Igbo, the ethnic community in which an acclaimed missionary maternity work based in Iyi-Enu was sited at the dawn of the twentieth century, the book's first chapter provides a framework for understanding the strategy by missionaries to target childbirth as an avenue for advancing a Christian missionary agenda. The traditional religious system among the Igbo in the first quarter of the twentieth century vested in women control over fertility rites and religious rituals associated with procreation. Upon becoming mothers, married women received their own homesteads from where they exerted control and ideological influence. Their membership in exclusive associations, as mothers, also granted them spiritual, judicial, and political powers in their communities. Missionary intervention in childbirth provided direct access to these women—these custodians of tradition—with a desire to interrupt the generational transmission of pagan rites and claim the souls of newborns for Christ. This local context also makes it possible to evaluate how local actors rejected, embraced, or inserted themselves in Western institutions of birth in efforts to navigate the unfolding political, social, and economic terrains brought on by colonialism.

Although various missionary groups were active in Nigeria, *Birth Politics* focuses primarily on the activities of the Church Missionary Society (CMS), the largest mission group to establish itself in Nigeria in the mid-nineteenth century and one that was considered to have "the greatest influence in Nigeria."[34] For decades after the CMS arrived in what became Nigeria in 1842, it did not undertake large-scale medical work and had no medical mission policy. However, the arrival of its fiercest competitor in this scramble for African souls, the Roman Catholic Mission (RCM), at the end of the nineteenth century compelled the CMS to adopt medical care as a deliberate policy to gain an upper hand over the RCM. In the Medical CMS Mission (under the Niger Mission), which the CMS established in 1898 and became Iyi-Enu Mission Hospital in 1907, large-scale maternity work unfolded earlier than it did among any other missionary group largely because this medical mission location was overseen almost exclusively by female European missionaries, resulting in full-scale maternity work that became lauded by European visitors and commended by the colonial administration. Iyi-Enu Hospital's reputation as "a woman's show" throughout the first quarter of the early twentieth century shaped decisions by CMS's London headquarters to send only female doctors to this location. This reputation and their impact in the maternity realm also attracted partnerships with the colonial governor of Nigeria, Donald Cameron, who launched his mobile Lady Doctor enterprise specifically in partnership with the Iyi-Enu hospital network. Tracing the missionary dimension of this contest primarily through the CMS and their famous Iyi-Enu Hospital, as well as CMS intersections with the Aladura, whose leaders were mostly former members of the mission group's Anglican congregations, offers detailed insight into the birth politics that unravels.

Government involvement in Nigeria's *birthscape* accelerated from the 1930s. Unlike the CMS, which jumped into the maternity realm at the end of the nineteenth century under the premise that relocating birth from traditional midwives and homes to hospitals would result in the conversion of mothers, their children, and entire communities, the colonial government's sidelining of women meant that maternal health care infrastructure or personnel was sparse in the colony, with long-lasting effects on the professionalization of midwifery. The government's realization that infertility, sexually transmitted diseases, and the generally high infant mortality rates in its prized colony threatened its future labor supply in Nigeria launched it into the bid to regulate birth and women's reproduction. To make up for lost ground, government partnered with missionaries, whose work it previously dissociated from, because most of the existing medical infrastructure beyond major cities belonged to missionaries. Locals, themselves, were not left out of these emerging contests but embraced, adapted, or rejected the various changes that missionaries and the government foisted on them.

Local agency, (re)appropriation, and adaptation, especially by independent African churches, become most visible in chapter 3, where the shortcomings of biomedicine and biomedical remedies led to the advent of a new site of birth—faith homes. Colonial correspondences, missionary magazines, and oral interviews show the emergence of faith delivery homes to be a product of an indigenous religious institution's insertion of itself in the colonial politics of birth and reproduction. CAC, the Aladura church that this part of the book focuses on, has been classified by Deidre Crumbley, who produced major studies of Nigeria's Aladura churches, as "the most institutionally self-aware" of its era.[35] CAC was the only indigenous church that institutionalized its faith homes, replete with its own school of midwifery and cadre of midwives. CAC's participation in Nigeria's *birthscape* first began due to the increasing concern by women in western Nigeria about (in)fertility, a problem that biomedical responses in the 1920s and 1930s could not readily fix. The movement's popularity among women, as well as the attention that it paid to women's maternity issues, put it and its foremost leader, Babalola, at a crossroads with the missionary and colonial agenda, leading to opposition from the latter parties. These assaults from missionaries and government officials against the Aladura helped push Babalola and the women's wing of CAC toward professionalization of the faith homes in 1959. Meanwhile, CAC women sought to use the emerging faith homes as a new and assured way to participate in the growing field of midwifery and private maternities across the country.

The latest actors in this politics of birth arrived on the scene in the late 1950s, shortly before Nigeria's independence. These international organizations, such as the Rockefeller Foundation, Population Council, and Ford Foundation, were primarily based in the US and heralded a politics of birth control from the 1950s through the 1980s that had been suggested to Britain but was rejected due to the British focus on boosting birth and infant survival for their own purposes. The international organizations whose influence multiplied in colonized or formerly colonized territories in the post–World War II era due to the financial resources that they often provided enacted a shift from the colonial-era goals of maximizing reproduction to the postcolonial goals of curtailing it. A combination of local resistance against what some considered as "pill peddlers" and a European attempt to undercut the African population, as well as global developments in women's health, compelled this birth control movement to coalesce into a family planning project that was tailored especially for Nigeria's local context.

Ultimately, these birth control efforts heralded a safe motherhood era in the 1980s that amplified the weaknesses of existing maternal health frameworks. The new politics of birth that emerged at Nigeria's independence, as well as broader economic developments in this era, impacted the postcolonial contest over birth and maternity and accelerated a proliferation of medical pluralisms and partnerships that shaped the maternity sector during this period. In the case of the Aladura and their traditional counterparts, the increased scrutiny that came with the safe motherhood era in the 1980s resulted in efforts to improve their services and remain competitive in a changing political and economic landscape.

These intersections and partnerships among the main actors in Nigeria's *birthscape*, some conflicting and others collaborative, especially come to the fore in the final chapter. The reactions and adaptations were not limited to local actors but included biomedical maternities and postcolonial squabbles with their traditional and faith home counterparts over influence and access to clientele. Biomedical maternities responded to local expressions of agency, including the continued acceptance of prenatal care but low utilization of hospital births. In the face of Nigeria's economic depression in the 1980s and the global shift from population control to interest in maternal deaths, these major maternal health care actors scrambled to adjust their practices to address internal and external concerns about maternal deaths. CAC faith homes adjusted their anti-biomedicine stance and implemented partnerships with hospitals to improve outcomes and avoid narratives of illegality. Traditional gynecologists and midwives underwent similar changes to claim legitimacy, resulting in what some traditional doctors described as "trado-western maternities" and the emergence of a new category of traditional midwives—Traditional Birth Attendants—whose practices sometimes combined traditional methods with elements of biomedicine. This era of blurred lines, blended practices, and a plural attitude to the choice of maternity care shaped contemporary Nigeria's maternal health landscape and is crucial to understanding the roles that religion, politics, and culture have played in maternal health care.

Researching Women: The Dilemma of Sources

The evidence for *Birth Politics* is drawn primarily from oral histories and written documents stored in a wide range of archives. During my initial visit to Nigeria's national archives at Ibadan in 2016, the limitations of archival research and the subjective choices over what histories are recorded or preserved in them quickly became evident. As I scoured through the three folders that I could find on Aladura churches or their prophets, I found no mention of faith homes.[36] Rather, the folder entitled "The Faith Healer Babalola" briefly spoke about the popularity of Babalola's revival services among women as well as the attention that he paid to reproductive health concerns.[37] This, however, was the extent of the discourse on their early involvement with reproduction and reproductive health.

At the Cadbury Research Library in the University of Birmingham, UK, later that year, boxes of the CMS documents as well as their yearly magazines further painted a picture of the prominent role that women and women's reproduction played in Babalola's early following. In one of these documents, CMS's Archdeacon Dallimore pointed out that Babalola gave particular consideration to women's maternity needs and offered "the good news for the soul; cure for the ills of the body; and knowledge and welfare work (pre-natal and post-natal) for the craving woman."[38] In Dallimore's opinion, Babalola's popularity partly derived from the views among locals that his revival meetings facilitated pregnancies and addressed infertility.[39] While these documents offered glimpses into Babalola's approach to faith healing and the number of women who sought attention in his revival services, they did not include information on the faith homes. This was partly because the faith homes became organized exclusively as a maternity facility in 1958 and 1959 but also because there was an established pattern in the colonial archives of overlooking or underreporting issues about women. By the time that CAC adopted its 1946 constitution that barred their members from using hospitals for birth and, thus, laid the foundations of an organized faith delivery home, colonial coverage of the Aladura had declined due to the decrease in government anxiety over the movement's potential to spur a political revolution. There was little incentive, therefore, for the continued government recording of Aladura activities to the extent that they did in the prior decade.

My knowledge of faith homes and their place in the history of childbirth in colonial and postcolonial Nigeria expanded, instead, as I visited CAC pastors, midwives, and church elders in Lagos, Ibadan, and Ede in an intermittent five-year ethnographic quest to Nigeria to seek out more contexts to augment the bits and pieces of information in the archives.[40] These journeys were crucial for piecing together a history, absent in official records, of CAC faith homes and their increasingly important role in Nigeria's contemporary *birthscape*. It tracked CAC faith homes' evolution throughout the 1980s and 1990s in the face of changing socioeconomic landscapes and a growing local and global attention on maternal deaths. The field research that ensued involved oral interviews and follow-up interviews of faith home midwives, their biomedical partners, CAC officials, faith home clientele, and all three surviving faith home matrons who presided over the training center in the 1980s, 1990s, and the present.

In Lagos and Ede, my research sometimes took the form of focus group interviews that involved women who had congregated for the weekly prayer meetings required of pregnant women registered in the faith homes. I had not planned these group sessions but had arrived unbeknownst to me on the weekday of the prayer meeting. After introductions to the midwife and the church's presiding priest, I was ushered into the meetings and, in this manner, became a participant observer in the prayer sessions that followed. This process of observation highlighted for me the persistent cultural outlooks of the Yoruba that had shaped Aladura pregnancy care, such as belief in *Abiku* (spirit children), evil eye, sacred water, and sacred words. It also highlighted women's search for protection from pregnancy complications that could lead to expensive cesarean sections or stillbirth. In many ways, it uncovered for me some of the motives that shaped women's choices of faith homes for birth.

The fieldwork among CAC congregations brought to the fore the gendered hierarchies among the CAC, as manifested in their recounting of the faith home's history. All interviewees, including members of the CAC Good Women, the church's department that was instrumental in the permanence that faith homes have enjoyed in the CAC structure, attributed developments in the faith home to males. However, the details of their narratives pointed to larger economic and political factors, explored in chapter 3, that CAC women sought to navigate in a manner that created for them careers in the burgeoning field of midwifery, within the CAC's confines of faith healing. With this realization, my narratives of CAC faith homes shifted from the male figures that the women signposted, one of whom was the church's most important figure—Babalola—to a look at the broader picture in this story of local agency in the politics of birth.

Although Babalola was an important and rather indispensable part of this story of faith delivery homes, my questions and analysis shifted to factors, beyond Babalola, that led to the professionalization of these faith homes in the late 1950s and their expansion in the postcolonial era. This shift in my analysis aligned the evolution of CAC faith homes to developments in the broader maternal health landscape. These external developments included the expansion of biomedical maternities as a viable field of employment for women and the government clampdown on the many auxiliary nurses and midwives whose limited education precluded them in the 1950s from government employment. A professionalized faith home, with its own training institution and locations where trainees could secure employment, ensured for CAC women a path to a new or continued career in midwifery. Here, the archives and the oral histories merged to produce a robust interpretation of local agency within a broader political setting.

Beyond the archival documents and the oral histories of the Aladura, I do a close reading of *Christ Apostolic Church @ 90*, published by Joshua Alokan, a CAC pastor who became a member of the church in the aftermath of the Aladura movement and witnessed a lot of the developments that he chronicles.[41] Although Alokan's text focuses mostly on the church's growth and was published for church members during CAC's ninetieth anniversary, it provides bits of information, including the author's firsthand experiences on certain developments connected to the faith home's history. This book, unavailable for sale elsewhere, was lent to me by a CAC pastor on one of my visits to his church. He had assured me that some of the answers that I sought in my oral interviews on colonial-era developments in CAC were addressed in the book, and when I returned this book to the pastor in the following year, he gifted it to me and it became an important resource to my research on twentieth-century CAC. Babalola's own teachings and publications, compiled and translated from Yoruba to English by Moses Idowu in 2000, also offer insight into the principles of health care that guided the faith home's model of maternity care and highlighted Babalola's emphasis on not only prayers but also cleanliness and nutrition for a positive pregnancy outcome.[42]

The challenge of finding faith homes in the archives reflected a bigger dilemma of locating women and women's institutions in colonial archives. Until the Women's War of 1929, in which women in southeastern Nigeria clashed with colonial administrators over the government's taxation policies, the colonial government largely sidelined women and wrote them into official records largely as marginal figures but rarely ever on their own merits as powerbrokers or influential actors in their communities. These British perceptions shaped outlooks of women in colonial Nigeria such that when the Women's War broke out, government officials failed to comprehend that women organized such a massive movement independent of their men.[43] In the aftermath of this women's uprising, the colonial government commissioned intelligence reports on southern Nigerian women. Beyond this measure, nonetheless, the outlook on women as marginal figures shaped the availability of documents on women in the archives.

When I set out to the National Archives in Enugu in 2013 in search of colonial-era data on traditional birthing institutions, the lack of any detailed documentation on the subject became immediately obvious. What was available were anthropological reports that addressed "native medicine" and sometimes offered brief glimpses into childbirth. C. K. Meek's anthropological report on Igbo customs included information on birth rituals sparsely distributed across its pages, but beyond this, data on childbirth among Nigerian cultures existed in scanty forms, often submerged under brief sections on marriage.[44] Amaury Talbot's ethnography, compiled during her journeys through the southeastern regions of Nigeria and published in 1915, also provided glimpses into fertility rites and practices around reproduction during the early twentieth century.[45] Beyond these brief coverages, childbirth among locals was not of importance to the colonial institution until the 1930s and did not feature in any significant way in archival records. Government records on matters surrounding maternity remained scanty until the second quarter of the twentieth century.

Mitigating this paucity of sources regarding the traditional birthing institution in government records meant drawing largely from oral history narratives on the subject. This paucity of written sources also solidified my decision to adopt a case study approach to the chapter on traditional childbirth. This case study approach allowed for conducting an in-depth analysis of traditional birthing practices without running into the problems of overgeneralizations across a culturally diverse country like Nigeria in a project that was not only about traditional childbirth but of four major actors in Nigeria's *birthscape*. The choice of this region as a case study was well fitting as conflicts between missionaries and their local hosts over birthing traditions were visible in this setting as it was here that one of the most lauded works of maternity care by any missionary group—Iyi-Enu Mission Hospital—was located. The search for these oral history narratives took me to the History Department Library at the University of Nigeria (UNN), where the department stored unabridged and unedited oral history transcripts of projects completed by its students. These transcripts became very useful in acquiring interviews conducted in earlier decades on various Igbo communities regarding traditional midwifery.[46] Beyond these transcripts, I visited various communities in Anambra, Enugu, and Imo between 2013 and 2016 to seek out midwives and community elders for their historical narratives.

In Nsukka, Enugu State, the search for traditional midwives took me to rural health centers and the Ministry of Health. There I found documents on the training of midwives and was directed to prominent traditional midwives that I could interview. Since there was hardly any contact information for these midwives, I embarked on trips to communities in the interior with no guarantee that I could meet with the midwives I sought. These journeys provided a different kind of insight into the challenges of maternal health care and the indispensable nature of alternative modes of birth for some communities. On many occasions, I trekked for miles with no hope of transportation back to the town. After the first few experiences of trekking, I contracted drivers to take me to my interview locations and stay with me throughout the duration of my day's sojourn to avoid being stranded with no means back to my lodgings. These companions proved very useful as they often inserted themselves into the interviews with their own questions or further clarifications.

The data from the interviews were augmented by missionary documents that I retrieved from the national archives in Enugu and Ibadan and UK's Cadbury Research Library in Birmingham, along with records from the British

Library, London; Wellcome Library, London; and British National Archives, Kew. Since childbirth was of importance to early missionary groups in Nigeria, especially the CMS, whose work in maternal health in the Niger Mission (which at one point extended to the Hausaland Mission in the north) had been hailed in 1927 as "one of the very best bits of medical works" in Nigeria, missionaries who viewed traditional midwives as the bastion of evil often recorded birthing practices that they viewed negatively.[47] Some missionary periodicals, notably the *Church Missionary Gleaner* and the *Medical Missionary*, were useful for discourses on the origins of medical missions and the mindset behind missionary involvement in maternity services.

The British Library, Wellcome Library, and the British National Archives provided minimal details on traditional birth but had ample documentation of medical developments in Nigeria. Relevant documents from these archives, dating from the 1920s, included data on maternal health as government interest in maternal health care expanded. Before this period, no maternal health section existed in the colonial government's annual medical reports, and the government did not build its first maternity hospital until 1929. By the 1930s, maternal health had become part of the rhetoric in the government's growing obsession with securing its future labor supply in the colony and building a more positive outlook on colonial rule. The British National Archives, for instance, had extensive records on annual medical reports, foreign and colonial office files, records on medical developments in Nigeria, and reports on various colonial districts. In particular, the Wellcome Library provided detailed annual medical reports on all the provinces of Nigeria from the early 1900s through the 1960s, as well as information on the birth control politics in which an independent Nigeria became immersed. In the British Library, the newspaper database on Nigeria was useful for highlighting colonial officials' views of women and women's education, especially between the 1920s and 1940s.

Beginning in the 1950s, shortly before independence, Nigeria, described as Africa's economic and numerical giant, featured prominently in international discourses of population control. To capture these perspectives on *Birth Politics*, I turned to the Rockefeller Archives Center (RAC) in New York, the repositories of foundations like Carnegie, Rockefeller and the Rockefeller-funded Population Council, and Ford, who were early participants in the 1950s population control movement. I first learned about the Rockefeller archives in September 2015 during a discussion with a colleague at the University of Texas, Austin, about my preliminary research at the British National Archives and Cadbury Research Library in Birmingham, UK, during the previous summer. This colleague encouraged me to contact an archivist at RAC about documents on Nigeria. I hesitated, thinking out loud, "What could an archive in New York have on early Nigerian history?" Ultimately, I consulted the RAC database and found a plethora of documents on health projects in Nigeria ranging between 1879 and 1999. These records helped advance this book's scope beyond the colonial era, demonstrating how the politics of childbirth developed beyond the colonial government and missionaries. In the case of Nigeria, the goals of US-based international organizations like Ford and Rockefeller on reproduction gradually replaced those of Britain as the country geared up for independence. The various documents on the origins of and rationale for the population control movement and the forms that it took in Nigeria highlight this increased role of international organizations in the politics of birth during the late colonial and postcolonial era.

All of these sources have shaped the various narratives explored in the pages of this book and demonstrate the indispensably interwoven relationships between the various key actors that are explored here. The book now opens with a look at the local contexts of birth, laying a background for understanding and analyzing all else that unfolds in the *birthscape* that emerges.

1

Local Mothercraft

Traditional Birthing Institutions and the Politics
of Reproduction

A child belongs to all because you don't know what the child would be or of
what use they would become to the society. A child is not only relevant to
the family but to the society at large.

Onyeugwu Nwa Ogwo, interview, April 6, 2015

The back that bears the black baby bears also the burden of
Africa's future.

The Nigerian Daily Times, October 31, 1928

Introduction

In 1928, an undisclosed British writer took to *The Nigerian Daily
Times*, a popular Nigerian newspaper, to write several articles on the need
for African women education. This writer, although nameless in the various
newspaper publications on African women's education, was clearly an
important personality in colonial circles as he wrote authoritatively about
education, referenced his decades of experiences in Britain's African colonies,
offered a keynote address at an education conference in Dar es Salaam in
October 1925, and received memoranda on this theme from missionaries. In
his articles, he argued that the social and economic development among
"the native races" rested on interventions in the lives of women and the
colonial machinery's ability to exploit such interventions.[1] "For the creation
of a healthy social system," the author wrote, "we must look to the home,
and the home is the woman's province."[2]

In a series from October 31, 1928, he wrote this assessment of the African woman's influence: "That 'The hand that rocks the cradle rules the world,' we have probably never doubted, as applied in Western civilizations, and yet it is not an uncommon assumption that the African woman is down-trodden, inarticulate drudge, without influence. This is far from the truth; she has influence and uses it."[3] His assertion was a reaction to a British educational policy that directed efforts at formal Western education in African colonies at male subjects at the expense of females whose roles were understood by British officials to be away from the public realm of sociopolitical affairs. He argued that it was understandable for male education to take priority over female education given the longstanding prejudices in the past "in other civilizations even more advanced than Africa is today."[4] Nonetheless, he reasoned, it was imperative that the colonial enterprise looked at female education albeit differently than the type of education that involved technology and "the machinery of teaching."[5] His ideal form of women's education would exploit "the vast educational power of the home" to make inroads into family life and the social fabric of the society.[6]

Throughout the 1920s and 1930s, this writer and other British officers argued that colonial health and social agenda would best be advanced where "an existing social system can be given its fullest economic expression with the assistance of medical and educational science."[7] Officials began to see in African women's motherhood and mothering the answer to colonial advancement and the success of health and social propaganda. Solutions to the problems of economic development, social advancement, and a reliable labor supply—which were frequently discussed in the context of local infant mortality rates—were increasingly connected to the home and the social and familial network that the home represented.

To back up their argument, colonial administrators cited missionaries and missionary work in Nigeria prior to the second quarter of the twentieth century. These administrators argued that missionaries, who had hitherto dominated the Western education of colonial subjects and had been closely connected with local populations, had proven the importance of advancing their agendas through a focus on the home front, "the woman's province."[8] In 1926, the superintendent of education in southern Nigeria, W. H. S. Curryer, made exactly this argument, highlighting missionary work in his region and arguing that the "peaceful penetration through the motherhood of the country," as advanced by missionaries, had proven to make significant inroads in reshaping attitudes within the home and raising a new generation that may be more amenable to colonial policies and agenda.[9] It was important, therefore, for such "peaceful penetration" to be replicated in the administrative approach to education and social services.[10]

To understand these social systems and spheres of influence in "mothering" as well as women's social networks, which colonial officials saw as an avenue for advancing colonial goals, this chapter utilizes a case study of the Igbo of southern Nigeria, of whom the colonial superintendent of education speaks to explore the local politics of motherhood as well as the connections of childbirth and birth rituals to the community's social fabric. Understanding this local context and its connections to sociopolitical developments in colonial and postcolonial Nigeria provides insight into why the spaces of birth were such contested spaces for the colonial government, the missionaries, and the local community. The discourse in this chapter offers a framework for understanding missionary, government, and African Independent Church (AIC) actions, as discussed in subsequent chapters, to target childbirth as a strategy for advancing their various agendas. It also offers a general understanding of the traditional birthing institution to better convey the adaptions that occurred later in the postcolonial era.

Any attempts at understanding the British colonial official's proposal to increasingly target women and the home for colonial propaganda involves understanding the dynamics in the home around the first quarter of the twentieth century. Among the Igbo, the successful attainment of motherhood bestowed on married women some religious power and social status and solidified women's positions in their marital homes and communities. It also strengthened the bonds between the two families involved in a marriage contract. Motherhood granted an Igbo wife her own *mkpuke* (house) over which she wielded control. This *mkpuke* was also the point of congregation and socialization for her children and was largely outside the direct control of husbands.[11] Motherhood, thus, gave women varying degrees of autonomy within their marital household and extended women's authority within their spheres of influence in and outside the home. For external actors like missionaries, therefore, controlling this space or wielding some sort of influence over its main character—the mother—potentially opened up the entire *mkpuke* and other affiliated spaces to the actors' ideological influence.

For the colonial government, intervention in women's reproductive lives was as economic as it was social. In the agricultural economies of the precolonial and colonial eras, the family was a significant source of labor supply, and the size of a woman's household determined the extent of labor from which she and her husband could draw for the cultivation of their lands. Married Igbo women received plots of land from their husbands from which they grew produce for sale and consumption while the whole family participated in the cultivation and upkeep of other family lands. Family size was, therefore, important to the social standing of married women and the prestige of their husbands. This correlation between family size and labor was not lost on the colonial government, whose officials connected the security of the colony's future labor supply to considerable infant deaths that they described as "wastages" and for which they blamed mothers.[12]

Increasingly in the 1930s, associations between birth and labor became more pronounced in colonial discourses such that controlling high infant death rates required more direct interventions in women's lives. These interventions were advanced through what government officials frequently described in the 1920s and 1930s as "mothercraft," the process of teaching "the African mother . . . the right methods and the sanitary methods" of tending to a household and rearing children.[13] Colonial proponents of direct involvement in the lives of women argued that the world needed the colony's agricultural and mineral produce, "for which labor, chiefly male, will continue to be needed."[14] Local women's indigenous mothercraft, according to colonial logic, stood in the way of ensuring this future labor supply. It was, therefore, thought that a joint intervention between educationists—almost always missionaries during the first quarter of the twentieth century—and the medical service "could tackle the problem in the home."[15] Regarding missionary impact on this subject, one writer stated, "We already have proof where natives have been brought under and have followed the guidance of Christian missions, that large and healthy families can be reared."[16]

For missionaries, mothers and traditional midwives represented the epitome of the very traditional practices and religious worldview that they sought to uproot. From the era of expanding missionary activity in the late nineteenth century, local birth practices and the rituals associated with them were considered backward heathen rites that needed to be uprooted for Christian light and Western civilization to thrive. Missionaries, therefore, targeted their efforts at eliminating these "bastions of evil" that they considered as sustained through women. In traditional Igbo society during the early twentieth century, childbirth had spiritual significance, embodied in various rituals associated with pregnancy and delivery. The spiritual powers that many Igbo mothers wielded were centered in rituals associated with *omumu* (fertility).

Due to the importance of childbirth in women's life cycle, the act of reproduction was well represented in many rites, ritual objects, and places of worship.[17] Deities associated with productivity, for instance, *Ala* (earth goddess), were portrayed as mothers, reflecting this female reproductive capacity. The spiritual component of a woman's identity as *nne* (mother) also raised her status from merely a daughter to a woman imbued with ritual authorities with which she could influence her community. For instance, mothers dominated public ritual ceremonies and rites associated with deities related to crop production. They also controlled rites of passage associated with fertility, including *Ebe* or *Nkpu*, both indigenous educational systems in which young girls who had reached the age of puberty received training from a group of women on private, public, and social conduct as well as instructions on family life and childrearing.[18] Institutions like *Ebe* were seen as propagating cultural practices and exerting ideological influences that colonial agents, including missionaries, sought to undermine.

Women's spiritual power also manifested in the reverence for women in various groups, such as the *Inyom-di* (patrilineage wives) and *Umuada* (lineage daughters), who controlled specific religious rituals in their lineages and wielded political and judicial power over men and women in certain circumstances.[19] These groups served as interest groups that preserved and perpetrated various traditions that missionaries and later the colonial administration identified as undermining the colonial vision of mothercraft.

Missionaries also focused on some of the birth practices of the Igbo as proof of the need for change and intervention. One of these practices, killing of twins, became a rallying point and constant part of missionary correspondence to their home countries to engender more support for missionary work and intervention.[20] Igbo cultures, like many neighboring cultures in southern Nigeria, saw twin births as an unnatural occurrence that could bring calamity to the community. As such, twins were left in forests to die shortly after birth. Their mothers were banished or required to perform cleansing rituals to avert any supernatural retributions against the community.[21] This practice buttressed to missionaries the need for intervention in local birthing institutions and women's traditional modes of socialization. By the late 1940s, both missionaries and colonial administrators agreed that "the situation [twin killing] can only be remedied by education and the consequent abandonment of current beliefs" and that the establishment and popularization of maternity homes "would help to eliminate the practice entirely as more cases of the birth of twins would come to light."[22]

In this chapter, I explore local ideas of marriage, conception, birth, and motherhood, reflecting on what colonial officials described as mothercraft—the act of motherhood and mothering—and why birth and motherhood among the locals became a convenient avenue for colonial intervention. Here and throughout the book, I treat the words "tradition" and "traditional midwifery" not as depictions of age-old practices but as porous constructions that are constantly negotiated as new cultural and geographic encounters occur.[23] Traditional midwifery is portrayed as a dynamic set of practices that have shifted over time in response to internal and external forces like urbanization, migration, colonization, religion, and geography.

Nwa Agadi: Marriage, Conception, and Pregnancy

Local ideas of mothercraft were well defined prior to the consolidation of colonial rule among the Igbo. These ideas traversed the periods of puberty, marriage, conception, and postpartum. The social and cultural lives of women in various communities revolved around two major rites of passage—marriage and motherhood—that were central to many religious, sociocultural, and political networks. In Nnewi and Onitsha, two Igbo communities where I spent my childhood, I constantly heard the term *Nwa Agadi* (old person) affectionately used by older community members to address pregnant women. This term signified that the woman so addressed had now fully joined the adult circle and had accomplished a major milestone in the life of a married female—pregnancy. The delight on these women's faces was always visible as they too understood that *Nwa Agadi*, a welcome salutation that signified impending motherhood, bestowed on them new degrees of public respectability that came with motherhood within the confines of marriage. In other words, motherhood was crucial for a woman's status, but marriage was just as important and ideally preceded motherhood.

The prospect of motherhood among the Igbo was both spiritual and biological, making the institution a fitting target for missionary and government intervention. In the first half of the twentieth century, motherhood was well

reflected in an Igbo religious cosmology that vested in women, female ancestors, and female deities the powers of procreation. Women's ability to harness
the spiritual forces of procreation lay in their activation of *omumu* (fertility/
reproduction) through sacrifices to their natal maternal spirits. Women also
made sacrifices to their *chi* (personal spiritual guardian) to clear any spiritual obstructions to conception. In matters of fertility, a woman's *chi* was not
considered very effective in maternity issues until the birth of her first
child. Therefore, her mother's *chi* or that of other maternal ancestors was invoked to protect her during a first pregnancy, a pregnancy that was frequently guarded jealously and, in some cases, involved the expecting mother
taking up residence in her mother's house to ensure that the pregnancy was
nurtured successfully. It was often a mother's responsibility to secure the fertility of a young female through fertility rites and appeals to the mother's
chi.[24] Obijelu Okpalaeze, wife of an Igbo monarch, describes this process as
one that at times required three weeks or more of residency in which an expecting mother stayed with her mother for an extended period, after which
she returned to her husband's residence.[25] This period was also a time of socialization in which rites and cultural practices surrounding birth and
motherhood were reinforced, highlighting the outlook that "a child is not
only relevant to the family but to the society at large."[26]

The importance of conception also featured in the ceremonies and rites
performed during marriage ceremonies. In Enugwu-Ukwu and the Afikpo
area, for example, Philip Nnatu, who spent some of his time in Afikpo as a
government dispenser during the colonial era and ultimately took up residence in his natal home of Enugwu-Ukwu as the community's *Dokinta*
(doctor), recalled that fertility dances were part of marriage ceremonies and
performed by the bride's *Umuada Ndikiride* (married female members of a
woman's kindred).[27] In some communities where *iyi*, an oath that dissuaded
men from engaging in sexual intercourse with an unmarried woman, was
placed on a woman by members of her family, the *iyi* was taken away by the
umuada relatives of the bride, allowing her to engage in intercourse, with
the aim of conception.[28]

Beyond the nuclear family, pregnancy was a matter of public health and
social continuity and, therefore, featured concerted communal efforts—
spiritual, medical, and social—to safeguard a woman's capacity to conceive
and deliver safely. In parts of Igboland, an indigenous educational system for
girls was in place until the 1930s when it began to give way to urban migra-

tions, a new class of educated elites, and growing Christian traditions. This institution—*Ebe*—inculcated in younger females the modes of conduct expected of them before marriage, after marriage, and during pregnancy or childrearing. When I first began to enquire about *Ebe* in 2003, my grandmother, Roseline, explained that this institution was crucial to marriage and motherhood. "Girls who did not perform *Ebe* could not perform *Ime Ezi*," a marriage ceremony that involved gift exchanges and communal celebrations, my grandmother explained.[29] "*Ebe* signaled to the entire community that a girl had attained the age of puberty and could now marry."[30] Girls, including those who may have gotten married during *Iso Ebe*, a process that occurred every two years and often lasted for three months, could not get pregnant until after this educational course and all marriage rites were completed.

Sexual etiquette featured strongly in this indigenous educational institution where acceptable motherhood was situated strongly within the confines of marital union and customary laws that colonial agents sometimes perceived to be at odds with their own missions. Older female instructors taught young women how to beautify their bodies and take care of the homestead. They also inculcated in their younger audience the shame of conception before marriage. According to a community elder in Adazi-Enu, "These girls were taught how to preserve themselves until marriage and learned that it was taboo to have premarital sex, not to mention giving birth outside of wedlock."[31] The girls also learned what types of births and babies were taboo, such as twins and children whose upper teeth appeared before the lower. According to my grandmother, those girls who "committed the abomination of conceiving outside wedlock, before *Iso Ebe* and *Ime Ezi*," invited priests to perform *Ikpu Alu*, a cleansing rite, before they could complete *Ebe*. Because previous generations of women had passed through *Ebe* and enforced the standards required of young women, mothers ensured that their daughters were raised following these ideals even before *Iso Ebe* and sent daughters of prepuberty age to perform *Ebe nwa afo* (junior Ebe) and be on track to perpetuate communal values.[32]

Once marriage occurred and conception followed, pregnancy was punctuated by ceremonies performed to ensure safe maternity and reinforce the communal nature of motherhood. These ceremonies frequently highlighted familial networks and served as pathways for religious and cultural transmissions, subjecting them to missionary criticisms as pagan practices. Following conception, it was typical for an expectant husband to visit his wife's natal village bearing a cock as gift for the priestess or priest of *Ala*, the earth goddess and most powerful deity associated with fertility. In the Owerri District during the first quarter of the twentieth century, it was common for the priest or priestess of *Ala* to invoke divine protection on the pregnant woman, notifying the goddess that the woman's husband fulfilled all marriage rites for their daughter and should, therefore, be blessed with safe delivery. Afterward, the husband proceeded to the wife's family to officially notify them of her pregnancy.[33] At the fifth month of pregnancy, the couple made a formal visit to the woman's family with palm wine and gifts for the mother-in-law. This visit lasted for a few days, after which the expecting mother received valuable gifts such as goats, fowls, water pots, and mortar from male members of her extended family. These gifts were practical items that every married woman needed to build her expanding home.

Upon delivery, a similar journey as that undertaken earlier in the pregnancy was embarked on by a husband to his wife's natal home to announce the arrival of a newborn. This formal announcement was punctuated with a celebration at the end of which the newborn's maternal grandmother, in the company of other relatives, visited the new mother with gifts of clothes, foodstuff, and other household items for the comfort of mother and baby. These types of formal visits were paramount in the first half of the twentieth century when families tended to live in relative proximity to each other and gave their children in marriage within their own towns or neighboring towns. As such, making these types of journeys, especially during an era when modern public transportation was sparse, was practical. Even in the changing landscape of colonial rule, such inter- and intrafamily connections persisted. The formality of birth announcements was held sacrosanct, and the lack thereof could prove injurious to relationships. As my mother's relatives often reminded us during our childhood, our natal home was bound to give us refuge or assist us due to our position as *Nwadiala* (child of the soil). Maintaining those connections from birth was, therefore, a crucial part of the social contract.

Beyond the religious and communal performances during pregnancy, certain taboos associated with pregnancy demonstrated connections that local communities made between the biological affairs of birth and spiritual or psychosocial elements, which missionaries saw as an obstacle to their Christian ideologies and "civilizing" efforts. These practices were not random acts of superstition but calculated efforts to protect the health of expecting mothers. They stemmed from local religious and cultural cosmologies and varied from one part of Igboland to the other. Some of these pregnancy-related taboos revolved around subjects like nutrition and the expecting father's conduct. In some communities, expecting parents were barred from eating the meat of animals killed in honor of a deity and sold in the market.[34] Since sacrifices were part of the normal course of pregnancy during this period, would-be parents freely partook of meats that had been used as part of religious rites or ceremonies but were discouraged from purchasing such meat from the market. One explanation for this practice could be to protect expecting parents from spiritual or physical consequences that could result from consuming sacrificial animals that may have been offered to unfriendly deities or those at variance with the family. Families would, therefore, not wish to unknowingly expose an expecting mother to the vengeance or anger of a deity not affiliated with the family.

In a similar fashion, C. K. Meek, a British colonial administrator who published an account of his observations among the Igbo in the 1920s, reported that pregnant women could not eat or touch the flesh of an animal that died on its own in order to avoid stillbirth.[35] This communal rule was possibly a public health measure put in place to protect the expecting mother from infection or contamination through contact or consumption of animal flesh ridden with diseases. In other communities, for instance, in Lejja, where Onyeugwu Nwa Ogwo, a traditional midwife, grew up in the 1920s, women avoided "bush meat" such as *Nchi* (grasscutter), bat, and similar meats due to the belief that these may cause difficulty in birth. Igbo communities also believed that infants could take on the characteristics of other mammals that were consumed by their mothers during pregnancy. For instance, there was the belief that women who ate *Nchi* could have difficult labor like the grasscutter. Those who ate snails may have children that drooled like the snail. Although such taboos were directly correlated to the characteristics of these animals, these may also have been a practical way of protecting pregnant women from exposure to harmful pathogens that may be associated with such "bush meat."

Taboos extended to husbands and offered psychological protection for the women. In various parts of the Owerri Province, husbands could not refuse food cooked by a wife who had recently delivered; otherwise, the newborn could refuse food and die. This requirement ensured the control of physical and verbal abuse from husbands. It offered emotional protection even for a disfavored wife. As children were a source of prestige and status for Igbo men, husbands were mostly bound to comply with such proscriptions placed on them. Communities in Imo State performed a festival, *Ajankita*, at the end of which the couple promised to be pleasant and "sweet mouthed" to each other. Expecting fathers also avoided carrying dead bodies, even those of animals, during their wives' pregnancies to avoid the death of the fetus in the womb.[36] This practice can be linked with hygiene and mitigating contagion of an infectious disease by the expecting parents. The taboos were not absolute laws, but any breach guaranteed the condemnation of the defaulting party if things subsequently went wrong.[37]

Iji-Nwa: Birth and the Midwife

The process of prenatal care and delivery was mostly controlled by women, including traditional midwives and female relatives of expecting parents. This gender dynamic was crucial in government and missionary bids later to control maternal health care. In the traditional setting, midwives were almost exclusively women, and men were generally isolated from affairs of childbirth.[38] In northern Igbo areas of Nsukka, Udi, and Abakiliki, various midwives and gynecologists who were interviewed from as early as 2008 and whose dates of birth fell between 1910 and 1925 recalled male *dibias* (traditional doctors) who primarily functioned as herbalists and diviners but also attended births. These practitioners were often popular in their communities for their treatments of infertility and other gynecological ailments, and it was in their capacity as gynecologists, herbalists, and diviners that they intervened in spaces of birth.[39] These *dibias*, male or female, were especially sought out to partner with midwives in the course of pregnancies or deliveries that were regarded as high risk. Evidence of this collaboration was depicted in an early twentieth-century artistic illustration of childbirth, situated behind the shrine of a deity, *Olugba*, in the Igbo town of Owerri and chronicled by Meek, a colonial officer. The sculpture showed a female attendant standing behind a woman giving birth and holding her shoulders. In front of the woman was the midwife positioned to receive the baby. At the side stood a *dibia* holding a bunch of leaves and other medicines to facilitate delivery.[40] The oldest woman in Lejja community, who became a midwife around the 1940s, also described this collaboration:

"When I am called to deliver babies and it is a difficult birth, I work with the diviner, Ugwu Asato. He divines, prays, and offers directions while I get to work. If there are complications, we both come together to save lives."[41] In a society in which male and female authority was clearly defined in the political and social realm prior to and during the early periods of colonial intervention, men's exclusion can immediately be explained as women's way of maintaining an intimately feminine domain of control and collective solidarity. Male exclusion could also be understood in terms of modesty and male gaze on the female body. In the decades before independence, female nakedness and nudity among the Igbo held various meanings. *Oto* (the state of undress) was a sign of health and public beauty for an Igbo child, and this outlook persisted until marriage. Upon marriage and with the conception of the first child, however, a woman's nude body became sacred, to be exposed only to her husband within a private space and to be wielded as a tool of protest against men.[42] This meant that the presence of men with whom a woman did not share marital or familial bonds during the intimate procedure of childbirth would have been unacceptable and considered a contravention of the rules of modesty. This concern trailed the encroachment of men into the field of midwifery across the world.

The exclusion of men in spaces of birth was more common in eastern and western Igboland. Here, women closely monitored the implementation of men's exclusion and sanctioned any woman who discussed matters concerning childbirth with men. In northeastern Igboland, on the other hand, older male family members, including a woman's husband, could assist during childbirth. Ogidija and Onyeugwu both recall that in some cases in their community and during their own practices as midwives, wives sat on their husbands' laps to deliver their babies. In this case, the husbands served as human stools and recliners for the expecting mothers.[43] Otherwise, husbands occupied themselves with making appeals to their *chi* through sacrifices and prayers for their wives' safe delivery, after which they waited in anticipation with other male members of the extended family for the announcement of a delivery.[44]

On the colonial end of the spectrum, traditional gender observances surrounding childbirth proved unfavorable as the realm of biomedicine during the early twentieth century was overwhelmingly male. Missionaries and colonial government officials up to the 1930s were also predominantly male. As such, they could not make inroads in childbirth with a largely male colonial and missionary staff. They were also at a disadvantage because missionaries who were in the position to engage with the locals lacked formal medical training that could have provided them some advantages in their attempts to penetrate the realms of childbirth. Until medical outreaches by various missionary groups in Nigeria expanded in the first quarter of the twentieth century, subverting the powers and influence of the midwife proved difficult without the corresponding trained medical personnel.

Many of the missionaries who dabbled in medicine were not trained medical practitioners. Some merely had knowledge of first aid, which they utilized in their dealings with the local communities.[45] In dire circumstances where these quasi-practitioners were invited to intervene, such cases were typically hopeless. Of this, Andrew Stirrett of the Sudan Interior Mission wrote in a manual first published in 1922 that "in such [abnormal] cases the European is not usually called until there is some trouble."[46] In one such case, a family in Onitsha sought out the missionaries—a male and a female—stationed in the town's clinic at an odd hour at night to intervene in a prolonged labor. Their assistance was not needed after all as the mother had delivered her baby before missionaries got there.[47] The conditions under which it became acceptable to summon them, despite the presence of a male missionary, is important to note.

Although traditional midwives in the first quarter of the twentieth century lacked the formal education akin to the Western institutional model, they received hands-on training through many years of apprenticeship to older and more experienced midwives. Onyeugwu described her training, which began with a grounding in purpose and ethics:

> It is like a school and you have to undergo some tutelage. In my own case, the person who taught me is Lolo Nwaeze. After observing me for a while, Lolo, a midwife in the community for many years, beckoned on me and told me that she wanted me to follow the path of midwifery so that it could help humanity. She advised me not to commercialize it, that my interest should be saving lives and not making money out of it. She trained me for a while during which I attended births with her until I had gained the knowledge of midwifery. My practice is over fifty years old and I am now about 100 years old.[48]

Like Onyeugwu, aspiring midwives ran errands for the senior midwife, assisted during delivery, and provided comfort and emotional support for pregnant women during labor. They also learned the act of midwifery itself during this period of apprenticeship and mastered the various remedies and techniques applied to different scenarios in childbirth.

For children of midwives who developed an interest in their mothers' work or were taken along to birthing sessions, such as Chizoba, who came from a lineage of midwives, their authenticity was easier to establish. They acted as junior midwives and were assigned the care of sick pregnant women. The community's trust in their abilities developed during this process until they could be relied on to handle more demanding responsibilities. Such young women who became part of the midwifery realm by virtue of their mother or grandmothers' roles could not practice independently until they became married and had children of their own. This was based on the reasoning that midwives would provide better and more humane maternal and infant care if they had themselves gone through the process of birth and delivery. Their legitimacy, as with other midwives, depended on the success of their practice and the community's confidence in their skills.

The midwife's influence and that of the *dibias* were far-reaching in their communities. This influence pitched them against missionaries who blamed them for steering prospective converts toward cultural practices that missionaries frowned upon. Colonial officials, too, were quick to cast communities' trusted health care providers as "medicine men" and "bush doctors" responsible for making community members disregard colonial health and social agendas. One official lamented that "the native doctors still have a strong influence and are very reluctant to relax it."[49] As such, any visits or admonishments by visiting colonial agents regarding the use of emerging maternity centers were counteracted by the presence and advice of the various community's traditional medicine practitioners. Any advancement of the colonial project, therefore, depended upon breaking this hold that traditional practitioners had on their communities.

The relationship between local women and their traditional midwives was hard to break, however. Expressing this sentiment, one medical officer wrote, "In bush villages, getting the mothers to call the [Western-trained] midwife to attend confinement is not so easy."[50] These women persistently chose to deliver at home with their traditional midwives irrespective of prior visits to government or missionary maternity centers. The traditional midwife was often an integral member of the expecting mother's kindred in ways that the clinic-based midwife, often an outsider and by the late 1930s typically a younger woman without an established family of her own, was not.

Culturally, childbirth occurred in the expecting mother's backyard or that of her father or grandmother, an intimate space over which the colonial machinery had little control. This familial location of birth was largely overseen by female members of a family, older women in the neighborhood, the midwife, and the expecting mother's female kin. Here, they controlled the rites associated with birth and delivery and enforced ideas about what were considered acceptable or taboo birth outcomes. This dynamic of control and regulation made it expedient for missionaries to relocate births to the hospitals and clinics, spaces that were dominated by senior European nursing staff, junior African midwives, and European doctors. This clinical space could afford them the opportunity to reeducate women without the oversight of their local kinfolks. In some communities, childbirth could occur in the midwife's backyard because the midwife had everything that she needed for the birthing process handy at home.[51] In this case, the same support system that would have been featured if the birth occurred in the expecting mother's home is featured here. Mary Ugwuanyi, whose mother was also a midwife, pointed out that even in her own days as a midwife up to the 1990s, she visited women's homes to attend their birth. She only started using her home because she was "too old to be walking about. Whoever knows me would come here to my house to give birth."[52]

Giving birth inside houses was considered a taboo in some parts of Igboland up to the 1950s, when Christianity and Western conceptions of sanitation had fully taken root among the people. Yet the midwives' practice of birthing outdoors was undertaken as a matter of sanitation. Birthing outside the house kept birth fluids from contaminating household items and food and made it easier to clean up after birth.[53] Chizoba was clear in her explanation:

> The reason why it [birth] is done outside is because of the blood and other things that comes out of the woman's body alongside the baby. After delivery, they used hoe to dig the ground and bury those things; then they carried the placenta gently and put it into the ground and buried it. These days, if you deliver inside the house, you must have pad and tissue, but these village people back then didn't buy those things. . . . The women needed ventilation too.[54]

Women's body fluids, notably blood, were also considered a spiritual contaminant, neutralizer of charms, and potential weapon that could be used to ensnare the new mother and her infant. As things evolved in Igboland during the twentieth century, however, deliveries routinely occurred in the home. Gloria Ozoani stated that "in our own time, after delivery, you lie down on the bed. If you didn't come with pad, you must come with cloth, old or new."[55] The pads or wrappers were used in absorbing the body fluid after delivery and facilitated the clean-up process.

In contrast to the British model during the early twentieth century in which a practitioner was called in during labor and delivery, the traditional midwife's care began as soon as pregnancy was ascertained by a couple, mostly through a combination of subtle body changes, including the state of the eyes, the lack of menstruation, and change in food habits. Skilled women had the keen eye to identify a pregnancy that had not become obvious. In my journeys through Onitsha during the later stages of my follow-up research in 2018, this skill was put to the test. Unknown to all but my immediate family members, I was pregnant. The woman that I was visiting announced to me that I was pregnant, despite the pregnancy's concealed state and the fact that only immediate family members were aware that I was expecting. According to her, I had all the tell-tale signs in the color of my eyes, my skin pigmentation, and other subtle physical features. Various interviewees explained that mothers and grandmothers of the older generation had keen eyes for identifying pregnancy, even at early stages. Gloria, a nurse and traditional midwife, explained that care for a pregnant woman, especially a first-time mother, began once such signs of pregnancy were detected.[56] For veteran mothers, it was not uncommon for the services of a midwife to begin much later in the pregnancy, unless the pregnancy showed signs of complications.

Although their role was largely advisory during the early part of pregnancy, the midwife influenced the patterns of care that were adopted by expecting mothers. She instructed pregnant women on appropriate nutrition, including the avoidance of fatty foods that would enlarge the fetus and, therefore, make delivery difficult or the avoidance of taboo foods that were believed to have negative impacts on the pregnancy.[57] Midwives also advised women on appropriate habits to secure the pregnancy. For instance, they believed that abnormal increases in body temperature during the early stage of pregnancy could induce abortion; therefore, they advised women against taking hot showers at this stage, and fever was promptly treated. They also massaged the back and abdomen of pregnant women to increase blood flow. This procedure was also an opportunity to bond with the expecting mother.

The beginning of the first genuine contraction was a crucial period for midwives and expecting mothers. Once the earliest signs of labor manifested, the midwife was immediately summoned. One such onset of labor was recounted by an elderly woman to whom a younger woman in her neighborhood turned to in 1926: "Wife came to my house crying one night and said she was in labor but it was too soon, so I said send for the midwife so I took her home and sent for the midwife."[58] In the meantime, another elderly woman in the same neighborhood was also summoned to stay with and monitor the laboring woman. Once summoned, a midwife encouraged the pregnant woman to stay mobile in order to speed up labor. She accompanied the woman throughout this process, offering verbal comfort and reassurance. The woman was considered ready for delivery once she felt the urge to excrete or had a distended perineum.[59]

In some Igbo communities, hiring the appropriate midwife at the onset of pregnancy was a crucial exercise. In such locations, a diviner was consulted to select the appropriate midwife that would carry out a successful delivery. In others, not all women consulted or engaged the services of midwives.[60] This category of women took care of themselves based on general knowledge. In time of labor, available elderly women or other women experienced in childbirth assisted in the delivery. In polygamous families, the senior wives and other mothers in the household assisted with childbirth. In these instances, the only requirement was that these women had firsthand experiences of childbirth. Midwives and herbalists were not involved except in complications or prolonged labor. Because pregnant women often went about their businesses, including trading and farming, some women went into labor on the way to or from their trading posts or farms. In this case, other women on that road formed an enclosure with extra wrappers and head gears around such a woman to secure privacy for her delivery.[61] Experienced mothers served as midwives in such births. Where possible, such an expecting mother was transferred to a neighboring household where she was cared for and then accompanied home with her newborn. At this time, there was inadequate transportation to ensure that a woman who suddenly went into labor was transported home to a midwife or *dibia*.

As colonial government interest in maternal health services increased gradually in the late 1920s and early 1930s, government officials portrayed midwives and *dibias* as one of the obstacles to reshaping birthing habits and improving maternity. Traditional practitioners' application of herbal medicines became part of the campaign against traditional midwifery as "dangerous midwifery" based on the arguments that the herbal solutions that midwives administered, even when effective, lacked scientific backing and could prove injurious to mothers and their babies. A medical officer who was involved in shaping midwifery policy wrote, "In bush practice there are very few abnormal cases and those there are, are often due to taking Native Medicine causing uterine inertia; or the results of manual interference."[62] He also recognized the reality of the situation and remarked of mothers, "The majority of babies have previously been taken to native doctors and will continue to be so unless given something to replace native medicine."[63] His reference to manual interference indicated some midwives' attempts to reposition the baby if the latter was in an unfavorable position toward the late stages of pregnancy. Skilled midwives prided themselves in their ability to conduct these maneuvers from the breech posture, for instance, to an appropriate one.[64] From the portrayals provided by locally renowned midwives, such as Chizoba, Mary Ugwuanyi, Onyeugwu, and Florence Odo, a narrative of this procedure emerges: the midwife added palm oil to a clay pot and warmed this oil in an open fire. Afterward, *Akpaigogo* (a part of the palm fruit) was added to the mixture and stirred into a paste. This paste was rubbed on the woman's abdomen while the midwife gently manipulated the baby. With the help of the mixture and the midwife's technique, the baby turned into the proper position and labor progressed normally.[65]

Unskilled or inexperienced midwives generally avoided this feat as it was well recognized that improper manipulations could lead to complications or rupture the uterus. While it is hard to rely on most data before the 1930s outside of urban and government-regulated Lagos due to their incomplete nature and lack of breadth, the British medical officer's mention of "manual interference" in his statement on "bush practice" affirms the point that these maneuvers occurred, albeit with unknown frequency. While some British officials acknowledged the traditional midwives' skills, their use of herbs and the manual interventions that they initiated, such as the repositioning of a baby or attempts to manually deliver a placenta, became the basis for blame and part of the argument for intervention. Such manual deliveries of placenta involved applying pressure at the top of the uterus and on the placenta to encourage ejection. This process, if not done with care, could exacerbate bleeding and invert the uterus. Delivery was considered incomplete and a birth was not announced until the placenta had been expelled and the baby had cried.[66] Although medical officers condemned the manual maneuvers by traditional midwives, a 1922 missionary doctor's manual for West Africa, based on his work in Nigeria, recommended a similar process as adopted by traditional midwives for the delivery of an unyielding placenta.[67]

In cases of prolonged labor, the midwife administered palm oil on the patient's abdomen to induce contraction. Her throat may be tickled for the same reason. The tender frond of the palm tree was inserted in the throat, contracting the abdominal muscle and aiding in the baby's expulsion. In northern Igboland, *Omu* (palm frond), *Akpa ido* (wasp bag), and *Akpaigogo* (a part of the palm fruit) were mashed together and administered to the woman to aid delivery.[68] Based on the Igbo belief that the characteristics of certain animals could be transferred, the wasp's aggressiveness was believed to be transferred to the medical properties of this mixture, therefore causing labor to speed up.

Pregnancy care and the application of herbs extended to culinary herbs or spices and general nutrition. Midwives and other elderly female relatives encouraged women to eat foods that contained common herbs like *Uda* (*Xylopia aethiopica*) and *Utazi* (*Gongronema latifolium*), believed to contract the uterus.[69] These herbs remain widespread in Igboland and are popular ingredients in a protein-rich soup—white soup—which are consumed by the general populace but specifically prepared for women in labor or new mothers, with a more generous addition of *Uda* and *Utazi*. These herbs aided not only delivery but also the discharge of the placenta. After delivery, the contractions that they promoted helped shrink the uterus closer to its prepregnancy size. Moringa leaves were used during pregnancy and after birth to promote general well-being. In the postcolonial era and following more scientific understanding of the benefits of this plant, midwives like Ngozi Ikwueze, who have learned to combine the traditional knowledge of their ancestors with biomedical training, apply Moringa specifically to regulate *obala ngbali enu* (high blood pressure).[70]

Since indigenous medicine among the Igbo did not include any surgical expertise beyond minor operations involving circumcision, bone setting, and body scarifications, complications requiring surgery were commonly fatal as the mother sometimes died of exhaustion before alternative approaches could yield results. It was in these scenarios requiring surgery that colonial doctors made their best inroads as the locals readily summoned them or referred the hopeless cases to hospitals when no path to a successful outcome was in view. In some instances, these cases were salvaged, and in others, it was too late for any interventions. Despite colonial interventions and criticisms of local birth, any large-scale success before the 1930s remained elusive. The strong female domination of the local birthing space, the overly male-dominated colonial service and missionary enterprise before the 1930s, and the lack of infrastructure or personnel to undertake women's medicine at a significant scale made the immediate colonization of childbirth all but impossible.

After delivery, the midwife or other female relatives massaged the mother's abdomen and pelvic region with hot water to stop blood clotting in the womb and allow for easy outflow of body fluid accumulated in the uterus. In many rural communities during the colonial era, families prepared a heated local bed made of molded clay and wood. Pounded piles of *igbegiri* (a part of the palm tree) were placed at a spot on the bed to absorb the bleeding from the mother's uterus. The baby was given a small amount of palm kernel oil and a little water and then covered in *odo*, a local powder. Visitors and relatives applied same powder on their face and neck to signify the arrival of a newborn. As talcum powder became more common in the cities in the 1950s and beyond, it replaced the local powder, *Odo*, as the preferred powder that was used in this cultural performance. The umbilical cord attached to the placenta was then buried and a tree planted on that location to mark the child's birth. This act of burying the umbilical cord was believed to tie the child to the land and the family, and it signified that wherever life took the child, they would stay connected to their homeland. In my grandfather's generation, my father explained, the trees chosen for a child were economic trees, such as palm trees, that the child became entitled to harvest and profit from in their adulthood. In many ways, this practice provided a head start for a newborn in an economy that was primarily based on subsistence and commercial agriculture. In some parts of Igboland, such as Ututu and Arochukwu, the cord's disposal took on more overtly ritual proportions and was placed in a special ritual pot made of clay, copper, or iron—*Ite ola okike* (pot of creation) after birth.[71]

In the days following birth, herbs were administered to the infant for common baby ailments. The herbal treatment of infants came under government scrutiny beginning in the late 1920s when government was becoming more concerned about infant health and mortality rates. Midwives and

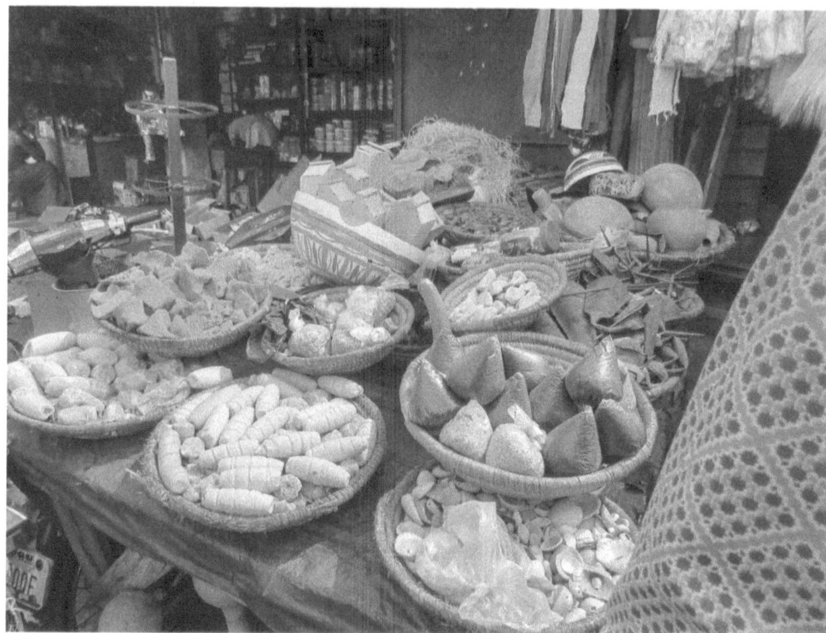

Display at a market stall showing the white Nzu, red Odo, and black poison repellant—nsi ulu enyi

mothers' use of herbal treatments were blamed for poor infant health and sometimes death, although the causes of infant deaths, which were high during this time, were many and varied and ranged from the results of tropical diseases such as malaria to the effects of other tropical infections. Some of the local treatments for certain infant ailments included massaging soap made of burnt plantain leaves, palm oil, parts of the palm fruit, and other natural ingredients onto the abdomen to address constipation and ease bowel movement. Children who suffered from fever were given a mixture obtained from *Akata*, a leaf whose properties were active against fever. Other childhood ailments like diarrhea and rashes were treated with home remedies or by the midwife. One such treatment for rashes was *ude aku* (palm kernel oil), which was rubbed all over the child's body as a regular lotion or to reduce fever and prevent convulsion. A small quantity was occasionally inserted into the baby's mouth. *Ude aku* was also used to treat the umbilical stump to prevent infection and ensure healing. It was a base for many traditional medical mixtures.[72]

At the end of childbirth, midwives' services were rewarded mostly through gifts. Since their work was considered crucial to the community's well-being, midwives generally began their training and practice with an emphasis on public service rather than money, a fact that made them more appealing to their communities to the detriment of missionary clinics. Onyeugwu emphasized this point about fees in her stories about Lolo Nwaeze, the female elder who trained her as a midwife and emphasized that her skill should not be commercialized into a profit-making venture. She recalled Lolo's final exhortation: "After she let me into the knowledge of midwifery, I took money and kola to her but she rejected the money and accepted the kola as it is part of tradition. She said that as she is rejecting the money, she is equally giving me an injunction not to make money my priority."[73] This de-prioritization of money and "in-kind" payments in traditional midwifery is still visible in the practice of contemporary traditional midwives, an element that makes their practice more attractive and accessible to women of lower economic status. When I walked into Chizoba's birthing center in Nsukka, she pointed out sets of items in the corner of the room and said, "These things that I brought back, I didn't buy them. Those women whose babies I delivered and whose lives I saved bought them for me."[74] In some communities in northern Igboland, the midwife was considered "blinded" by the birthing process. In order to open her eyes, the family of the new mother offered different gifts and food items.[75] In places like Mboo in Imo State, if the child was male, the midwife was presented with a cock a few days after childbirth. She pressed this cock on the mother and child, saying, "I remove from you all evil spirits."[76] Then, she killed the cock at the threshold of the compound and took the meat home for her use.[77]

In the Awgu division of Igboland in the 1930s, the midwife had one final role after delivery. One month after a child's birth, formal rites of purification were performed in which the midwife played an active role. The new parents invited the women of their kindred to a feast. The midwife attended and waved a yam over the head of the mother and child, saying, "May everything that comes into this compound be pleasant like this feast. The evil spirit shall not assail the mother and child, for I am now removing all evil spirits from this household." She then threw the yam on the ground.[78] Afterward, a young boy made the following utterance to the infant: "If your father or mother sends you on a message, do not refuse to go. But if a spirit (*ndi mmuo*) sends you, do not go."[79] This latter injunction was a nod to the common belief among the Igbo that the spiritual and physical worlds were inter-connected, and spiritual beings, including neglected ancestors, were capable of intervening in the lives of the living, for better or worse.

After Birth: *Omugwo* and the Postpartum Period

For a new mother, the postpartum period was a period of rest and education on motherhood and family life. It involved a network of women who became responsible for the mother's care and that of her household. At the top of this network was the newborn's maternal grandmother whose chief responsibility was to nurture her daughter back to good health, usually over a period of one to three months, and to ensure that she learned proper childcare techniques. This interval was known as *omugwo*, a time when the new mother rested and recovered from pregnancy and childbirth and was released from the burdens of household responsibilities.

This *omugwo* period commenced following the new father's visit to his wife's family to formally announce the birth of a child. The customary drink that he brought along was palm wine, which eventually changed to other Western-style alcoholic and nonalcoholic beverages by the latter part of the twentieth century. Upon this formal announcement, the baby's maternal grandmother prepared a trip to her daughter's house. She brought with her a wide range of gifts for the newborn and mother from her side of the family network. She also bore choice food items like stacks of dry fish, meats, and a wide range of delicacies that would help nourish the new mother back to good health. Her primary responsibility was to care for the mother and the newborn and ensure that the mother was properly fed.

Good food during the postpartum period was a priority for many families. How well a woman was fed during this period brought praise and honor to her husband. For affluent families, protein-rich soups paired with pounded yam was freshly made at each meal. Such soups were not reheated or consumed twice by the mother. At the next meal and upon her request, a fresh pot of soup was made.[80] Onyeugwu emphasized the importance of food in the postpartum period by recounting a story that had been passed down in her community and a neighboring community:

> In Lejja around the 1920s, a woman from a neighboring community who was married to a wealthy man had a baby. This presented an opportunity for the husband to showcase his wealth, and he left an order for fresh okra soup and pounded

yam to be prepared routinely on demand for the wife. This woman desired a different type of food and another type of yam that was considered inferior but could not demand this of the husband because such a request would displease him. While the husband was away, the woman's father visited and found his daughter roasting and eating this inferior yam. Upon the husband's return, the father confronted and insulted him about reducing her daughter, a new mother, to the status of eating such lowly food in her delicate postpartum state. This disagreement became a matter that involved the communities of both parties and a source of humiliation for the man. In anger, the husband lashed out and hit his wife for reducing him to scorn, resulting in her death. This incident and its outcome resulted in a scenario in which both communities barred members of their communities from intermarrying. It's been over a hundred years, and this ban on intermarriage is still upheld.[81]

Extended families of all economic statuses sought to provide nutritious meals for the new mother, at least during the weeks following delivery. The preferred food in many parts of Igboland was *Ogbono* or *Okro* soup, a vegetable-based soup made with assorted types of meat. Lower-income families fed the new mother whatever foods were available but tried their best to provide meat in the first few days after delivery. In her reflection on this subject, Chizoba remarked that "it is not everyone that had meat, but one tried to provide meat as soon as a woman delivered."[82] In other parts of Igboland, new mothers ate yams cooked in herbal vegetable sauce or pounded yam and *nsala* soup, a delicacy rich in proteins and herbs that aided healing.

During this *omugwo* period, the baby's grandmother frequently administered a hot water therapy that involved squatting over a large bowl of hot water infused with herbs. The steam from the water was believed to heal the womb as well as tears from birth. She also massaged her daughter's lower abdomen to loosen up any "bad blood" retained in the womb. She was helped in her role of caretaker by other females in the new parent's extended family household, including co-wives, the new father's aunts and his brothers' wives, and other women in the extended family network. Before the 1930s, urbanization had not become a large force that stretched families across large geographical areas. Instead, families lived closer together, and entire kindreds and extended family networks lived within walking distance of each other.

Polygamy was also the norm, especially in an agrarian society where wealth was tied to the land and, therefore, value was attached to family size and a family ability to lay claim to communal land, work the land, defend the family unit, and produce a sizable number of heirs to lay a reasonable stake in the community both in decision-making and inheritance. Where they existed, such co-wives offered assistance and became responsible for a new mother's household and other joint family responsibilities until the end of *omugwo*.

Polygamy, although condemned by the British colonial government and missionaries in Nigeria, served another role for women besides increasing the number of children and potential labor force that the family and community could draw from. It released women from sexual obligations to their husbands during the period of *omugwo* up to two years after delivery. The traditional length of breastfeeding was two years, and it was frowned upon for a woman to have intercourse with her husband while breastfeeding. It also reflected poorly on the husband and wife if the woman became pregnant during this period as many communities believed that her body needed time to heal. This extended breastfeeding became a form of child spacing that women relied on and that dissuaded husbands from engaging in intercourse with their newly postpartum wife due to the belief that such intercourse could lead to the malnourishment and withering of the child. Those women who sought to regulate their birth, therefore, stuck with the generally accepted mode of extended nursing for two years, during which time they could legitimately thwart unwanted advances from their husbands.[83]

The *omugwo* period was an important process in the socialization of mothers and the reinforcement of local ideas of mothercraft, including childrearing. It was during this process of *omugwo* that new mothers became very conversant with the locally accepted methods of infant feeding, care, and dressing that had been in place for generations. Missionaries frequently condemned traditional mothering as cruel, just as they described traditional birthing practices as neglectful and inhumane. As a missionary put it, "The poor thing is frequently put on the floor with exposed skin while the cold got the better part of them."[84] In many instances, these kinds of assessment were a matter of perspective. In the early twentieth-century British setting, babies were swaddled immediately after birth, so the lack of swaddling immediately after birth, albeit in a tropical setting in which high temperatures and humidity were the norm, seemed to the British observer neglectful and irresponsible. Igbo mothers had similar divergent views of their Western counterparts' childrearing skills. Church Missionary Society priest G. T. Basden describes, for instance, the reaction of some Igbo people to a missionary who laid her baby in a cot in the early 1900s: "[This] raised grave doubts as to whether she cared for her child. To put the baby 'upon a shelf' as if it were a common utensil, was utterly incompatible with the local ideas of affection. To neglect the child thus showed a complete want of love, and a scant respect even for duty."[85] These various perspectives highlight the importance of understanding practices on their own terms and within particular cultural settings.

Ejima: An Unwanted Outcome of Childbirth and a Basis for Colonial Intervention in Birth

As discussions about mothercraft proliferated in colonial conferences about education and maternal welfare in Africa during the 1920s, missionaries in Igboland converged on one practice—twin killing—which they used to buttress the image of savagery.[86] Up to the 1940s, when missionary efforts to eliminate this practice had yielded visible results, the birth of *ejima* (twins) or any set of multiple babies was considered sacrilege and a sign of spiritual uncleanliness. The rationale behind the practice of twin killing has been related to a distinction between humans and animals. In the Igbo local logic at the time (as well as that of some of their southern neighbors), animals were known for multiple birth, not humans; thus, a multiple birth among humans was interpreted as abnormal and offensive to nature. The Igbo made a clear distinction between animals and humans, and to act like an animal was a curse. Similarly, to be called an animal (*anu ofia*) was a form of insult. In 1939, for example, when a mother discovered that she had borne twins, she lamented to the doctor in the mission hospital where this birth occurred, "Am I a dog," and dejectedly turned her face to the wall.[87]

This phenomenon of multiple births has historically elicited multiple reactions in different African cultures. Among the Yoruba of Nigeria and Nyoro of Uganda, for instance, twin births were a cause for celebration.[88] In Igboland and surrounding areas, however, they were interpreted as "a calamity of the first magnitude, and spells disaster for them [the babies] and the unfortunate mother. . . . ; for a woman to bear more than one child in a birth is to degrade humanity to the level of the brute creation."[89] Women who gave birth to more than one child were in some cases banished. In most circumstances, they were considered to have soiled the land and were subjected to cleansing rituals (*Ikpu Alu*).

Households where twins were born were also ostracized by their communities until cleansing was completed. One Igbo officer of the Native Court in Ogbu, for example, confirmed the birth of twins in the town of Mgbidi based on his observation of the new mother's postpartum treatment. He stated, "I personally went to the house of No. 2 accused and found him in a small annex house with his wife in another so I knew the report [of twin birth] was true to Native Custom."[90] The mothers were especially penalized as the harbingers of such evil while the twins were put in earthenware pots and left in the community's *Ajo Ofia* (evil forest), a large forest dedicated to deities and the disposal of unwanted things, to die of exhaustion, starvation, or dehydration.[91] New and tender palm fronds were tied around the pots to signify the unwholesome nature of the pot's contents. A witness in a 1926 court proceeding on twin deaths described the scene of such disposal: "We saw a broken pot and two tiny babies lying on palm leaves. No 2 accused said the children were first put in the pot and the pot was broken in the bush."[92]

During the *Ikpu Alu* (ritual cleansing) process, some communities required the mother of twins to confess the "abomination" for which *Ikpu Alu* was being performed. The ritual involved sacrificial animals, specific leaves, and eggs, believed to be useful for appeasing angry deities. The sacrificial animals, as well as the subject of the cleansing, were tied with palm fronds, a traditional symbol of the sacred or taboo, and the eggs were broken on the bare earth and mixed with soil in order to ease the anger of certain deities, including the earth goddess—*Ala. Ntu Egbe*, believed to protect from evil spirit, was then sprinkled around the mother while some prayers were made on her behalf to rid her of any evil repercussions of her twin delivery. Afterward, the compound in which this cleansing was performed, if it was a private space, was swept thoroughly. In some communities, this cleansing was a public affair and involved public performative ridicule of women who had born twins. After this public display of shame, absolution through *Ikpu Alu*, which varied from one community to the other, was then performed, after which the mother's period of ostracism ended. As government and missionary campaigns against this practice increased, this cleansing became a more private and subdued affair to avoid attracting government attention.

In the efforts to combat twin killings, missionaries and government officials identified midwives as among the "class of African women amongst whom this work is most required," for it was the midwives and other womenfolk in the community who indoctrinated the expecting mothers regarding the dos and don'ts of birth and childrearing.[93] A letter from the district officer in Nsukka to the resident officer of Onitsha Province remarked of midwives, "The native midwives make sure that such children [twins] as well as all breech deliveries and abnormal children are 'still-born' and no report is made to anyone."[94] This act of concealment through traditional midwives was identified by government agents as one of the ways that families evaded any accusations of twin disposal. If the children were born dead, then no question arose as to suspicions of infanticide. Archdeacon Basden also wrote in his 1926 publication recounting his experiences among the Igbo in the early 1900s that a midwife could connive secretly with a mother to preserve the life of one twin while concealing the other's birth.[95]

It is hard to determine how frequently midwives may have participated in these efforts to prevent the delivery of two living babies. Colonial officials had no proof of the midwife's participation but speculated even as late as 1955 that twins were stillborn "probably with the cooperation of the native midwives" since it was midwives who delivered the babies.[96] It is clear, however, that by the 1920s and with growing colonial attention and prosecution of twin deaths, it was more likely that midwives did not want to be caught in the middle of the possible arrests and litigations that ensued over a suspicious death of twins. From a midwives' own account of the birth of a twin in 1926, she and another female assistant concluded the delivery and immediately left the home as soon as it became clear that the expecting mother had borne twins.[97] In the midwife's own words, "She [new mother] said the children ought to be dead and I being afraid ran away."[98] The more likely scenario was that such decisions to preserve one twin were in the hands of the pregnant woman's family members, including her female kin. One report to the district officer of Udi described how hard it was to look out for the birth of twins, stating that families "do not permit anyone into the homes where birth is taking place, and only close family members are allowed into the compound."[99]

The practice of preserving the life of one twin was common as early as 1903 and became the norm in areas where there were early contacts with colonial administrative oversight and missionary presence. A female British missionary in Onitsha, Mary Elms, recounts this practice in a report from 1903 in which she detailed a family's disclosure of the birth of twins and admission that one twin had died.[100] Elms accused the family of poisoning one twin, although she could not conclusively prove this. Another missionary,

Miss Jewitt, recounted being summoned to assist a woman in delivery only to be told upon arrival that "all was well." Upon further inquiry as to the nature of the initial trouble, Jewitt learned, "While we had been coming, twins had been born, but one babe was already dead. These people were not Christians, and although now the mothers of twins were not ruthlessly driven out into the bush and her babies killed, yet both children are never allowed to live."[101] In these cases where one twin was allowed to live, *Ikpu Alu* was quietly carried out to ensure that the act of the birth itself as well as the preservation of one twin from certain death did not result in any spiritual backlash.

Nurse Jewitt wrote, "It is the spirit of Christ alone which can move the hearts of men and women and so completely fill them that all dread of evil spirits may be driven out" and thus help abolish the practice of twin infanticides.[102] The spread of the gospel within local households and among families was in this way articulated as the solution to the practices surrounding the birth of twins. Female missionaries targeted a reeducation of the female population but also recognized that women were generally not the imposers or upholders of this widespread practice and that they needed the colonial machinery to enforce its eradication. Missionaries began to threaten local chiefs and the male heads of families with arrest in cases where twins were known to be discarded. In the previously mentioned case involving the nurse, Mary Elms, the twins' grandfather, who also happened to be a powerful chief in the important town of Onitsha, was arrested until Elms wrote a letter for his release in the hope that such a release might induce the community, who had come daily to ask for her assistance in securing the chief's release, to change their attitudes toward twins.[103]

Some communities avoided conflict with colonial representatives and potential spiritual backlash by willingly turning over twins and their mothers to the care of the church. In the early days of heightened missionary activities in Igboland during the late nineteenth and early twentieth centuries, missionaries often secured land that was considered deadly to humans, for instance, the *Ajo Ofia* (evil forest). When they defied death and instead thrived in these lands that were marked for deities and all that were considered evil and polluted, locals became accustomed to relinquishing unwanted taboo objects to missionaries in the hopes that such transfer absolved them of spiritual repercussions. As such, various communities were willing to relinquish twins and their mothers to missionaries rather than deal with them or risk government prosecution should the twins die.

With increased government clampdown on this custom of twin killing, including criminal prosecution for murder, towns and villages readily agreed to build houses close to missionary stations or hospitals dedicated to the care of twins and their mothers. This served the purpose of preserving the lives of the twins but also removing them from within the community for fear of spiritual backlash. The churches and church shelters became the new evil forest in which polluted objects were deposited. In 1903 and 1906, for instance, two towns readily built shelters near mission stations to care for twin mothers and their babies by missionaries.[104] One town near Onitsha agreed to feed the shelter's residents. In Onitsha, the king, a nominal Christian and a benefactor of the missionaries in his community, was convinced by Elms to construct a large building that served as "a twin-rescue home."[105] For the communities, they were able to avoid government retribution as a result of twin killings but also any spiritual backlash that could occur from harboring such children within their own homes and communities. Missionaries, on the other hand, were suspicious of local intentions and wanted to keep a close eye on twins and their mothers to avoid poisoning or other kinds of "malpractice" from community members eager to circumvent colonial opposition.

Locals had still other motives for acceding to the construction of twinneries. It minimized the risk of government prosecution for lack of proof if twin children died, even under suspicious circumstances, in the twinneries. To elaborate this point, a set of healthy twins were born to Onitsha parents in 1909. The infants and their mother were immediately transferred to the twinneries, where they appeared in good health until they died suddenly within hours of each other, shortly after their relatives visited them in the twinneries. Since there were no capabilities for a postmortem, poisoning or other foul play could not be proven. Nonetheless, a suspicious Elms accused the king and his chiefs of using the twin homes as a guise to shield a continued and subtle practice of infanticide.[106]

Accusations like that of Elms were hard to prove throughout the campaign to eradicate the practice of twin killings as multitudes of other circumstances stood against the survival of multiplets. For one, these births typically occurred earlier than the normal duration of pregnancy and were likely to be preterm. These premature deliveries undermined the infants' chances of survival and exposed them to negative outcomes of childhood ailments. In a country in which high infant mortality from a wide array of tropical ailments for children under five was a recurring complaint, twins were likely to perish quicker than singletons. The district officer from Nsukka remarked, for example, that "the fact that most twins are inevitably somewhat 'weedy' makes detection of conscious neglect of them almost impossible."[107] There were also challenges posed by malnourishment, resulting from a woman's inability to provide the proper amount of nourishment for the multiple infants at a time. This was especially so in an era in which powdered milk was an alien idea. According to a letter from the resident officer of Onitsha Province to the Ministry of Welfare in the Eastern Region, some mothers who were ostracized by their family and communities suffered from low morale and possibly depression and, under such circumstances, "neglect[ed] to suckle the children," leading to death.[108]

The colonial administration tied interventions in childbirth to any successful eradication of twin killing and other unwanted cultural practices surrounding birth. A report from the Catholic mission in Iwollo Oghe to the district officer of Udi highlighted this correlation, stating that "more maternity homes, I think, would help to eliminate the practice entirely as more cases of the birth of twins would come to light."[109] The district officer himself recommended to the resident of the entire area, "I would unhesitantly put first the provision and encouragement of more maternity homes."[110] What colonial administrators described as propaganda against practices like twin births was not hugely successful at the individual level because of the social process that childbirth entailed among the Igbo. It was not enough to address individual families, including Christian ones, as it was sometimes the extended family that exerted influence to uphold certain practices. As such, tackling infanticide entailed limiting or eliminating the influence of these parties, including the local midwife, who was speculated to be complicit in the act of twin killings, from the birthing process through the relocation of birth to maternity homes.

Twin killing died a slow but sure death, and by the late 1940s, it had significantly declined due to the expanding growth of churches and colonial prosecution of such cases. During the same period of this pronounced decline, however, the stigma against twins remained, albeit at a significantly reduced scale, as expressed in this nurse-midwife's report from the 1940s: "The case of twin babies is still looked upon as an abomination. People dreeded [*sic*] the parties [twins] . . . this custom is gradually dying out."[111] A missionary doctor writing in 1946 similarly remarked of the practice, "Much of these superstitions about twins and other 'abominations' still exist even in these days, but the influence of the church and the examples of many Christians are gradually undermining it."[112] By the time Roseline, who was born in the Onitsha Province in the late 1920s, had her youngest child in the early 1960s, it was becoming the new norm to celebrate a twin birth rather than despise it. According to Roseline, "Eliminating twin killings was the highest thing oyibo [white people] did for us."[113]

Conclusion

The birth of a child was a celebrated moment in Igbo life, one that shaped the social status of married men and women. Its connections to the sociocultural and spiritual affairs of the people made childbirth a subject of interest and a targeted avenue for reform by both missionaries and the colonial government. Motherhood and childbirth have long been at the heart of local and global politics of gender, power, religion, and nationhood. In the local Igbo sphere, narratives around gender and motherhood shaped power dynamics and social status. It also featured in the narratives of legitimacy and illegitimacy. Among the Igbo, "legitimate" motherhood, one that was created within the confines of marriage, secured for married women a firm footing in their marital homes and improved their social standing as full adult citizens of their societies. Childbirth was, itself, a rite of passage that these married women had to fulfill as proof that they were true women and useful members of the society.

Childbirth was crucial and central for various reasons. Beyond ensuring continuity in the society, women's reproductive bodies were essential in an agrarian environment in which labor was drawn from the family unit and a large household directly correlated with greater economic output. As such, birth and birth rituals reflected the cultural, social, and spiritual priorities of the people and reinforced ties that ensured social support to expecting parents and their babies. These rites of pregnancy and childbirth also demonstrated the saying, "*otu onye anaghi azu nwa*" (a single individual does not raise a child), an assertion that signified the communal nature and collective importance of childrearing.

With the advent of the colonial and missionary encounter in Igboland in the late nineteenth and early twentieth centuries, birth and motherhood once more became important to the imperial actors as an avenue for advancing their agendas and reshaping society. Missionaries hoped to utilize the sociocultural connections that childbirth facilitated and the important spaces that mothers occupied in their homes, extended families, and communities to advance Christianity. In this case, if they converted a mother, she would, in turn, raise her children in the Christian tradition and influence others in her social network, including the young people over whom she wielded influence, to become Christians. She and her children would also break free of the control and instruction of traditionalists, an act that would disrupt the indigenous educational systems on which various societies relied for cultural continuity.

For colonial government officials, interest in childbirth, fertility rates, and infant mortality was tied to concerns about the economy and labor supply. As conversations increased about the need to ensure that African colonies could give birth to the future labor supply and, thus, guarantee the extraction and exploitation of agricultural resources across the continent, government officials and missionaries identified mothers and midwives as the problem and obstacle to infant survival due to their birthing and childrearing practices. For them, these practices were propagated by midwives and the network of older women who regulated the affairs of younger women in indigenous educational networks like Ebe and Nkpu, as well as in the tightly controlled spaces of reproduction. Infant feeding, dressing, and care came under attack at every turn, and there was a determination to replace the midwives and the groups of older women who perpetrated these practices.

Training in "mothercraft," a buzzword from this era, became the focus of many colonial gatherings, including conferences, to retrain the mothers to become better childrearers and mothers of a healthy nation. Controlling motherhood and "mothercraft" meant ensuring that women raised their families along the lines of acceptable colonial principles but also guaranteed that their childbearing and rearing practices preserved the government's ability to harness an abundant labor supply with which it would exploit agricultural production and natural resources in the colony. As colonial scrutiny over motherhood and childrearing increased, it sparked off a rivalry and a series of intersections and adaptations that shaped Nigeria's landscape of birth beyond the colonial era. In the case of twin killings, officials explicitly stated that its eradication was expressly tied to the expansion of maternity centers and their replacement of traditional birthing institutions.

2

Instruments of Propaganda

Colonial Maternities, Medical Missions, and Colonized Women

No service rendered by a mission to a community is more appreciated and brings more vital contact with the people than does midwifery.

Clement Chesterman, *In the Service of the Suffering: Phases of Medical Missionary Enterprise*

Introduction

On the eve of the twentieth century in 1899, Dr. Arthur Clayton, a medical missionary for the Church Missionary Society (CMS), wrote in *Mercy and Truth*, the CMS publication on medical missions, that over a hundred people passed through the CMS's little hospital in Onitsha on the eastern part of Nigeria. He lamented, however, that the salvation of their souls during medical care was not sustained because 75% of the patients were from the interior and returned to their various distant locations at the end of their care.[1] His publication was a rallying call for missionary doctors to join the CMS's work in Nigeria and advance the society's medical missions. In 1905, Dr. Druitt, another medical missionary who had worked in northern and southern Nigeria, echoed Clayton's interest in medical missions as a means to evangelism and reported that missionaries believed that medical missions would result in the rapid conversion of non-Christians.[2]

Like Dr. Clayton, Dr. Druitt believed that the greatest obstacles to medical mission work were the lack of adequate missionary staff and the inability to reach former patients who lived further away from hospital posts where there were no churches and no Europeans.[3] These doctors' discussions, along with those of other medical missionary workers, dominated CMS pamphlets in the early twentieth century in a manner that was hitherto absent. Their presence indicates a shift toward medicine as a path to the Africans' soul. At the turn of the twentieth century, medical work in Nigeria was of a limited scale in both the number of medical staff and the number of biomedical facilities. What existed during this period was limited to the coastal areas, such as Lagos, Badagry, and the Calabar area, where there were concentrations of Europeans and a longstanding missionary presence.[4] Inland, the existence of biomedical work depended on the unlikely availability of European medical staff or the presence of missionaries who had formal or informal medical experience. There was little colonial interest in the development of health infrastructure for Nigerians during this era.

As more Europeans ventured into Nigeria, the government concentrated its health facilities around their urban outposts.[5] In many instances, these foreign personnel resided in separate parts of town, often in areas known as Government Reserved Areas (GRAs). As such, medical infrastructure was concentrated there to safeguard the health of government employees. The impact on access to care is evident in this CMS archdeacon's description of the availability of government medical care in a portion of Nigeria during the first quarter of the twentieth century: "In this area . . . as large as England and Wales, there are perhaps four or five government doctors [but] their time is largely taken up with ministering to the scattered groups of [British] officials and government servants."[6] As a result, realms of medicine such as women's and children's health that affected large portions of the rural populations were neglected in Nigeria until the late 1930s, when the British government was under pressure to demonstrate its dedication to colonial development. In 1931, for instance, four officially recognized midwifery training centers existed in the colony of Nigeria, and only one government training center, Massey Street Hospital, Lagos, was in operation.[7] This government institution trained a limited number of Nigerians (seven pupil-midwives in 1930) for midwifery positions.[8] In fact, a formal medical policy for the colony did not exist until 1942 when colonial administration issued a policy document, *Medical Policy in the Colonial Empire*, to address this problem and guide medical development.[9]

Similar to government's initial disinterested approach to health care provisions for the local community, CMS, the missionary wing of the Anglican Church and the largest missionary group to set up operations in Nigeria in the mid-nineteenth century (1842), enacted a policy that dissuaded the adoption of temporal means to achieve spiritual ends. Missionaries upheld the principle that salvation could only come from the desire to be saved and not from physical benefits that Christianity might offer. The CMS shifted its policy, however, when it saw how successfully their main rival, the Roman Catholic Mission (RCM), utilized the provision of medical care as an opportunity to baptize children and, thus, claim their souls for the Catholic Church. By the late nineteenth century, the CMS had fully embraced medicine as an evangelical tool, triggering a race between the two missions to claim converts through baptism.[10] Having arrived late to the scene in 1885, RCM sought to establish their influence in areas that had already been dominated by the CMS and, to a lesser extent, other Protestant missions through the provision of medical care. In the process, they indiscriminately baptized children in the name of the Catholic Church. This baptism, they believed, gave them a claim to the individual's souls and signified that the baptized person could be counted as Catholic.[11]

These baptized patients included members of the Anglican church, a trend that the CMS found provocative. A. C. Strong, a CMS missionary, described the situation in 1886: "Parents did not take their children for baptism but for medical aid and the priest seized the opportunity of administering holy baptism first and then medicine afterwards."[12] In another report, he wrote, "Medicines and presents of various kinds were benevolently and liberally given and by these they are hoping to become strong. . . . Five infants whose parents are full members of our church were baptized by one of the priests."[13] RCM action caused panic in CMS ranks, especially because they lost members to the Roman Catholic Church who had become sympathetic to the Catholic cause due to the latter's provision of medical care and, in some cases, other forms of assistance.[14]

Increasingly in the 1890s, CMS leaders appealed to their London headquarters to open medical missions across Nigeria to counteract RCM activities. These appeals were the CMS's first steps toward adopting maternal health as an arena for evangelism.[15] The CMS abandoned their longstanding policy of not using temporal means for spiritual ends and instead hailed the work of mercy, notably medical work, as a worthy Christian pursuit. Jesus's work on earth, they argued, included the saving of souls and healing of bodies.[16] In 1897, the CMS dedicated its maiden quarterly medical mission publication *Mercy and Truth* to drawing an analogy for its supporters in the United Kingdom on the strong connections between the physical body and the soul as well as the connections between mercy (health care) and truth (the gospel).[17]

To advance Christianity amid the personnel shortages that threatened to stall missionary work in the first quarter of the twentieth century, CMS and other missionary groups placed local women at the center of their medical mission agenda. Childbearing women, they believed, could be a conduit for spreading mission propaganda among other women in districts beyond the grasp of mission hospitals. As established in the previous chapter, missionary societies like the CMS directed their attention to maternal health care based on the view that providing care for pregnant women gave missionaries access to not only women but also their children and extended families. Midwifery and child welfare services were, therefore, seen as a way to penetrate local communities and, through local women, advance Christian propaganda. This outlook is aptly captured in a colonial official's commentary that "this peaceful penetration through the motherhood of the country" afforded colonial agents and missionaries an effective way to advance into the country and spread their agenda without the use of violence.[18] Dr. E. Downes, another CMS medical missionary, conveyed a similar sentiment about the tactic in his call to "make friends through the wives, mothers, and sisters of the people."[19]

Government and missionary reports reveal the nature of and rationale behind missionary and, later, colonial government involvement in the development of biomedical maternity services at diverging moments in Nigeria's history. They also show the extent to which these rationales determined the scope and pace of women's medicine, education, and the professionalization of midwifery. What tactics did government and missionaries employ to achieve their goals, and how did local women navigate these policies and the consequent new landscapes that they created? From the early 1900s, CMS doctors and nurses began deliberate medical mission work in connection with maternal and child health. In the first quarter of the twentieth century, the mission group intentionally recruited female doctors from the United Kingdom to advance this work. It also recruited widows and older women in the local community as auxiliary nursing staff.[20] Unlike their married counterparts, widows could carry on mission maternity work without the encumbrance of marriage. As twinneries—facilities that were set up to accommodate twins and save them from certain death—expanded, missionaries also utilized the services of teenage female twins as nurses and midwives due to their low likelihood of marriage. In this way, these twins, raised and catered for by a mix of local and mission funds, became a valuable part of the colonizing mission.

Missionary interest in positioning women as agents of social conditioning, as well as the general view of women as inactive political and economic observers, shaped the nature of educational and professional opportunities that were made available to them. Since the colonial government largely excluded women from colonial politics and economy, there were limited opportunities for women in professional fields and a lack of investment in women's education. Instead, women's education before the 1940s focused mostly on domestic subjects, such as cookery and needlework, and training that was considered essential for grooming a successful Christian family in which women were submissive housewives. One of the missionaries' key tactics involved opening marriage training homes to spread the gospel among local women and educate them in Western etiquettes and mothercraft. Some local women readily enrolled in these homes or were sponsored by fiancés and husbands—not for their salvation or "civilization" but because it improved their chances of attracting educated spouses or laying claim to a spot in the emerging elite class of Westernized locals. More women, including auxiliary nurses and mothers, found ways to participate in the emerging medical landscape in ways that were not originally envisaged by the colonial administration.

As government interest in large-scale women's welfare work increased in the 1940s, additional educational opportunities gradually opened to Nigerian women in the fields of nursing and midwifery. The British government had realized that an efficient system of colonial economic extraction and political pacification in a postwar era of rising nationalist movements required a reasonable degree of intervention in public health initiatives. One government officer said of this, "Such inroads into family life would be led by first and foremost the medical service."[21] As in the case of missionaries, maternal health care was viewed as the fast track to making such advances. Nonetheless, the decades of neglect of maternal health infrastructure and female education meant that there was a shortfall of women with the required level of education or years of experience to qualify for the Grade I midwifery certificate, a rank that was dominated by European staff. The number of certified training centers that could accommodate the growing demand for midwifery training was far too few. Government's late intervention in this branch of health care and in women's education had left a severe and intractable shortage of midwives, maternity hospitals, and training schools. These shortages remained acute at independence and shaped the politics of childbirth for the rest of the twentieth century.

Centering Women in Mission Propaganda: Medical Missions and Maternity Work

Before the twentieth century, maternity work was very limited by the absence of a sizable female missionary population. Few European women accompanied their husbands to Nigeria, and even fewer ventured out independently.[22] This circumstance gradually changed in the first half of the twentieth century as more female missionaries accepted postings to Nigeria. To balance the shortfall of qualified medical doctors and fulfill missionaries' growing requests to rely more on trained medical personnel, the CMS recruited European nurses, mostly women, for its missionary outposts. These female medical personnel began to advance maternity work as a deliberate means to penetrate local households. Making mothers and maternity homes the center of medical missions ensured the continuity of Christian work as converted women were expected to raise Christian children in the faith and expose members of their multigenerational households to the gospel. "Civilizing" the woman meant "saving" the family and ultimately the nation. Here, motherhood and mothering were deployed as the ultimate tool for Christianizing the colony.

Nowhere in Nigeria were maternity services more clearly the core of an early twentieth-century medical missionary enterprise than in the Medical CMS Mission, later renamed Iyi-Enu Mission Hospital, a major hub of operations for medical work in the Niger Mission, an administrative territory that covered parts of northern and southern Nigeria and included the Hausaland Mission in northern Nigeria (from 1890 to 1905). The history of Iyi-Enu Hospital dates to 1890, when it was first established in Onitsha as a dispensary without a doctor. It became a full-scale medical mission, the Onitsha Medical Mission, in 1898 with the arrival of a doctor.[23] The CMS relocated the medical mission to its present location in neighboring Ogidi in 1907 after access to adequate water supply was secured at Iyi Enu (High Spring), a spring in Ogidi after which Iyi-Enu hospital was named.[24]

The development of women's medicine and maternity work at Iyi-Enu was driven by the shortage of doctors at mission outposts across Nigeria. The

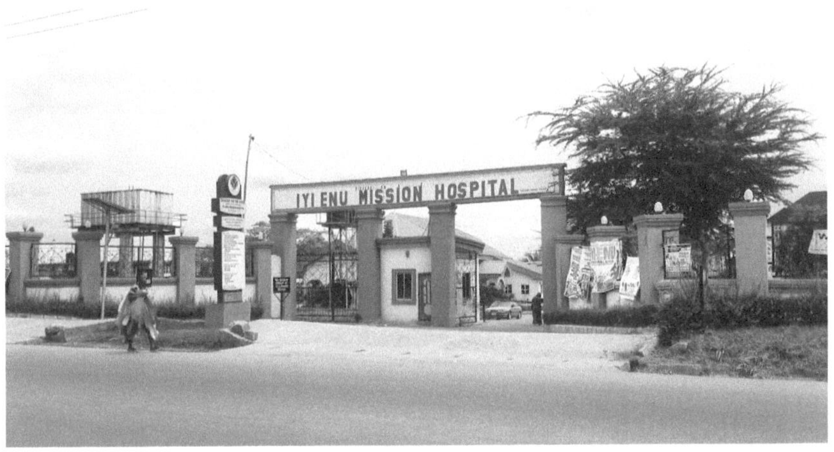

Entrance to Iyi-Enu Hospital, Ogidi, 2016

doctor at the mission hospital, for instance, had to cover other locations and would travel from places like Asaba, west of the River Niger, to Iyi-Enu, east of the Niger.[25] The doctor also routinely made other necessary medical trips further afield. Between 1903 and 1907, the CMS ameliorated the situation by sending more trained nurses, all women, to their medical mission on the Niger rather than take on the more expensive prospect of securing additional doctors. This increased presence of women in the mission enabled the expansion of maternity work. Under the initiative of the nurses—L. M. Maxwell, Miss Warner, and Miss Wilson—a women's inpatient ward was added to the Onitsha Medical Mission in 1900, and women's medicine began to advance.[26] By 1918, the hospital had two large wards for locals, one small ward for Europeans, a dispensary, three houses for European staff, and an unfinished theater and had established a legacy for its work in maternity services.[27] Of Iyi-Enu's reputation, an English man touring Nigeria in 1927 reported, "[The work at Iyi-Enu] was one of the very best bits of medical works I saw in Nigeria at all."[28]

The encouraging level of patient visits to the female ward at Iyi-Enu was a source of satisfaction to the nurses, who soon expanded their services to include midwifery. Notable among these nurses was Mary Elms, who joined the Medical CMS Mission in 1901 and whose work in midwifery and child welfare influenced the outlook of Iyi-Enu and other medical missions in the region for the next twenty-five years. By 1930, the medical mission at Iyi-Enu

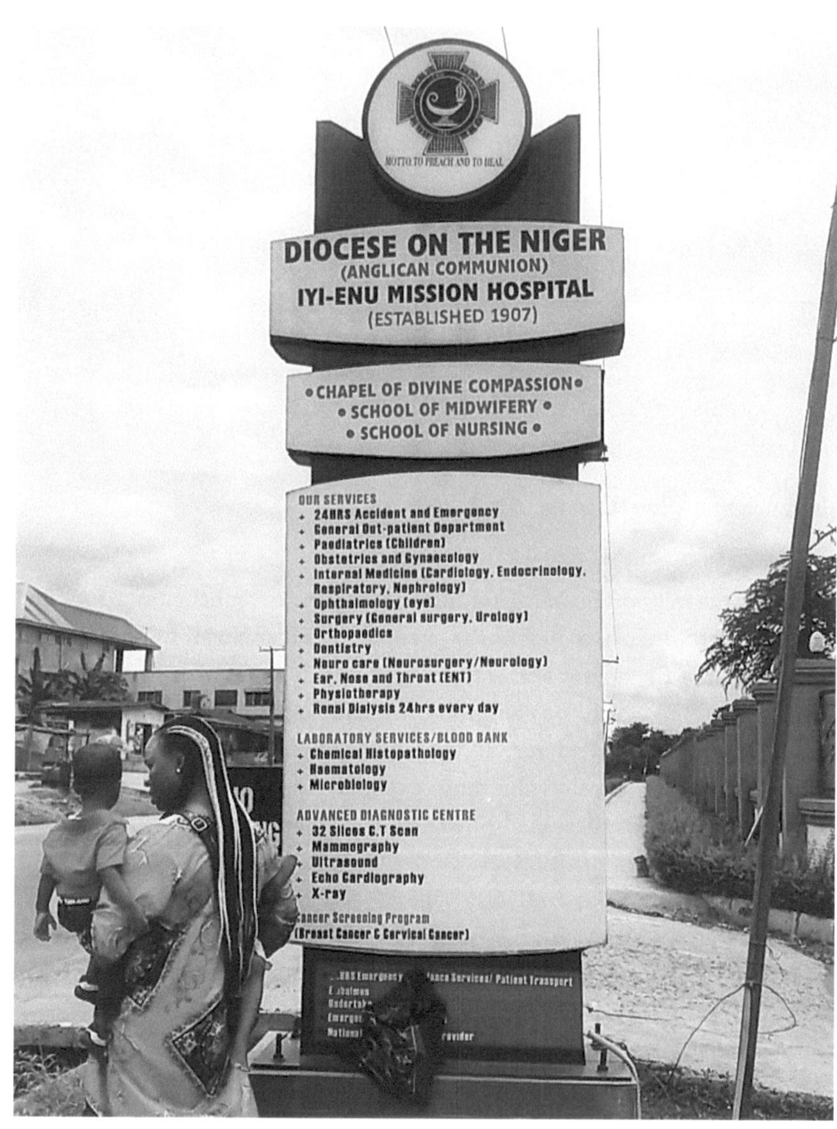

Signpost displaying Iyi-Enu hospital services, 2016

was dominated by female health workers and considered a "women's show" in official circles.[29] In 1932, the hospital was recognized by the colonial government as one of only four centers in Nigeria for the training of midwives.[30] From Iyi-Enu Hospital, maternity work expanded to other medical outposts in Owerri, Nsukka, Ogwashi, Ebu, Aba, and Isokoland.[31]

According to Archdeacon Basden of the Niger Mission, the CMS maintained Iyi-Enu Hospital as a predominantly women-run establishment because the female composition of the doctors and nurses would stir up more sympathy in England and move more people to provide financial support for the mission.[32] However, this was only part of the story. In line with the agenda of medical missions, Iyi-Enu Hospital's female staff rapidly expanded the scope of maternity and child welfare work to create a medical platform for evangelism that became central to CMS evangelism. Missionaries not only aimed to promote Christianity through healing but also sought an efficient way of doing so through maternity work. They believed that these hospital encounters "were the most favorable environment in which to win the confidence and disarm the prejudices of those opposed to it [gospel]."[33]

Later appointments of doctors and nurses at Iyi-Enu between 1926 and 1940 deliberately maintained the mission's status quo as predominantly female-staffed to exert continually greater influence on local family life through its direct contact with the mothers, children, and families in its maternity care ministry.[34] This approach, according to one missionary, was a "particularly effective Christian side of medical service" that connected evangelical, educational, social, and medical work together for the purposes of saving souls and altering cultural practices unwanted by missionaries.[35]

As mission outposts expanded and their reputation grew, so did their desire to undermine what were considered pagan customs, a category that covered broad subjects like "native" dance, dressing, marriage customs, naming, medicine, and birthing traditions. These efforts were stalled due to staff shortages exacerbated by the onset of World War I, when medical staff were called into military service or were unable to secure transportation to their posts after vacationing in their home countries. From 1915 to 1919, mission societies in Nigeria resorted to recruiting local staff to advance their influence. To leverage the general lack of European staff and the mission's inability to reach women in distant local communities, medical missionaries targeted their recruitment efforts toward certain groups of women who appeared to be unencumbered by marriage alliances.

In parts of southern Nigeria where the killing of twins was common, European missionaries recruited twins for training as mission and maternity staff. Although the practice of twin killing had come under missionary assault in the nineteenth and early twentieth centuries and had declined by the late 1930s in areas with prominent colonial administrative presence, the stigma associated with twins persisted into the 1940s.[36] As such, the twins who were raised as government or missionary wards in twinneries became prime candidates for work as missionaries, nurses, and midwives due to the likelihood, as late as the 1940s, that twins were unlikely to get married because of prospective suitors' fears of stigma and spiritual retribution.[37] Twin girls were sent to female schools and trained as midwives and nurses to prepare them for their most viable social role as medical missionaries.[38] Missions also recruited widows and older women whom they trained informally as evangelists and nurses or midwives because they, like twins, would be un- encumbered by marriage and families over the course of their lives.[39] In Enugu District, church councils sent four elderly Christian widows to Iyi-Enu in 1927 to train as midwives for a period of four months and to start work- ing in the district immediately afterward.[40] Other branches of the Niger Mission adopted this trend.

This initial focus on older women reflected traditional views of midwifery, as discussed in chapter 1, in which midwives were required to be women who had themselves experienced childbirth. Communities rebuffed girls and younger women in those early days, refusing to follow their instructions out of a belief that women who had not given birth were ignorant of birth and birth pangs and, therefore, had no basis for instructing laboring women on the subject. Missionary assessments blamed this resistance from local com- munities on familiarity between the midwife and the patient, the former having grown up in the same locality as that of their midwifery training.[41] While this missionary interpretation cannot be discounted, this challenge was more emblematic of traditional views of childbirth in which trust in the midwife was established over years, sometimes decades, of proving compe- tency as an apprentice and then as an independent midwife.

Mission hospitals made a public spectacle of their maternity work to at- tract the broader public to their stations and elicit interest in their medical and evangelical work. One tactic for doing so was by hosting "baby shows." In these shows, mothers who gave birth in mission hospitals were invited to display their babies for inspection by medical missionaries. The best-looking baby was selected by a medical worker, and both mother and baby received prizes. These baby shows had a history from Britain during World War 1 where a Baby Week was initiated in 1917 to promote the proper rearing of healthy babies and curb high infant mortality rates.[42] *The British Journal of Nursing* reported of these infant deaths, "Of 800,000 babies born in England and Wales, 100,000 die before the year is out, so that a soldier at the Front has a better chance of life to-day than a baby under a year old in this country."[43] The Baby Week, which included baby shows, became popular at the time as a tool for social education and realignment of mothercraft and was transported to British territories during the post–World War I era by missionary nurses.

In Nigeria, the earliest recorded baby show occurred in November 1926 when nurses at Iyi-Enu Hospital organized an "Ibo [*sic*]" Baby Show in which about fifty mothers who gave birth at the hospital in a three-year window displayed their babies to the public. In return, they were each given gifts, such as soap, baby clothes, lotions, and cots.[44] Cots were alien to these parts at the time and became one of the new items that missionaries introduced as part of their attempts to "civilize" the delivery and childcare process. In fact, the cots used by some missionaries, including a West Indian couple, had some Igbo women wondering if the missionaries cared at all for their babies or had any respect of their duties as a mother by putting "the baby upon a shelf."[45] These Igbo women instead had babies sleep next to their mothers after birth. Over time, however, cots became one of the curious attractions at baby shows and maternity wards, as well as a class symbol for many in the emerging urban areas.

Iyi-Enu Hospital's baby shows garnered much community interest in the work of the mission hospital. They were publicized in mission outposts and among the local communities through town criers, an indigenous means of circulating information to the public through public announcements in village squares. To build momentum and boost attendance for such shows, missionaries made them public spectacles by extending invitations to local chiefs and government officials and, therefore, ensuring that the constituents of these local and foreign dignitaries would show up, as is customary among the locals.[46] The shows were calculated to influence public opinion regarding hospital births, hygiene, and health care. In addition to witnessing the presentation of awards, attendees received the occasional demonstration of hygiene, cookery, and grooming. The ceremonial air that was associated with these baby shows, boosted by the attendance of chiefs and European officials, as well as the gifts received by mothers and their babies, attracted the curiosity of the populace and ensured attendance. This early stage of the baby show focused not on the obsessions with baby scales and weights that marked later events but on drawing attention to the activities of the maternity wards and hopefully increasing the attendance of women at the mission stations. A nurse wrote of another baby show that occurred in Iyi-Enu two years after the first one, "There were some very bonny specimens among them," highlighting the focus on a public show of the numbers of successful births in the hospital as opposed to a baby's robustness.[47]

By the late 1930s, baby shows became common among both missionaries and government health departments across the country as a tool for influencing public attitudes toward delivery and infant care. In Abeokuta in 1938, for instance, more than five hundred expecting mothers and six hundred babies attended a baby show hosted by the Infant Welfare Center.[48] Whereas every contestant received prizes for presenting their babies during the first years of the show, winners were chosen in subsequent years based on the baby's weight, evidence of good grooming, and a robust appearance. The babies were judged as specimens of what an ideal hospital-delivered and well-groomed baby should look like and were held up to the community as an honor and public recognition to aspire to.

In addition to baby shows, mission outposts instituted regular tutoring sessions on health and hygiene that targeted the female population. As missionaries like Mary Elms and Miss Jewitts reasoned, these sessions at women's conferences would be carried on by women to their children and communities, thereby influencing the attitudes of the future generation.[49] By the late 1920s, biweekly health sessions in which doctors and nurses addressed patients on health, hygiene, and the Christian faith were commonplace.[50] Local girls who could be coaxed into visiting the hospital for training or those who were presented by their parents to medical missionaries became exposed to maternity work in mission hospitals. It was not uncommon for parents to leave feisty or headstrong daughters with missionaries. During the first decade of Mary Elms's work at Iyi-Enu, an irritated father showed up at the mission hospital with his adolescent daughter whom he described as headstrong, defiant, and combative. Since this daughter was supposedly useless to him due to her strong will, he reasoned that Elms might have better use for her.[51] In this way, the girl entered missionary services and became a competent assistant to the European nursing staff. Around the same time, more local girls independently applied to Iyi Enu to be trained as nurses for reasons that will become clear shortly.[52]

By the mid-1920s, missionaries were educating young girls on health, hygiene, maternity, and other domestic subjects in "marriage training homes" that they had opened across the Niger Mission to mold the young women into suitable Christian wives and mothers.[53] In some cases, girls were taught enough reading skills to study the Bible. The rest of the curriculum focused on needlework, "African cookery, laudry [sic] work, housewifery, and the mothercraft."[54] By 1939, these marriage training homes were commonplace and had more than 900 females enrolled in them in that year.[55] A missionary report from the same year stated that the schools produced, "year by year a number of Christian young women well prepared for Christian marriage."[56] These various avenues of contact with local women increased attendance at mission hospitals and promoted dissociation from traditional medical practices and other cultural norms, such as local naming and dress patterns or indigenous educational systems like those described in the previous chapter—Iso Ebe and Ikwa Mkpu.[57] They also sustained debates over polygamy, traditional marriage rites, and frictions over the implementation of colonial ordinances that were sometimes at variance with local customs.[58]

As more churches grew in various communities, women's organizations, notably the Mothers Union and Women's Guild, emerged to promote the views of Christian missions and mission hospitals.[59] These arms of the church effectively indoctrinated its members against associations with traditional medicine practitioners and monitored members' participation in all of the cultural practices that missionaries campaigned against. The Mothers Union, for instance, advanced the church's view on polygamy and served to sanction or proscribe members who acted outside what was considered Christian norms, such as marital unions with married men. The same shaming and sidelining applied in the case of members who utilized traditional medical systems.

The success that the marriage training homes enjoyed during this period was not entirely a result of missionary efforts or because local men and women sought Christian marriages. In the 1930s, the economic and social landscape in Nigeria was changing. Many young men who attained any level of Western education sought work as clerks, drivers, teachers, school masters, and public servants. Others relocated from their villages to the city to insert themselves in the urban economies that were expanding across the country. In describing these new changes that were occurring across Nigeria, the missionary Margaret Roseveare wrote, "Changes were taking place very rapidly in Nigeria at this time . . . great developments were taking place commercially. Numerous roads had been made, bridges erected, and a system of lorry transport begun. The 'wire road', so named because of its telegraph fittings, linked up Onitsha with Iyi-Enu, Awka, and Enugu, a new town. . . . Some of the more wealthy Africans owned cars, and bicycles abounded on the roads."[60] Women were largely left out of these new colonial occupations, and while missionaries aimed to civilize them and bring Christianity through them to their extended families, the women and girls sought to improve their chances of securing a marital union with the urban or Western-educated men by acquiring basic knowledge of the English language and the trappings of European etiquette. The Marriage Training Homes offered exactly the advantage in the emergent social order sought by mothers for their girls and by women for themselves. It also provided excellent opportunities for those who embraced Christianity to become proficient in the Western etiquette that was associated with missionaries.

In other cases, according to a retired dispenser whose wife received training in nursing and home economics, men also sent their fiancés and wives to the training homes or mission hospitals for short courses in nursing.[61] One colonial administrator wrote of this arrangement, "These girls are the betrothed of the advanced men in the District, school masters, court clerks and others who desire as wives something better than the mere manual laborer and automatic producer of children that surrounding bush woman very largely is."[62] For missionaries in the southeast, this interest in missionary and European facilities meant that "the whole attitude of the Ibo [sic] people towards spiritual teaching had changed," and there seemed to be "a widespread and eager desire for knowledge."[63] For families, participation often meant an avenue to achieve upward mobility in a changing society. Young Christian men, often educated, frequently married Christian women or those who had been exposed to some Christian or Western instruction, and both went hand in hand as missionaries were in the habit of baptizing the nurses, midwives, and students that they trained.[64]

Progress in maternity work at the Niger Mission was slow, but it maintained a steady growth. At Iyi-Enu Hospital, attendance at prenatal clinics expanded each year, although most patients still preferred a home birth surrounded by their midwife and family members. As a result, many cases handled by the hospital in the 1900s to 1920s involved emergencies and difficult births. An estimated 50% of those who visited the hospital for delivery did not attend prenatal clinics or were difficult or emergency cases that could not be handled by the traditional midwife.[65] Low utilization of the hospital by prenatal patients during labor and delivery remained the case throughout the 1940s and 1950s as most women continued to receive prenatal instructions in the hospital and deliver at home.

One practical speculation about this trend, especially in the early years, lies in the fact that many women had active lifestyles during pregnancy and engaged in agriculture or trade up to the onset of their birthing time. Women, therefore, went into labor at odd periods and had no choice but to deliver their babies at home or other location at the time of labor. Hospital outposts were, after all, few and far between and modes of transportation inadequate. In the Isoko District where the Niger Mission had sent delegates from Iyi-Enu— nurses Jewitt and Sheath—to begin a maternity hospital, the swampy terrain and lack of good roads meant that many patients with complicated delivery "preferred to stay at home and die."[66] According to Roseveare, "The nearest hospital was two or three days journey by canoe, or a long journey by stretcher across rough tracks through forest and swamps under a tropical sun."[67]

Local women's calculations of the risks and benefits of birthing options are telling of the motivations behind women's participation in colonial medical spaces. The fact that prenatal attendance and home deliveries persisted for decades suggests that it was a deliberate pattern set by local women. These women perhaps chose to take advantage of the health education and monitoring provided during prenatal care while birthing in a culturally sensitive or familiar environment. Within the confines of their own homes, women and families could observe postbirth practices that missionaries disregarded, such as the proper disposal and burial of the placenta and umbilical cord. As discussed in chapter 1, local communities placed as much importance on these postbirth practices as the birth itself. The monetizing of birth that became a part of maternity care in the 1920s and beyond also cannot be ignored. Iyi Enu's annual report for 1928 indicated, for instance, that "normal cases have decreased in numbers possibly on account of a confinement fee of one guinea having been introduced."[68] As emphasized in the previous chapter, traditional midwives during the early to mid-twentieth century practiced as a matter of public good rather than monetary gain. Thus, women who had no complications made the calculated efforts to utilize hospitals' free prenatal services but retain the services of their midwives for delivery.

The community health education work performed by nurses played a critical role in enhancing medical missions' reputations. At the end of 1926, Dr. Batley, the medical superintendent at Iyi-Enu, reported that families were more open to utilizing the hospital for prenatal and maternity services.[69] By 1929, the number of hospital births had grown from 102 in the previous year to 129, although more prenatal clinic attendees still chose home birth. Of this figure, eighty-nine were normal cases, reducing the stigma on hospitals as the place for abnormal cases.[70] The Isoko district saw a similar increase in the number of expecting women receiving prenatal care, with less than 50% of the women utilizing the maternity ward for delivery. Of the 673 prenatal cases in 1934, for instance, only 246 patients had their babies in the hospital.[71] This pattern persisted as late as 1942 when the medical superintendent, Dr. Anderson, reported that an estimated 50% of women who birthed in the hospital were not prenatal patients, although not necessarily emergency cases, and most of those who faithfully attended prenatal care for eight months did not utilize the hospital for birth, highlighting women's agency in this emerging maternity landscape.[72] As prenatal care and hospital birth became popular, demand for midwives also increased across various districts. By the mid-1940s, many local governments scrambled to hire trained midwives for service in their districts or to sponsor a midwifery candidate in the few available training centers.[73]

Colonial Politics, Female Education, and the Professionalization of Midwifery

Until the late 1930s, maternal and child welfare work remained mostly in the hands of missionaries. A professionalized or nationally recognized midwifery sector was still nonexistent. As the colonial government faced heightened international and local criticism of its colonial enterprise during the interwar years, Britain redoubled its public health and welfare measures to gain the support of its colonial subjects and ward off criticism from abroad. The League of Nations, which was formed in the aftermath of World War I, convened the Pan-African Health Conference and an African Commission in the 1930s to push colonizers to institute comprehensive plans for health care in African territories. They also began to compel colonial rulers to connect the economic status of the colonized to the attainment of improved health conditions.[74]

According to a 1933 letter by a CMS official on this subject, "government feels there is great scope for such a piece of welfare work and realizes that no one can do this better than missionaries."[75] Several dialogues occurred between missionaries and the government in the 1930s over the nature and extent of their collaborations in health care provision. In 1932, the colonial governor of Nigeria, Donald Cameron, authorized an experimental project that tested the potentials of such collaboration in maternal and infant welfare.[76] In conjunction with the Niger Mission and its medical missionaries at Iyi-Enu, the governor proposed the hiring of Traveling Lady Doctors for itinerant work across various districts. These female European doctors were selected from the corps of Iyi-Enu's medical missionaries as "a specific gesture towards the Mission based on real appreciation [by the governor] of the work done at Iyi-Enu."[77] The doctors provided general care where necessary but were most committed to the medical needs of women and children. According to Archdeacon Basden, who worked to solidify this collaboration between CMS and the government, the doctors' responsibilities "would lie entirely outside the hospital and consist in travelling round the surrounding country and working at dispensaries, schools, etc."[78]

Under this mission–government partnership, government provided all of the financial resources for the operation while the mission contributed medical personnel and infrastructure.[79] These doctors continued to fulfill the medical mission's core agenda—conversion through health care—and were instrumental in the continued operation of the mission's marriage training homes. These were two primary motivations for accepting this government partnership, considering CMS and other missions' suspicion of government motives for partnerships prior to this time.[80] Mission skepticism was clearly referenced in Basden's 1933 letter to the Niger Mission's medical committee in an attempt to secure their agreement to work with the governor:

> The Government is arranging to start welfare work among women and children. . . . As you will observe, it is not a case of government trying to get a piece of work done on the cheap, a complaint which has often been alleged when there has been co-operation between government and missions. Full salary is being offered in this case. . . . I can say unhesitantly and emphatically that the offer is a sincere and genuine one from both H.E. the Governor and the Director of Medical Services. They both value highly the work done by our medical missions and are prepared to extend its operations.[81]

In addition to the traveling doctor scheme, government offered grants to missions to aid in the development of more maternity wards and the maintenance of medical personnel. By 1946, the work of the Traveling Lady Doctors had burgeoned and resulted in the proliferation of maternity homes and infant welfare centers.

The newfound partnership between government and missionaries in maternal and child welfare work extended to the education sector. As has been established earlier, women's education prior to the 1940s aimed at grooming proper homemakers and mothers rather than competitive professionals. While some colonial officials, including the superintendent of education of the southern provinces, had begun to contemplate improving women's education in the late 1920s, no concrete action was taken. Since colonial rule emphasized the domestication of women, the type of education afforded them differed from that of men and revolved mostly around domestic sciences. While these types of domestic service–oriented schools were established independent of the government, their existence was lauded in official circles. A British official had remarked of this type of education in 1927, "Normally speaking, an education department would not consider such work under them, but it is real education in this place and alive."[82] Where female education lacked a curriculum centered on cookery, laundry work, and infant care, as in Ibadan in 1933, colonial administrators questioned such education. In their opinion, the future of these female students was marriage and not much else.[83] Formal domestic science schools that provided a "female-centered" training for women became standardized by the colonial government across Nigeria.

As the need to address socioeconomic welfare and expand maternal health care services grew, so did the desire to open more opportunities to women than were previously available to them. However, the impacts of prior policies that privileged the professional training of men since the beginning of the colonial era posed an obstacle to this endeavor. There was a chronic lack of female staff to take on what was considered women's work. A British visitor in Nigeria captured this shortage of trained female staff when he described the condition in a girls' school where teachers were entirely male until a new chair, a woman, became head of the school. One of her first acts was to sack the entire male staff and begin the training of female teachers who did not have the formal certifications of their male counterparts.[84] Such issues were widespread in mixed-gender schools across the country, where the lack of certified female teachers meant a higher rate of male admissions due to beliefs that the nature of the education did not suit female training.[85]

This scarcity of trained female personnel manifested itself more acutely in the realm of medicine, midwifery, and maternal welfare from the onset of colonial rule and medical missionary work. A missionary observed in 1900, for instance, that their "little hospital" on the Niger employed four or five medical helpers, all of them male. Dressers—people who treated wounds and other minor injuries—were men as well.[86] The professional field of nursing also favored men over women. Nurse Dorothy Ross reported in 1924, for example, that local nurses in Iyi-Enu Hospital during that year were all male.[87] Where female nurses existed, the extent of their practice was restricted. In 1929, at Iyi-Enu, female nurses were limited to appointments in female wards, which implied that male nurses existed in sufficient numbers to preside over nonfemale wards.[88] Men, on the other hand, practiced as dressers and served in the dispensaries. Nurse Lee Pronger wrote in the same year (1929) that, "for the work in the men's ward and the dispensary, male nurses are trained, while for the women and children we teach African girls."[89] This predominance of men in the medical sector, including the field of nursing, remained the case until the late 1930s and 1940s. The Colonial Social Welfare Advisory Committee reached the conclusion in 1945 that the government's efforts to recruit women for enrollment in the newly established Yaba Medical School were fruitless because too few girls had even a preliminary science education. One committee member wrote, "At present only one girl's secondary school in Nigeria teaches science and even there only up to School Certificate standard. The project, therefore, is dependent on the development of secondary education for girls."[90]

Government partnership with missionaries accelerated even more in the 1940s. On the one hand, international attention on the health and economic status of colonized territories expanded with the establishment of the United Nations (UN), the League of Nations' successor organization, in the 1940s. In 1949, for instance, the United Nations Trusteeship Committee put Britain in the spotlight by demanding it explain its policy of unequal education in its colonies.[91] In a similar incident, the US Economic Co-operation Administration requested a detailed inventory of Britain's development projects in its colonies in lieu of possible American aid.[92] Although the secretary of state for the colonies argued that the UN committee did not have the right to interfere in colonial administration, Britain was being held to account for the shortfalls in the governance of its colonies and grew increasingly concerned about further criticisms that might come from the UN and other countries. It was under these circumstances that the colonial government in Nigeria adopted a "Medical Policy for the Colonial Empire" in 1942 as the blueprint for the coordination of medical development.[93]

The colonial government also needed the partnerships with missions to overcome the distrust that they encountered in local communities. Despite government efforts at public welfare measures in the 1930s and 1940s, decades of distrust were not easy to erase. Communities were suspicious of government motives for very clear reasons. Considering the oppressive and extortionist nature of colonial occupation and the "native administration" that they installed across Nigeria, government medical intervention was not always welcome. Government officials grew increasingly doubtful that they could gain sufficient trust to clear this atmosphere of suspicion. Therefore, they embraced partnerships with medical missions to create and promote their social welfare programs in local communities.[94] Government's new policy in the 1940s stated, "Not only should there be the closest co-operations between government medical departments, medical missionaries and other unofficial workers in the medical field, but there should also be intimate collaboration between medical workers on the one side and Educational, Agricultural, and Veterinary staff on the other."[95] Prior to this "intimate collaboration," the government mostly dissociated itself from the medical missions. Missionaries, too, kept their distance out of their belief that the government only paid attention to medical missions when it wished to "execute a project on the cheap."[96] Since missionaries performed an array of community health services and enjoyed the goodwill of many communities through years of persistence and perseverance in these stations, government sought to ally with them to expand its capacity for welfare work, specifically in the realms of maternal and child health. Government administrators also recognized that setting up separate institutions for maternal health would result in personnel stretch and understaffing due to the shortage of trained midwives.[97]

Like missionaries, the colonial government identified women's welfare work as an avenue to boost morale about the government and promote government's social welfare agenda in the World War II and postwar era. There was, after all, an established history in the United Kimgdom and in Nigeria, of viewing women and children as cause and effect of a healthy and economically robust nation, or the opposite.[98] It made sense, therefore, that attempts to generate support for the colonial administration and foster a sense of nation-building on their part were couched in interventions in the lives of women and children. In a 1942 memorandum on its medical policy, the colonial office observed that certain tropical conditions exacerbated maternal and infant mortality, creating a disproportionately high ratio of maternal deaths in comparison to the general death rates.[99] Colonial policies advocated for emphasis on preventive medicine with a particular focus on tropical diseases like malaria and the health of mothers and children.[100] For the latter goal, the government focused largely on maternity work, building upon the groundwork that was already established by missionaries.

The future of government welfare programs in the 1940s—and all of the public relations benefits that came with them—also depended upon the administration's reevaluating of its negligence of girl's and women's education. The lady superintendent of education for the southern provinces who favored broadening female education argued that local communities would see this change as necessary and welcome: "As I said in my Annual Report, I believe that girls' education is now at a critical stage, and if financial reasons do not forbid, that the time has come for a real advance. It has become clear to me that the people wish education for their girls, and are willing to send them to school. . . . If an adequate supply of trained women teachers is not available, these girls will be educated by men, or by untrained women."[101] Starting in the 1940s, government expanded its partnership with missionaries from the provision of maternity care to the professional training of women in recognition of what the Colonial Office described as "the influence they [women and girls] have on the social life of the community" and the need for "the female social worker on whom reliance must be placed to secure a full measure of improvement in social welfare."[102] This World War II era of increased government involvement in women's reproductive health measures was thus a defining moment in the development of maternal health in colonial Nigeria and the gradual expansion of training schools for midwives.[103]

It was also in this era that the government perceived medical missions' social welfare objectives as an extension of the government's scheme.[104] This reorientation of the church–state relationship caused a change of attitude toward government funding of medical mission projects, including the expansion of missionary training institutes for midwives. Government objectives included diminishing the number of untrained or informally trained female personnel, the latter being typical of mission trainees, in favor of professionally certified ones.[105] Earlier in 1930, the colonial administration implemented a Midwives Ordinance, which made midwifery a formally recognized profession in colonial Nigeria, with codes of conduct and requirements for certification. However, it was not until the 1940s that government began to pay closer attention to enforcing this ordinance and revising its requirements based on the realities of circumstances in Nigeria, including the low numbers of educated women and the lack of adequate training facilities.[106]

The effect of this 1930 ordinance was double-edged. On the one hand, government recognized midwifery as a certified and officially recognized career path in public service, with the benefits of public service work. The ordinance and its increased implementation in the 1940s also boosted the number of women who entered to train as government-certified nurse-midwives. On the other hand, there were not enough certified midwives and women with the requisite standard of education to fill the new and expanding ranks in midwifery. Thus, a field that was already struggling for qualified staff entered more dire straits because auxiliary staff could not advance beyond a certain level and could not practice by law, although this law preventing them from practicing at this time was nearly impossible to enforce across the country because the majority of existing staff trained before the 1940s had auxiliary status. The Midwives Ordinance further put the government at odds with itself by restricting a midwife's jurisdiction, only permitting midwives to practice within a small and clearly defined area, usually the community in which they trained.[107] In an unstable field in which prospective and certified midwives moved outside of their training areas due to marriage or other family dynamics, this restriction worsened an already bad situation.

Missionaries routinely complained that midwifery personnel were lost to marriage due to the 1930 law that tied their services to the communities in which they trained. As a result, trained midwives who married and moved to their husbands' locations could not practice professionally as midwives if their spouses lived outside of their training locale.[108] An Akure medical officer depicted a typical scenario for pupil-midwives in a 1942 correspondence: "Native law and custom, and public opinion deter girls from the unmarried state. Most of the girls who would and do take up this work are betrothed in infancy or before they leave school and a prospective husband might be willing to wait 4 to 5 years before claiming his wife."[109] This restriction did not work well in practice as nurses and others with Standard 6 elementary education were desirable spouses to Christian men and other educated or semi-educated people who were likely to seek colonial service work far afield from their hometowns and relocate with their wives. Their motivations for joining the nursing and midwifery profession, as described earlier in this section, were frequently at odds with missionaries' objectives of service and evangelism.

Before the 1940s, two grades of midwifery—Grade I and Grade II certificates—took into account the shortage of educated females. Grade I midwives had higher requirements for qualification and trained for three years.[110] Grade II midwives, on the other hand, required minimal qualification and little education and were set up to be higher than traditional midwives and lower than Grade I practitioners. Their training period was shorter and varied based on the applicant's learning pace.[111] As will become apparent in the next chapter, government efforts later to consolidate the two grades became crucial to subsequent developments in the private health sector. Table 2.1 on the training of midwives in Nigeria displays the difference between Grade I and Grade II training prior to 1942.

Despite desires among colonial administrators to standardize training and qualifications for midwives, standardization was impractical due to the nonuniformity in women's level of education in various parts of the country. In the northern region where Western education was still in its infancy in

Table 2.1. Requirements for Grade I and II Midwifery

Grade I	Grade II
Must have had a good education, passed Middle IV Secondary School or equivalent.	No particular standard of education required. Syllabus states "may be quite illiterate."
Must train for at least three years. Must have delivered at least fifty women and attended at least fifty lectures.	Must have been under instruction for at least six months and delivered personally twenty women.
Must be willing to serve in any part of Nigeria. Need not be "local" inhabitant.	Should be local women by birth or long residence, taught (locally) and registered to practice locally.
Written paper required as well as oral and practical examination.	Examination entirely oral and practical. No paper required.

1942, for example, there was a lack of candidates with the qualifications to be trained as Grade I midwives, thus limiting midwifery personnel in these locations to Grade II certificates.[112] In the Wusasa Training Center, a major nursing and midwifery training center in the region, for example, only one in six nursing and midwifery candidates anticipated passing their exams.[113] There were insufficient northern indigenes, male or female, who could advance the health and educational schemes being adopted in other parts of the country.[114] The number of children enrolled in schools remained extremely low compared to southern provinces. In 1949, this number was 2.5% in the North and 20% in the South.[115] In the southern provinces, circumstances tilted toward the opposite as more women had higher levels of education to qualify in the Grade I category. The limited availability of training centers and Grade I midwives across the colony meant a heavy reliance on the retention of the Grade II status.[116]

As female education gradually improved, a more unified requirement for Grade II midwifery that was closely in line with Grade I standards was proposed by a medical officer:

a. That they shall have passed standard vi. (elementary school) and that they hold a School Leaving Certificate to this effect. <u>Must be able to understand English.</u>

b. That they are at least sixteen years of age.

c. Need not be local inhabitants but must be able to speak the language of the patients among whom they will work.

d. May sit for the CMS examination at any time after the completion of their second year provided that they have reached examination standard.

e. Must be willing to stay on for at least a year after they have qualified [This was to circumvent married students leaving immediately after their training].

f. Must be willing to go where sent provided it is in the Area under which they are registered.

g. Must have attended at least fifty lectures and delivered at least fifty women, before taking the examination.[117]

The government approved these new standards shortly after they were proposed in 1942. References in several medical and missionary correspondences show that they were in effect by 1948, although they could not be applied evenly in many provinces due to the persistent lack of qualified personnel.[118]

To address the issue of staff continuity caused by loss of trained midwives upon marriage, the new guidelines for Grade II certificates made it easier for newly trained nurses and midwives to continue their midwifery practice outside their place of registration. These guidelines eliminated the earlier restriction and stipulated only that midwives should be competent in the local language of the community in which they wished to work. Supporters of the new policy argued that marriage could advance mission and government agendas rather than deter it. Official sentiment at this point was that "if we are to get anywhere with medical development in this country, we have got to encourage the private practitioner."[119] Married women could extend their knowledge to their new families and the remote communities in which they sometimes settled with their husbands. These interactions would in turn undermine the influence of traditional medicine practitioners in these communities and strengthen the reach and impacts of the government's maternal and infant welfare policies. The contributions of these married midwives to the Nigeria Medical Service were felt by the 1950s when they increasingly opened private practices and maternity homes in urban and rural residences, making midwifery services accessible to a larger proportion of the population than previously.[120]

As maternal health infrastructure expanded and the medical service hired more nurse-midwives to improve the pre-1946 level of female staff, conversations arose within the ranks of nursing and midwifery associations about reserving this field exclusively for women, an idea that made its way into the 1950 Nigerian Nurses Conference agenda but did not materialize.[121] In Ondo Province, the medical officer proposed a scheme to replace most African dressers, predominantly male, with women who doubled as midwife-dressers, a reversal of earlier policies in which dressers and dispensers were almost exclusively male.[122] In this way, communities would simultaneously have the basic medical services of a dresser and a midwife. These midwife-dressers were attached to dispensaries, and a few beds were added to the dispensaries to accommodate maternity cases.[123] Programs like these were already in force in parts of the southern region and were well received by the local administration and patients.[124] For local women, it meant more opportunities to participate in the colonial economy as medical service workers.

Based on a belief that local medical recruits understood the community's lifestyle better than foreigners and that trusted community members could best advance colonial and Christian agenda among their families, friends, and relatives, the colonial regime proposed "Nigerianization" policies in 1946 to decrease the number of European staff in Nigeria's medical department and replace them with more African staff.[125] Colonial officials had also begun to consider the possibility of an independent Nigeria as nationalist movements and requests for self-government were on the rise during this decade. A ten-year plan was developed in 1947 to expand educational and medical institutions and improve local participation in them.[126] By the mid-1950s, more Africans occupied major positions in the medical service. Among the most notable examples is the leadership of the Ministry of Health in the eastern region, whose Nigerian leader, Dr. Michael Okpara, was succeeded in 1954 by another Nigerian, E. P. Okoya. Parliamentary secretaries to the ministries were also Nigerians.[127] By 1955, the Senior Service staff, previously dominated by Europeans, was 62% Nigerian.[128] In 1956, the number grew to 71%, and by 1957, only thirty-five foreigners remained in the senior service corp. Out of a total of 155 service members, 120 were Nigerians.[129] In the Lagos territory where 45.8% of Nigerians held senior appointments in the medical service in 1954, this number rose to 62.6% in 1956 and 73.5% by 1958.[130] The directorship of the Nigeria Medical Service also passed to a Nigerian, Dr. Samuel Manuwa, in 1951. He became the inspector general of the Medical Service three years later.[131]

More Nigerians were also elevated to Grade I midwifery posts in the 1950s, a level that was previously dominated by Europeans. Nonetheless, the professional field of midwifery was relatively new compared to other medical sectors in Nigeria and did not have the adequate number of qualified Nigerian staff with the required years of experience for the Grade I certificate. Up to this time, colonial policy favored hiring European personnel in high-ranking positions while paying local workers with equivalent qualifications less and assigning them to less important posts.[132]

Despite the government's Nigerianization policy, the problem of adequate personnel persisted. There remained a shortage of nurses and midwives even in the southern provinces, where much progress had been made compared to other parts of the country. The health minister reported at the dawn of 1958 that many hospitals remained understaffed and were especially in dire need of midwives.[133] In the often-lauded eastern region, in which the famed Iyi-Enu Hospital and most of the Niger Mission were located, a total of 610 nurses, midwives, nursing sisters, and superintendents, including temporary staff and those in training, served a region of an estimated nine million people.[134] There was a clear realization by the colonial office that "to enable this [medical] work to be carried out effectively larger staff of women workers of all grades will be required"; however, decades of neglecting female education and inclusion in the colonial machinery could not easily be undone.[135]

Conclusion

The colonial enterprise in Nigeria and its concentration of social services in the urban centers created an unintended consequence. Many "urban women" who had been exposed to life in the towns appeared to be less receptive to the demands of missionary motherhood, a vision of the "good Christian wife" and the colonial nurturing of bodies on whom the responsibility lay to birth a plentiful and healthy labor force. As one officer complained, these women's "mother instinct" became jeopardized due to "the enervating and vicious influence of the town."[136] Some local woman had remarked to him of "mother responsibility": "babies make you look old, we can only be young once, so let's have a good time."[137] While missionary and colonial intervention in local economies and landscapes was meant to advance colonial governance, the new cultures and spaces that they created, especially in emerging urban spaces, created new sites of contests in which the women themselves, now exposed to the pace of life in the cities, began to negotiate new ways of being and new ideas of motherhood, womanhood, and personhood that undermined the ideology of a pliant, submissive, and reproductive body. Many of those who entered the colonial medical service as midwives and nurses did so because such training improved their chances of success in the emerging urban landscape through elevated social status, financial freedom, and prospects of marriage to the emerging Western-trained local elites.

The lopsided system of education that disfavored girls for training in science and arithmetic-related subjects and instead focused on domestic education in subjects like cookery and needlework backfired especially for the colonial government in the 1940s and 1950s, when it had the desire to expand maternal health infrastructure. The personnel shortage that resulted in the midwifery sector because of this neglect was worsened by the unwillingness, especially before the 1940s, by missionaries to train and utilize Nigerian staff for higher positions in the medical service. Missionaries showed a reluctance to place locals in independent or supervisory posts, often arguing that they were incompetent, were dishonest, or simply lacked the mental capacity to carry on any reasonable degree of medical work without supervision.[138] As such, Grade I midwifery posts were reserved largely for European staff, though there would not have been enough qualified locals to fill these posts due to the big gap in educational qualifications.

Although women were at the heart of colonial and missionary propaganda as a means to evangelism and the path to a healthy reproductive nation, the avenues through which these agendas were carried out marginalized women not only economically but in the intimate arena of childbirth that they controlled prior to colonial and missionary intervention. As explained earlier, removing women from the traditional places of birth to hospitals was meant to disrupt the control that local women exerted in upholding birth rituals and determining normal versus abnormal deliveries. When viewed alongside women's marginalization in the colonial educational system and the limiting of their education largely to domestic sciences, women's control of the space of birth as birth practitioners and objects of care declined in the emerging biomedical landscape. While more women became nurse-midwives and increasingly rose to these positions in the 1950s, fewer women had the educational qualifications to train as doctors even when government medical schools, such as the one established at Yaba in 1945, sought to recruit them. In this way, biomedical birth came under the firm control of male doctors in the hospital setting even as more Nigerians took up roles in the health sector during the 1950s.

Notwithstanding, local women sought ways to create new forms of agency within this emergent medical landscape. This agency manifested in the ways and the extent to which women chose to engage with colonial maternities by assigning more value to aspects of it and less to others. As this chapter has pointed out, women enjoyed the benefits of the prenatal care that mission hospitals provided but chose their own homes for delivery, except in the cases of abnormal deliveries. This became a pattern that the colonial government could neither fully comprehend nor overcome. Similarly, some women who entered the services of missionaries as nurses or sought training as midwives had their own motives that sometimes varied from the agendas that their trainers had set out for them. Some women sought economic empowerment while others desired upward mobility through education and a career marriage. To missionaries, the training in nursing and midwifery was mostly a Christian calling, while the locals that entered these spaces were interested in Christian duty as well as the economic benefits that such training offered them.

When government and missionary partnership later in the late 1940s led to the harmonization of requirements between Grade I and Grade II midwifery, the latter being previously an informal training program that required little educational qualifications, even fewer female candidates could meet the requirements for midwifery training or pass the necessary exams. This standardization had rippling effects in the private and independent medical sector. Women in these sectors, the majority of whom lacked the qualifications to become Grade I midwives, embraced an informal auxiliary field in midwifery. Individuals who were affiliated with African Independent Churches, such as those discussed in the next chapter, embraced these churches' faith-based delivery homes and sought a career in the new and independent training institutions that they instituted.

Personnel shortage both triggered and hampered the Nigerianization policies that government sought to implement in the 1950s. This problem of inadequate staffing was widespread in every region of the country, including the southern provinces, whose numbers of educated women were higher than in the rest of the country throughout the colonial era. Training institutions were also lacking at this time and could not accommodate demands, especially in southern Nigeria. Although the government adopted policies, such as the midwife-dresser programs, in parts of the country and launched rural health care initiatives that were rapidly expanded by Nigerian ministers of health in the 1950s, these projects faced an acute staff shortage, especially in midwifery.

On the eve of independence, traditional midwives persisted but were vilified rather than uplifted and incorporated into colonial maternity programs. An increasingly educated and urban population viewed them, in accordance with missionary teachings and the growing attachments to Westernization, as backward and fetish, a stigma that became associated with traditional medicine in general. Simultaneously, the urban areas, which typically removed women from the established social support embedded in the process of birth, were rife with overcrowded hospitals and maternity wards with inadequate staff and infrastructure while nurturing a marginalization of traditional birth that had been institutionalized by years of vilification. These inadequacies in the maternal health care setting created an environment in which women—as nurse-midwives, traditional midwives, auxiliary health staff, or aspiring health workers—charted various courses, as will be explored in subsequent chapters, to appropriate the emerging landscape of birth. Despite all of the changes at the governmental level, traditional midwives remained the closest maternal health care providers who were accessible to the bulk of the population in rural communities. In western Nigeria, an alternative birthing platform that emerged in the 1930s and was based on the principles of faith healing rapidly expanded in the 1950s to confront some shortcomings of the biomedical system that had been present throughout the colonial era. It is to this subject that we now turn.

3

"Attendants Mostly Women"

The Indigenous Aladura Faith-Healing Movement and the Advent of a New Space for Childbirth

His [Babalola] attraction has lain in his intense earnestness, his claim to cure sickness and to give children. He has offered the good news for the soul; cure for the ills of the body; and knowledge and welfare work (pre-natal and post-natal) for the craving woman.

Archdeacon Dallimore, *Church Missionary Outlook*, 1932

Introduction

One dusk in August 1930, the assistant district officer of Ilesha, H. Childs, disguised himself as a member of the local Yoruba community to spy on a revival service organized by Joseph Babalola, a former steamroller driver for the government's Department of Public Works and son of a Church Missionary Society teacher who had triggered a massive faith-healing movement known as the Aladura (prayer people) movement.[1] The religious movement that Childs spied on began in 1928 but gained momentum across the region in 1930 as Babalola's fame as a faith healer spread beyond his community. Childs's goal was to gather information about a faith-healing movement that the colonial government viewed as potentially dangerous due to its large scale, growing momentum, and potential to become politicized as an anticolonial movement. In his report to the resident officer of the Oyo Province where Babalola was most active, Childs described "a crowd of many hundreds of people, including a large contingent of the halt and lame and blind" proceeding into Ilesha town in search of healing and divine intervention at Babalola's revival services.[2] The religious movement that he described was popular among locals, including members of the civil service and the native administration.[3]

Based on Childs's observations, much of the crowd at Babalola's revivals were women. Colonial reports from 1931 indicated that out of 7,656 Aladura converts during that year, 1,596 were men while 6,060 were women.[4] Childs himself wrote, "I had been surprised by the extraordinary number of people, mostly women, pouring into Ilesha."[5] As the number of women in the revival services steadily increased, Babalola began to give particular attention to women's health-related concerns, such as infertility and maternity-based issues. His rhetoric and that of other Aladura leaders who were mostly former members of the Church Missionary Society (CMS) mirrored the tactics of CMS in utilizing maternity services as a crucial element of their Christian ministry, although this was not a deliberate tactic but one that developed due to the predominantly female attendees and the issues of fertility that they brought to Aladura revivals.

According to the British colonial government's *Demographic Survey of West Africa* and other reports from the 1920s and 1930s, sterility was a growing issue in Lagos and surrounding Yoruba territories, areas that were proximate to Babalola's realm of operations.[6] The medical officers in charge of the African Hospital in Lagos, for example, stated that "80 per cent of the attendances of women are for sterility," attributed to the expanding and widespread infection of gonorrhea and syphilis.[7] In the areas around Lagos, notably the Oyo Province in which Babalola operated, high infertility rates were recorded well into the 1950s.[8] Although the government-commissioned survey remarked that "gonorrhoea is an old disease and was known long before European occupation of Nigeria," syphilis, which was believed to be more prevalent among the Yoruba than elsewhere, threatened Yorubaland due to "closer and longer contacts with Europeans at the seaports."[9] By the 1930s, the effects of these diseases on fertility in this part of the country began to receive more attention, and the medical officer, Dr. Turner, suspected that "probably both disease and diet play their parts" in the varying fertility rates.[10]

Throughout the 1920s and 1930s, the birth rate continuously declined in the Yoruba region, and in Lagos, Dr. Turner reported in his medical census that these rates went from 33 per 1,000 in 1920 to 28.6 per 1,000 in 1930.[11] This decline in number of births due to sterility was a problem for not only the colonial government but also the locals due to the importance of family size in a predominantly agrarian society and one in which a greater number of children was a source of wealth and pride. Babalola and his promise of faith healing, therefore, came at an opportune time in which women were seeking solutions to reproductive health concerns, solutions that they did not readily gain in the biomedical realm in the 1920s and 1930s. According to government's own account as of 1935, "little progress can be said to have been made in the elimination of syphilis."[12]

Just as women sought succor in the hospitals for their sterility, they also trooped to Babalola's prayer sessions when news about his miracles, such as the raising of a dead child, cure of the blind and crippled, and delivery of a long overdue pregnancy, spread. Based on Babalola's own accounts, one of the events that increased his popularity was his ministration to a woman who was well known in the town for her prolonged pregnancy of close to four years. Following Babalola's ministration, the woman delivered successfully to the amazement of her family and the town.[13] Another incident involved the pregnancy of one Hannah Fapohunda, who could not conceive for seven years until Babalola prayed for her.[14] Cases like these attracted crowds to Babalola's stations. Archdeacon Dallimore acknowledged in his 1931 report to London the impact of Babalola's provision of maternity care, stating, "His attraction has lain in his intense earnestness, his claim to cure sickness and to give children . . . and knowledge of welfare work (pre-natal and postnatal) for the craving woman."[15] Many colonial administrators believed that Babalola's religious movement would be short-lived. Childs's assessment of the movement was that Babalola's popularity "would wane as quickly as it had risen when the people come to appreciate the true value of his blessing," in other words, his inability to heal or provide solutions.[16] This expectation did not materialize, however, as the movement grew into enduring independent African congregations and posed a serious challenge to European missions, notably CMS and Wesleyan Mission, the two foreign missions most active in the vicinity of Aladura operations. Local converts left churches and hospitals in large numbers and moved to Aladura rallies in search of healing from all manner of ailments.

In a move that was resented by European missionaries and thrust the Aladura into the evolving colonial politics of birth and maternity, Babalola admonished attendees at his revival services against the adoption of biomedicine and traditional medicine for healing. While he directly associated traditional medicine with idolatry, biomedicine was positioned in his teachings as a medical practice whose failures and inadequacies, which were plenty at the time, could drive people toward traditional medicine and, therefore, idolatry. True believers, he argued, must rely on God absolutely for cures.[17] As a result of this antimedicine stance, expecting mothers who were keen on successful pregnancy outcomes frequently returned to Babalola's congregation for birth, and he, in turn, created an ad hoc system in which evangelists' wives and elderly prayerful women in the Aladura congregations cared for expecting mothers. By the 1940s, Babalola's church, the Christ Apostolic Church (CAC), had created a formal policy prohibiting pregnant church members from utilizing hospitals for birth.

In the 1950s, during an atmosphere in which women's education, expansion of nursing and midwifery, and proliferation of private maternity homes were the norm, Babalola and the women's wing of the CAC created a formal institution that trained midwives based on the concept of faith healing and natural birth. With the development of trained personnel, the CAC created faith homes or faith delivery homes, staffed by a trained faith home midwife and an assistant, as distinct components of the CAC congregation to serve expecting mothers, including non-CAC members who chose to utilize their services for childbirth. In postindependence Nigeria, these faith homes or faith delivery homes became a significant part of the reproductive health landscape.[18]

This chapter explores the emergence of faith delivery homes as a product of the Aladura movement and how an Aladura church inadvertently inserted itself into the colonial politics of childbirth and reproduction. Contrary to the belief among British officials that Babalola's movement would efface, it thrived due to the growing importance of medicine and women's health during the colonial era. Since the Aladura movement and the foremost church that arose in its wake—the CAC—filled a need in the important realm of childbirth for its predominantly female membership, it found a niche that ensured continued local patronage and resilience, creating a site of birth that challenged the established influence of traditional and biomedical spaces. When faced with opposition from the government and biomedical practitioners, as well as changing socioeconomic realities, Babalola and his supporters pivoted in 1959 to create a formal institution of faith-based delivery, replete with a training school for midwives and a set of systematic practices.

The Makings of a New Site of Birth: Aladura Origins

The Aladura's early emergence and stronghold in western Nigeria was a result of the long history of European presence around the coast of Lagos, dating back to the fifteenth century. With Britain's increased colonial ambitions in the region around the 1840s, Lagos and neighboring cities like Abeokuta, Badagry, and Ibadan became important to traders and imperialists but also a stronghold of missionary groups. By the 1900s, Yoruba Christian converts had become disgruntled by the various discriminatory treatments that they faced from missionaries at a time that missionaries were still making inroads in other parts of Nigeria.[19] This deep-rooted encounter laid the foundations for the early emergence of independent African churches as offshoots of European missionary societies and what became known as Aladura churches in this region.[20]

The immediate seeds of the Aladura movement were sown during the World War I era when economic depression and disease outbreaks, combined with a weak medical infrastructure, provided fertile grounds for apocalyptic teachings, prophetic movements, and promises of divine intervention. One major event that contributed to this development was the influenza pandemic of 1918, which spurred the founding of various local prayer groups that ultimately became independent African congregations. On September 3, 1918, the influenza disease penetrated Lagos through the SS *Bida*, which dispatched 239 passengers, including infected people, from the Gold Coast to Nigeria without notifying the Lagos port authority of outbreaks in the Gold Coast.[21] The disease spread across the coastal city and made its way to surrounding Yoruba towns despite attempts to slow down the infections through quarantine, segregation, church and mosque closures, elimination of large gatherings, and disinfection campaigns.[22] In Lagos, with an estimated population of 84,684, the influenza disease was calculated to have killed 3% of the population, and more than half of the population were estimated to have suffered the disease in a mild or severe form.[23] The number of casualties was conservative and did not include infections that were untreated by the medical department and, therefore, unreported to the medical officer.[24]

As part of the effort to curb the influenza outbreak, church closures were enforced by the colonial government, forcing locals to move prayer groups and prayer meetings underground to members' houses. During this period, the biomedical infrastructure was inadequate. As described in chapter 2, government hospitals focused on medical care for European personnel, the civil service, and the military. Where hospitals were available to locals, they were expensive and mostly accessible to those elites who could afford them. The colonial medical infrastructure also largely focused on preventive sanitary measures that were concentrated in the urban areas, with little outreach in rural communities. This limited medical infrastructure and a shortage of medical staff due to emigrations and redeployment of medical personnel worsened an untenable situation.[25] The colonial medical service was ill-equipped to curb the disease outbreak while the local community could not find much respite from the biomedical system. The attitude of the colonial government by the end of 1918 was that "the Epidemic was too overwhelming for treatment to have much effect. Matters had necessarily to be left to themselves."[26]

The influenza pandemic was just one of several disease outbreaks of epidemic proportions to strike Lagos and surrounding provinces like Ijebu-Ode Province and Oyo Province between 1918 and 1926. There were at least two epidemics of bubonic plague in 1924 and 1925 and various smallpox outbreaks throughout the 1920s.[27] According to official medical records, the plague persisted over several years and considerably increased the death rates in the affected areas.[28] In Ijebu-Ode Province, it posed such a problem that a separate medical report was issued on plague cases in the annual medical report for 1925.[29] In the absence of answers for the sick and the grieving, prayer meetings proliferated where prayer groups relied on dreams, visions, and revelations to guide them.[30] It was under these circumstances that Faith Tabernacle, a notable African Independent Church (AIC) that became connected to Babalola and eventually assumed the name Christ Apostolic Church, came into existence.

Faith Tabernacle, which was first known as the Diamond Society or Precious Stone, was founded by members of St. Saviors Anglican Church, Ijebu-Ode, in the house of J. B. Sadare, the church's people's warden, during the pandemic of 1918. At the end of the pandemic, the group continued to thrive and was formally inaugurated into the Anglican Communion in 1920.[31] In 1923, the group severed ties with the Anglican Church over Diamond Society's rejection of infant baptism, reliance on dreams and visions for guidance, and belief in faith healing and founded an independent congregation, Faith Tabernacle.[32] Similar religious groups also emerged in response to other disease outbreaks. For instance, the Seraphim, later known as Cherubim and Seraphim, was founded during Lagos's bubonic plague of

1925.[33] Although the number of independent African churches and self-proclaimed prophets expanded during the 1920s, their activities were confined to small areas and did not trigger a large-scale religious movement until the arrival of Babalola in Ilesha as a prophet.

Babalola's religious call began in 1928 in Ekiti, where he worked as a steamroller driver in the Public Works Department.[34] One day in October, his steamroller ceased to function, and he heard a voice that commanded him thrice to embark on Christian evangelism or forfeit his life. After initial resistance, Babalola abandoned his job and commenced the work of evangelism as a prophet. Part of Babalola's mandate was to preach absolute reliance on divine healing. In his early teachings on faith healing, Babalola wrote, "In all the towns where I went, the Voice will teach me to tell the people to desist from the use of herbs and all native medicines but to trust in the Lord for their healing. . . . The Lord is coming to render useless and powerless all herbs and leaves being used for medicine."[35] A literal reading of Babalola's description of his vision specifically pinpoints core components of traditional medicine—herbs and leaves—for condemnation; there was no mention of biomedicine. However, Babalola's interpretation of the message later on categorized the use of all medicine, traditional and Western, as demonstrating a lack of faith. Babalola capitalized on the failures of biomedicine to protect the population from influenza, smallpox, and other disease outbreaks to condemn medicine as a worldly and temporary recourse that signaled a lack of faith in God and to promote faith healing as the remedy for both spiritual and physical ailments.

Babalola's message was well received in many circles partly because the faith healing that he offered was free of charge, contrary to the fees that mission and government hospitals charged for care. Many of his supporters argued that his religion was a free one as opposed to that of European missions, which required membership dues and service fees from church members for the maintenance of European priests, mission schools, and hospitals.[36] His reputation as a faith healer also attracted crowds to him. In his own writings and in missionary records, several miracles, including the curing of the lame, raising of a dead child, and delivery of an unusually extended pregnancy, were attributed to him at the onset of his prophetic ministry and carried his fame across Yorubaland.[37]

Babalola attracted the colonial administration's attention in 1930 when he traveled to Ilesha and drew a huge crowd following the public resurrection of a ten-year-old child and a man.[38] By this time, he had gained popularity as a faith healer and an Aladura whose model was absolute reliance on faith healing through prayer, psalms, and the administration of blessed water.[39] According to a CMS report, his method included "to pray, to quote the psalms, . . . to call people to the surrender of idols and magic, and to the confession of witchcraft, and then to bless water brought by people in the calabashes and bottles. This water was later drunk by them to the healing, as they believed, of disease, or the making of childbirth possible. It was a wonderful sight to see hundreds of idols and magical instruments surrendered, and to witness the crowd swayed by the personality of the prophet."[40] The same report stated that there was nothing special about Babalola's emergence as a prophet because it was common during that era for individuals to declare themselves prophet. What was special about Babalola, the report argued, was that "he had both personality and power."[41] His humility, simplicity, and belief in his mission, as well as the crowd that he commanded, were equated by one missionary account to Jesus's mission on the road to Palestine.[42]

Up to 1932, Babalola's revival services received some positive coverage in European mission circles because it brought many new converts to the doors of the CMS, Wesleyan, and Methodist missions.[43] By 1932, however, he officially left the CMS, to the chagrin of the European missionaries, and affiliated himself with the Faith Tabernacle, whose membership in turn increased significantly due to his activities. A 1932 report to the Resident of Oyo Province stated that "Faith Tabernacle before his [Babalola] arrival was a very small concern, and was more or less negligible. Its large increase, however, because of Babalola's teaching, made it a factor to be reckoned with."[44] Other Aladura congregations, such as Church of the Lord-Aladura and Cherubim and Seraphim, also received a boost in membership.

The growth of Aladura churches had a negative effect on mission revenue as hospitals emptied out because patients departed for Aladura revival services in search of healing.[45] A colonial report emphasized, for instance, that Wesleyan and CMS missionary activities were at the risk of shutting down because of the Aladura movement's growth.[46] In their own reports, the CMS pointed out that their loss of revenue due to Aladura activities amounted to one-third of the year's annual income. The unavoidable salary reduction that followed in CMS missions was put at 25%.[47] The challenges that Babalola's activities and that of other Aladura churches posed to missionary presence brought him into direct conflict with missionaries, who increasingly saw him as a source of competition. In order to check this Aladura growth that increasingly interfered with the missionary agenda of Christianization and of fundraising through local church membership, mission societies barred their members from associating with Aladura churches.[48] Those members who erred were fined, threatened with arrests, and denied positions in the churches.[49] Their children suffered retribution too and were denied enrollment in mission schools or expelled in the event of the slightest provocations.[50]

Government perception of the Aladura as a potential political threat shaped the ways in which Aladura institutions were received and set the stage for government reactions to their practices of faith healing. As concerns increased that the Aladura movement might have political repercussions, including the potential for uprisings, district officers and their assistants assumed a more aggressive stance and blocked attempts by the Aladura to secure land for the construction of churches and meeting grounds. They also charged the Native Administration, consisting of kings and local chieftains, to monitor Babalola's group for any signs of political activity.[51] In 1932, when Abigail, an Aladura who became popular in the course of Babalola's movement, instigated a tax riot in Akure following teachings that the colonial administration could only collect a fixed amount of tax from the people, she was imprisoned, and the events in Akure and elsewhere in Yorubaland were monitored very closely.[52] Colonial officers also embarked on what they described as "propaganda against 'faith-healers' and 'prophets.'"[53] In the Yoruba town of Esa Oke, for instance, a senior resident officer traveled around town admonishing traditional rulers that the Aladura were the Oba's (local ruler) enemy and sought to usurp the authority of the chiefs, destabilize towns, and wreak havoc on families.[54] Wherever he went, he also recruited locals to mock and laugh at Aladura members with the aim of discouraging membership.[55]

Babalola, who was acutely aware of the increased surveillance, strategically avoided any politically charged statements and encouraged his followers to abide by government laws. He also distanced himself from teachings arising from any Aladura quarters that involved or were perceived to involve political assertions.[56] Following Abigail's public statements about taxation, Babalola visited Akure to condemn these teachings and order Abigail to desist from them.[57] When Oshitelu, founder of Church of the Lord-Aladura, published some prophecies that were considered by colonial officials as antigovernment teachings, Babalola embarked on a tour to condemn the prophecies contained in Oshitelu's *Awon Asotele* (book of prophecies) and distance himself from Oshitelu's pamphlet.[58] These kinds of adaptations became a pattern in the ways that Babalola responded to government or institutional opposition or criticism, up to the institutionalization of faith homes.

Though Babalola's religious movement did not assume any obvious political dimensions, it represented a subversion of a larger scale. Considering the thin veil between colonial politics and missionary work—a fuzzy line between church and state in the colonial empire—Babalola's religious activities had initiated a disruption that the colonial government was unwilling to tolerate. For the first time since the advent of colonialism in Nigeria, a sizable portion of the local population asserted control within a relatively new colonial Christian religion and founded a widespread movement that resulted in the proliferation of African Independent Churches.[59] Though Babalola himself refrained from challenging political authority, his religious movement affected other aspects of colonial rule, notably European missionaries and their medical and educational institutions. It placed Aladura church members outside of a religious and social space that was neither controlled by the government nor European missions.

As demonstrated in chapter 2, medicine and women's health were avenues through which missionaries and the government sought to advance their various health, religious, and social propaganda and consolidate colonial rule. Because the movement existed outside the realms of Western Christian missions and opposed the use of biomedicine, which would have brought individual Aladura members into repeated contact with the colonial establishment, Aladura churches removed a part of the population from the direct control of some instruments of state control, such as clinics and European mission facilities, hence government's discomfort with their existence. For Faith Tabernacle, which became the CAC in the 1940s, one of those contested arenas that they carved out for themselves was their new sites of childbirth—the faith homes.

"You Shall Deliver Like the Hebrew Women": Faith Delivery Homes in Nigeria

As Childs observed in his 1931 tour of ten Yoruba towns, many participants in Babalola's revival meetings were women.[60] In his 1931 report of the Ilesha District, Childs had remarked, "Attendants mostly women," an acknowledgment of the large presence of women at Aladura meetings and during Babalola's revival services.[61] Other accounts from mission reports support Childs's observation but point out the comparable presence of men and women during the early periods of Babalola's ministry of healing and evangelism before 1932. *The Church Missionary Outlook* reported in September 1932 that "great numbers of men were originally attracted," although many Aladura revival attendees at the time of the publication were women.[62] Reports from the colonial office also indicated that the movement "seems to have attracted people of the clerk type" and was popular among African government workers, clerks, the police force, and members of the Native Administration, including local chiefs.[63] That this group of government and Native Administration workers were overwhelmingly male highlights how deeply rooted and popular the movement was in the larger community, including among men.

Notwithstanding, there is enough evidence from missionary and colonial government records that women and issues surrounding female reproduction were very visible in these Aladura meetings. In addition to Childs's report, there were multiple references in mission documents to the work that Babalola and his team of evangelists did among women, especially regarding reproductive health matters, which became a core of his health interventions.[64] As established earlier in the Introduction, various annual reports of the 1920s and 1930s also pointed to growing concerns about infertility in Yorubaland, which was attributed by medical officers largely to the prevalence of gonorrhea and syphilis. These two venereal diseases were common in urban centers where trade and migrant labor were well established. Lagos, Ibadan, and neighboring territories fit this description. Lagos was particularly known as a transit city that attracted traders and travelers from outside Nigeria but also from other parts of Nigeria. The 1931 census report explained that the persistence and spread of these venereal diseases, particularly syphilis, among the Yoruba is "partly to be expected owing to closer and longer contact with Europeans at the seaports and to the large number of Hausa traders who are found all over Yorubaland. The Hausa is believed to be generally infected."[65] Dr. Turner, the author of the Medical Census conducted in 1931, connected the prevalence of these diseases, particularly gonorrhea, to miscarriages and a decline in fertility.[66] It only makes sense, therefore, that women, on whom the burden of conception, successful pregnancies, and childrearing were placed, would gravitate to the Aladura movement. "If in a way the couple fails to have children, more blame is given to the woman," explained a Nigerian editorial on childless marriages, or as Tola Olu Pierce puts it, "Childless women have historically been held in great contempt in Yorubaland."[67]

These women were drawn to an Aladura healing platform that promised divine protection. It addressed their physical, spiritual, and cultural concerns about pregnancy, such as evil eye—the idea that one's neighbor or a stranger could project evil against an individual, stillbirth, and *Abiku*—born-to-die children caught up in a cycle of birth and death. The women also sought to protect their fertility and their place within an agrarian society in which a man's wealth was often judged by the size of his family, and a woman's worth was connected to her ability to procreate and expand the family's agrarian resources. Two columnists in a Nigerian newspaper surmised the situation: "In fact, in most customs, it is believed that a marriage that is not blessed with a child is not sanctioned by the ancestors."[68] Such childless marriage boded unfavorably for a woman and her position in the nuclear and extended family unit.

Rates of infant deaths in the mid-to-late 1920s should also be taken into consideration when attempting to understand the predominance of women in Babalola's revivals, especially because Yoruba women who repeatedly lost their children ran the risk of being labeled witches.[69] Although statistics from the early colonial era, especially in the first quarter of the twentieth century, are highly unreliable and incomplete, data from the medical report of 1925 and 1926 showed a high infant mortality rate for the western provinces between 1922 and the end of 1926. In Lagos, which usually had the most reliable data in the entire colony, recorded deaths of infants under the age of one were 809 in 1922 out of 2,843 and 948 out of 3,203 births in 1925.[70] The 1925 data were alarming enough that they were reported to the Lagos Town Council for immediate action in the form of a Health Week.[71] These numbers looked similar to the influenza pandemic highs of 830 deaths out of 2,514 births in 1918.[72] By contrast, in 1929, the infant death statistics was 345 out of 2,788 births. However episodic, incomplete, or overestimated the high infant mortality data may be, they point to some ongoing concern about this trend prior to the Aladura movement.

The role that reproductive health solutions played in Babalola's long-term success, as well as the broader importance of reproductive health care in colonial Nigeria, is reflected in missionary responses to his healing services. Since the CMS, from whom many Aladura leaders emerged, structured maternity services as an avenue for the conversion of women and their children as well as their extended family networks, Babalola's popularity threatened this technique. A CMS report attributed Babalola's fame to "his claim to cure sickness and to give children" and capitalized on the large-scale response that Babalola received to campaign for the expansion of maternity services in the region.[73]

Beginning in 1932, when Babalola officially broke ties with the Anglican church and joined Faith Tabernacle, which assumed the name Apostolic Church in the same year, missionaries in the western region sent urgent reports back to the United Kingdom through their publication, the *Church Missionary Outlook*. In these reports, they decried the dangers of the new religious movement and advocated for the expansion of medical care in the region as a counter to the Aladura.[74] The overwhelmingly positive response that Babalola received among local communities was relayed by missionaries to potential sponsors and medical mission recruits as proof of the people's desire for the expansion of missionary medical work. The CMS in the western region described the urgency of the situation to their readers: "In the affected area of 40,000 square miles, there are at the time of writing one European missionary and his wife. Two others and their wives and one West Indian and his wives are at home on furlough. In addition there is one Wesleyan missionary and his wife. Such is the whole staff!"[75] Across southern Nigeria in the late 1920s and early 1930s, prenatal visits and hospital births, carried on mostly by the CMS, the Roman Catholic Mission, and the Wesleyan Mission, were increasingly popular as part of missionary services. Yet, it was still out of reach for many, especially following the severe personnel shortages that assailed mission and government hospitals from the onset of World War I until the mid-1930s.[76] In the course of the war and its aftermath, missionary personnel were dispatched outside Nigeria to various warfronts. Some were called home in anticipation of the war, and others who were on furlough or other business outside Nigeria could not make their way back. For years after the war, some of these personnel were not dispatched back to their original posts, and since the organization of missionary work, including medical missions, relied heavily on European personnel, medical mission work suffered, leading to the scenario that the above quote from the CMS report described.

Arguments made by Babalola's followers and other Aladura preachers that people should not pay for God's work, as evidenced by Babalola's non-imposition of fees for his services, resonated in an era of postwar economic hardship and global depression in which the price of palm oil, cocoa, and other cash crops dropped. This sentiment resounded in the local communities, as evidenced by the empty hospitals that plagued mission hospitals following Aladura services, and among European mission groups who petitioned the colonial government to stop the Aladura.[77] For European missions, such teachings were particularly harmful because the missions relied heavily on funds raised from local membership dues, hospital bills, and related fees to pay mission workers and maintain mission stations, hence the opposition that they mounted against the Aladura.[78]

Government hospitals barely filled the needs unmet by medical missions. As of 1929, only one government maternity hospital, Massey Street Hospital in Lagos, existed in the region.[79] In 1931 and 1932, the government introduced more maternity wings mostly in partnership with existing mission hospitals, as was the case with Sacred Heart Hospital, Abeokuta, a Catholic-owned establishment where the government created and funded a maternity ward, or as part of several "African Hospitals" that were constructed in some urban areas mostly by Native Administrations.[80] The government was gradually turning its attention to what it described as the low standards of maternity care in the hospitals and "a further step in the reduction of the present high [maternal] mortality rate."[81] However, the demand in maternity services far outpaced supply.

Following the considerable number of women at his revival meetings, Babalola created a system of maternity care that was premised on the biblical promise in the book of Genesis, "You shall deliver like the Hebrew women," a term that became widespread in Aladura churches and referred to Egyptian midwives' statements that Hebrew women delivered their babies so quickly before a midwife's arrival.[82] In the Aladura context, safe delivery was the reward of any faithful and spiritually diligent Christian woman. Deviations from a positive outcome during pregnancy and labor were attributed to the presence of sin, unhygienic or careless living, a lack of faith, or an act of God.[83] This attribution of negative outcome in pregnancy to sin was neither new nor unusual in this community. In many cultures in southern Nigeria, prolonged or obstructed labor was sometimes attributed to a woman's unfaithfulness to her spouse. In such cases, only a full confession was believed to ease delivery. It was, therefore, easy for the families in Babalola's congregation to embrace the idea that sin could result in negative delivery experiences. Babalola also taught his congregation that any recourse to worldly medicine—traditional or biomedical—signified a lack of faith in God and could result in negative health outcomes as divine healing could not be achieved without *Igbagbo* (faith) and *Igbekele* (trust).[84]

At revival meetings, Babalola arranged special prayer sessions for pregnant women and employed the recitation of specific psalms and the use of blessed water to invoke spiritual protection on them.[85] These psalms included Bible passages with themes ranging from thanksgiving, affirmation, healing, and protection. Expecting mothers were assigned a psalm for each month of pregnancy, to be recited in daily prayers. This psalm was to be repeated according to the number of times that corresponded to the month of pregnancy. Hence, a woman who was three months pregnant recited Psalm 23 thrice daily while one in the fifth month of pregnancy recited Psalm 121 five times every day.[86] This schedule of psalm recitation served the dual purpose of helping women monitor the advance of their pregnancy and the expected day of delivery.[87]

After the services, Babalola consecrated water for the women's use, a practice that came to symbolize his mode of healing and that of many Aladura churches. His followers believed that the water was capable of eliminating diseases and "the making of childbirth possible."[88] Various CAC members explained that pregnant women and those who sought relief from infertility or other ailments went home with the blessed water, which they infused in their baths and drank in portions with the belief that it was a conduit for healing.[89] Babalola's own rationale for this adoption of water was based on the indispensability of water as a life force and cleansing instrument that posed no harm to the users.[90] Babalola's use of water for divine healing during this period became a widespread practice among the Aladura and has remained an enduring component of CAC liturgy. One CAC elder recalled a common song that was passed down from the older generation of the Aladura movement: *Omi la o mu ye Aladura, Omi la o mu ye* (As Aladura people drink water, they will always remain alive and well).[91]

Although Babalola's teachings expressly condemned the use of traditional medicine, his practices of using water and blessed words as a conduit of healing derived from the Yoruba medical traditions. Some instruments of healing in Yoruba culture included the use of *Ohun ife* or *Ofo* (blessed words or incantations), which were believed to compel compliance from the object to whom it was directed.[92] In childbirth, these blessed words were combined with the application of herbal medicines at various intervals during pregnancy to achieve positive outcomes. They were also used by traditional doctors, who sometimes doubled as priests, to ward off the evil eye, believed to be projected by an ill-intentioned person against an individual. Toward the end of pregnancy in the traditional setting, the expecting mother took baths infused with herbs and *Ohun ife* to prepare for birth.[93] These spiritual baths were also taken when necessary to ward off bad luck and misfortune.

Similarly, at the onset of labor, the *Iya Agbebi* (midwife or elderly woman who played a similar role) worked hand in hand with the traditional doctor to ensure safe delivery. The traditional doctor recited specific *ohun ife* made for this occasion to provide spiritual protection for the expecting mother in readiness for birth. A similar recitation took place following the rupture of the amniotic sac and the onset of active labor.[94] *Ohun ife*, spiritual baths, and divinations were deployed to address pregnancy-related issues such as *Abiku* (spirit children), a phenomenon in which a child died shortly after birth and was believed to return repeatedly to the same family through subsequent pregnancies. The Yoruba believed that unless relevant sacred words, prayers, and rituals were offered, this born-to-die cycle continued.[95] These cultural interpretations of health and well-being became the basis around which the practice of faith healing and maternal health care was organized. The parallel healing tradition that the Aladura created integrated cultural interpretations of health and illness, Christian belief in the boundless power of God, and biomedical explanations of sickness and health to gain credence in a rapidly changing society. In his reports in the *Church Missionary Outlook*, Archdeacon Dallimore described a conversation with Babalola regarding his rationale behind the use of water for healing: "He simply allowed the people to bring the water, and to hold the belief that, after blessing it, it assumed [healing] powers, in order that he might get the people to come and listen to his preaching, and thereby to throw away their idols and accept the gospel teaching. The water could at least do them no harm."[96] Dallimore's observation buttresses the argument that Babalola was deliberate in his attempts to gain local support for his prophetic mission by drawing on well-known cultural practices to tend the physical and spiritual concerns of people.

Due to Babalola's teachings against the use of medicine—traditional or biomedical—expecting mothers returned to Aladura congregations for childbirth at the onset of labor rather than visit the traditional midwife or a hospital. Throughout the 1930s and 1940s, these expecting mothers were cared for by female evangelists, minister's wives, and prayerful older women who generally had more experience in childbirth.[97] These caregivers relied on their own experiences of birth, including experiences gained from attending the birth of other relatives, as well as natural processes for augmenting labor and relieving pain, such as increased mobility and the use of palm oil for massage. As in traditional midwifery, massage with palm oil was believed to have soothing effects. When blessed through prayers, the oil doubled as a spiritual tonic imbued with divine protection. The women also relied on the administration of blessed water, the utterances of psalms, and relentless prayers to address any perceived spiritual and physical symptoms of the expecting mother. Prayer groups, known as *Egbe Aladura* or *Egbe Afadurajagua* (the Praying Battalion), were also in hand to offer prayers of protection and intercession against any negative outcomes or spiritual attacks.[98]

Beyond prayers, Babalola emphasized the importance of nutrition, hygiene, and exercise to maternal health outcomes. As a core part of his teachings and essays on maternal health care, he underscored the connections between dirt and diseases, arguing that pregnant women should take daily baths to cleanse themselves from pollutants.[99] He also advised women to keep contaminants from their homes and immediate environment, notably the kitchen, because "a dirty kitchen is the forerunner of death."[100] Otherwise, he reasoned, germs from these contaminants could penetrate the body through pores and reproduce inside, causing ill health and possibly death.[101] He encouraged pregnant women to exercise daily by taking walks in the morning or early evenings but discouraged afternoon walks because of the belief that some evil spirits, including spirit children (*Abiku*), were active during this time in the day and could affect pregnancy outcome.[102]

As the son of a Church Missionary Society teacher who received missionary education, Babalola could read and write and, as was the practice among early leaders of Faith Tabernacle, likely received and read literature from abroad. In one of his teachings, he wrote, "In other parts of the world it is believed that it is not good for a pregnant woman to eat the fruit of the tree. But this is not bad. Fruits and a measure of work will keep the body exercised."[103] Although he does not specify what part of the world he references, he was demonstrably comparing his teachings with developments elsewhere. His teachings regarding nutrition were that foods rich in fruits and vegetables were crucial during pregnancy.[104]

Babalola also advocated against the lithotomy birthing position that was adopted in hospitals and by mission-trained midwives, which required expecting mothers to lie flat on their backs during labor. He argued that this position was dangerous for mothers and did not facilitate birth.[105] He also condemned the standing posture, possibly because the baby could hit the ground during delivery and sustain injury. He had reasoned earlier in his writings that some people did not know how to hold a pregnant woman during labor. Instead, he promoted the kneeling and sitting position, as was practiced by many traditional midwives. His regimen detailed practical steps for the care of pregnant women during pregnancy, childbirth, and the postnatal period, including a requirement that those assisting in childbirth must wash their hands regularly with soap and water.[106] Most important to his stance against the employment of traditional medicine, he argued that herbs posed a danger to expecting mothers because they made the women lean and anemic and could introduce germs and evil spirits (such as spirit children) into the body if not properly cleaned. He proposed, instead, that the women should "drink plenty of water especially the sanctified water that has been prayed upon."[107] His practical approach to pregnancy care arguably promoted better birth outcomes in his congregation in an environment with limited health care infrastructure and formed the basis on which the faith homes became organized.

At the beginning of his prophetic ministry, Babalola made no claims on expertise in pregnancy and focused on whatever ailments or conditions that followers presented before him. However, as the needs of his largely female audience in the 1930s revolved around reproduction, it only became expedient that he garnered more knowledge and protocols for birth. Unlike other Aladura leaders operating at the same time as Babalola, who believed in the syncretic use of traditional medicine, biomedicine, and faith healing, Babalola adopted an unequivocal stance against the use of any type of medicine, including during childbirth, an inevitable event that typically involved intervention by traditional midwives and other birth attendants or hospital attendants. His position against medical intervention required the creation of an alternative space of birth that conformed with his principles of faith healing and that his followers could utilize.

Beginning in the 1940s, Babalola's maternity services began to advance toward an institutionalized phase. Between 1938 and 1940, a rift occurred in the Faith Tabernacle over divine healing. A segment of the church that advocated a loose application of faith healing and the complementary use of biomedical care for healing formed The Apostolic Church (TAC) while those in Babalola's camp who favored absolute reliance on faith healing formed the Christ Apostolic Church. After this rift, CAC moved to formalize its stance against the use of medicine as an official part of its doctrine. In a 1940 letter explaining their refusal to compromise on the practice of absolute faith healing, CAC leaders argued:

- That the use of medicine, drugs, quinine or other human remedy, either for protection or healing of the body in this country will only lead people back to idolatry and will absolutely remove their confidence and trust in Christ as Saviour and Healer.
- That this practice of going back to idolatry is prevalent in West Africa with the denominational Churches where converts have been allowed free use of medicines, drugs, quinine and other human remedy, either for protection or healing of the body, with the result that they have become disgusted with Christianity as if there is no virtue therein and the power in the Blood is trifled and nullified.
- That Denial of Divine protection will only send our people back to idols and witch doctors, etc., and it is our common experience here that fetish priests and witch doctors have both good and bad medicine.[108]

In connecting the use of biomedical therapies to a return to idolatry, they highlighted the past failures of biomedicine to protect or preserve life during periods of epidemic or endemic outbreaks throughout the 1920s and 1930s.

In the church's first constitution, released in 1946, the CAC took a rigid stance on childbirth and explicitly condemned the use of hospitals for birth, stating, "Expectant mothers of our church ought not to go to any hospital/maternity home either for check-up or childbirth since the Bible has promised us good care and safe delivery. . . . Anyone found guiltily of the above shall be suspended from sharing of the Holy Communion for a period of six months."[109] It was now a mandate for CAC women to rely solely on prayers, psalms, and the use of the church's ad hoc midwives during childbirth. Developments in Nigeria from the late 1940s through the 1950s, however, compelled the CAC to consider the creation of a professional class of midwives whose services were dedicated solely to the care of pregnant women. This and other attempts to solidify its structure and establish long-lasting administrative frameworks were mostly a response to colonial antagonism that they lacked elaborate structures and were, therefore, not respectable.

Beginning in the late 1940s, the colonial government had ramped up its focus on improving maternal and infant health. It was also attempting to expand the educational opportunities available to women to create a female workforce that could make the expansion of nursing and midwifery possible.[110] As a result of this expansion in maternity services, nursing and midwifery became popular among Nigerian women as a platform for participating extensively in the colonial public service. Nigerian newspapers during this period were filled with calls to expand the place of women in the country's economy.[111] CAC women were not detached from these developments and sought training as nurses and midwives in the biomedical setting. Those who became nurses and midwives offered counsel and assistance during childbirth in their local CAC churches, although they could neither administer tablets nor injections, per church rules.[112] They also brought with them ideas about the organization of the church's maternity services as a more coherent whole. Because Western education was viewed in Nigeria as a means to escape poverty and uplift one's family, CAC leadership did not outlaw the participation of members or their children as workers in the health sector. Such a move to prohibit health work could cause another rift in the church, similar to what had occurred in the Faith Tabernacle, due to its economic repercussions and implications for social mobility.

From 1948 through the 1950s, when the government began to implement a proposal to integrate academic requirements for qualification into Grade I and Grade II midwifery, the new and more rigorous qualification standards for Grade II midwives left many CAC women unable to explore nurse-midwifery as a form of economic empowerment.[113] The annual medical report of 1958 for Lagos and surrounding territories complained of "wastage" in the nursing program due to higher requirements for which many women did not have the educational background to surpass.[114] According to this report, only twenty-five people qualified as nurses out of the fifty-five recruited.[115] Those with Grade II qualifications from the preintegration era also found it harder to get employment in government hospitals. *The West African Pilot* reported, for example, that teaching hospitals in Ibadan and Lagos refused to employ nurses or midwives who had Grade II certificates and had qualified as nurses due to the belief that "their standard of education is not high enough to be admitted therein."[116]

As a result of these developments as well as the need to consolidate care for expecting mothers, CAC women, who had become organized in 1944 under the CAC Good Women Association, began to consider supporting a dedicated midwifery unit in the CAC that would comprise career midwives trained in basic health education, maternal health care, and the practice of faith healing. Such a unit would provide its women an alternative form of economic empowerment. Since its debut in 1944, this organization had served to elevate women's roles in the CAC beyond wives and mothers to administrators and active participants in church development.[117] It became an internal publicity wing of the church that circulated the church's version of appropriate Christian and secular teaching, family life, academic curriculum, and health care.

In 1958, when Babalola decided to establish a Faith Home Midwifery School that would train career faith-based midwives whose occupation would be as midwives in various CAC congregations, the CAC Good Women supported this initiative and provided financial and logistical support to realize this vision. Babalola had first built a faith home at Efon Alaye, a community whose traditional ruler had always shielded Babalola and his congregation from colonial persecution. In 1959, at the suggestion of pastor Samuel Akande (Baba Abiye) and in partnership with the CAC Good Women, Babalola relocated this faith home to Ede, where the CAC secured larger expanses of land through Oba John Laoye, Timi of Ede, the traditional ruler of Ede and an ardent supporter of CAC.[118] Beyond the economic importance of establishing a training school for faith home midwives, Babalola and those who succeeded him believed that they were making a crucial intervention in improving maternity services and the chance to reduce maternal deaths. During this period in the 1950s, the government was well aware of recurring maternal deaths due to inadequate care and the lack of sufficient biomedical facilities. Those government facilities that existed were sparse, overcrowded, and poorly staffed. Expecting mothers who attended the Oko Awo clinic in Lagos complained in 1950 that they queued under the sun for hours before they received any medical attention. An average of 360 women attended prenatal clinics in this location daily, but only about sixty new cases could be addressed due to the lack of space and staff.[119] These concerns echoed in the CAC and among its leaders who lived with, heard of, and experienced stories of maternal deaths and near misses.

The growing government concern about maternal deaths also meant increased scrutiny from the government on faith-healing practices among the CAC and similar congregations and how the prohibition of hospital care resulted in preventable deaths arising from pregnancy complications that required urgent medical attention. Since the 1930s, the colonial government had been wary of Aladura influences and their rigid faith-healing beliefs and had unleashed what CAC pastor Alokan described as "unyielding persecutions from detractors and government health officials . . . regarding the welfare of pregnant women in the church" in the 1940s and 1950s.[120] In some cases, medical officers denied death certificates to families of CAC members who sought care among CAC congregations prior to their deaths.[121] This move by government agents prevented family members from claiming a deceased's pension or other financial accounts or utilizing public cemeteries for burials. It was part of a tactic to dissuade patronization of the CAC and similar churches during pregnancy or illness.

Babalola's vision was that creating an institution for training dedicated faith home midwives who could then practice in local CAC congregations in the communities would address the issue of growing maternal deaths and provide affordable access to care. In her reflection on the rationale behind the establishment of the faith home, faith home matron Funmilola Awoyongbo pointedly argued that Babalola was taking action to stop the growing maternal deaths.[122] "Faith birth attendance is a good response to the need of saving women from avoidable untimely death," she stated.[123] A former matron affirmed, "I was told that FH was established by Baba Babalola who received divine inspiration to establish FH to ensure safe delivery of pregnant women from the hands of evil doers."[124] Taking into account the timing of the changes in the faith home, it is also logical that Babalola's strides in creating a more institutionalized faith home also targeted addressing a major government criticism in the 1950s that CAC institutions lacked structure.

Babalola died on the same night that he commissioned the faith home training center in Ede on July 27, 1959, but the support and investments of

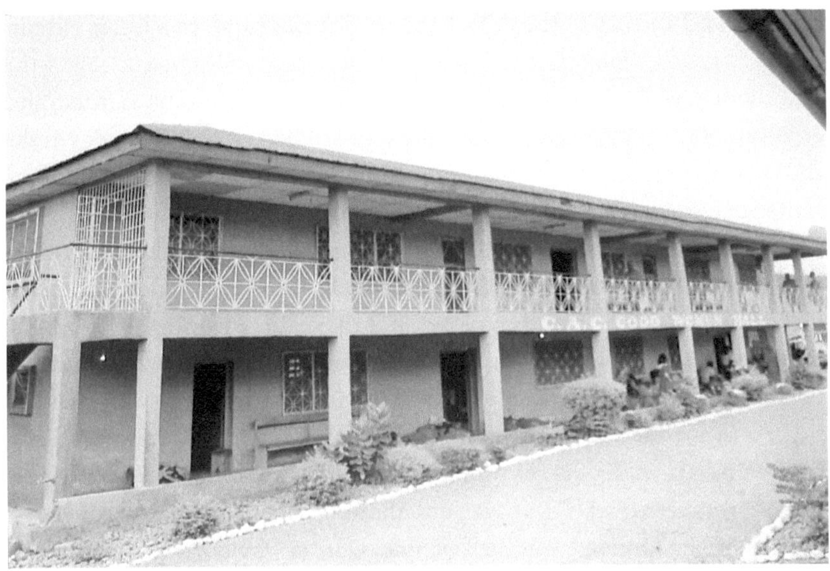

One of the earliest structures in the Ede training center for midwives, named after CAC Good Women

the CAC Good Women ensured the project's success and longevity.[125] The group went on to establish and maintain a residential building for the home's matron and a dormitory for enrolled students.[126] Its members, including those without any form of Western education and who were excluded from Nigeria's medical service for falling short of the educational standards for admission, took advantage of the faith home training school as an alternative avenue to build a career and provide service in the evangelical ministry as midwives. Adeleye, who trained under the faith home's first matron, recounted how individuals who could not read and write were admitted, "and when you get there, they will teach you how to read and write."[127] Many indeed claimed that they received a divine call to serve in the Christian ministry as midwives and viewed their entry into this field both as service to the public, akin to traditional midwifery, and as a professional career.

Babalola's interest in maternity care throughout his prophetic ministry is undeniable; however, the role of the CAC Good Women in the establishment of codified and institutionalized faith home services is understated, even by CAC women themselves. Over the course of my interviews, CAC women, including midwives and leaders of Good Women, attributed the creation and success of the faith home to Babalola and, to a lesser extent, Samuel Akande, who was instrumental in the siting and construction of the faith home in Ede. This trend of putting men at the forefront of important achievements provides insight into the well-studied gender dynamics in the CAC and was critical to the success and support enjoyed by the faith home center in a patriarchal religious environment that mirrored the sidelining of women in the leadership of colonial mission churches and the colonial establishment.[128] To succeed, influential women in the CAC who desired to make headway in the church took secondary positions under the leadership of men. One of these women, Mama Ogunranti, a popular figure in the CAC who qualified as a Grade I nurse at the first University Hospital in Nigeria in 1949 and was known for establishing many CAC congregations, had to operate under the cover of her husband, who was elevated to the role of pastor in her stead.[129] She was not allowed to lead any of the congregations that she founded. Another woman, Dorcas Olaniyi, also a biomedical nurse who became a renowned prophetess, refused to operate under the restrictions of the church's patriarchy and broke away from the CAC to lead her own congregation and maternity home.[130]

In the quest to successfully advance maternity services in the CAC, the church's women thus needed some of their influential men to be at the forefront of and adopt their campaign to systematically organize and develop the faith home, hence the recurrent attribution of this work to key male figures, Babalola and Akande. The women's imprint on the faith home training center in Ede was obvious. Their collective financial contributions sustained the new faith home training center's mission, especially after Babalola's death, and funded other agendas, including the establishment of a women's theological school for training female evangelists in the same location as the midwifery school. The continued association of the faith home to Babalola's final act and legacy, however, ensured its pride of place at the forefront of the CAC's mission.

The Institutionalization of Faith Homes, 1959–1979

The service that the faith home provided in Ede was twofold. First, there was a school of midwifery that trained prospective midwives on how to practice midwifery along the lines of faith healing. Second, there was an active faith home that catered to church members and members of the public, irrespective of religious affiliation, for prenatal care and child-

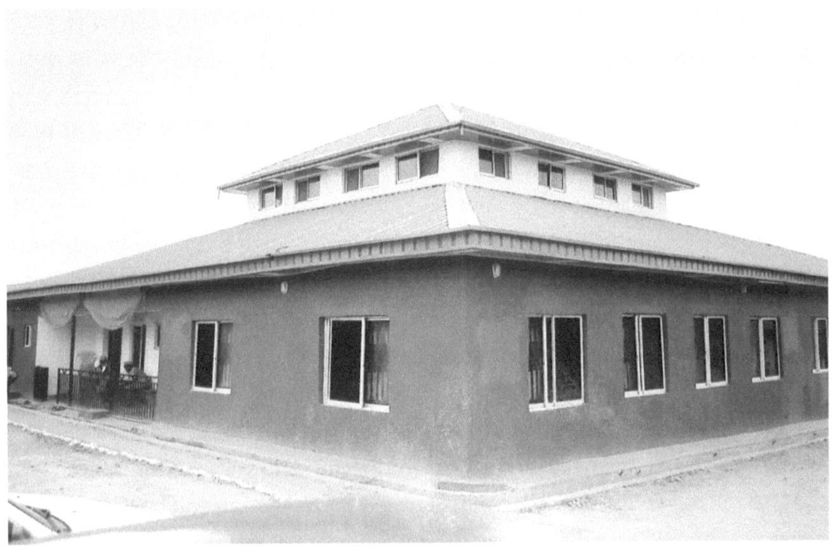

Newer Labor Unit at Ede, 2018

birth. The delivery home also doubled as an avenue for midwives-in-training to experience practical aspects of delivery. At the time of the Ede faith home's establishment, the CAC was subjected to persecution by government officials who accused them of meddling in health affairs—childbirth—for which they had no qualifications and were bound to cause a public health nuisance. To overcome such criticisms, Babalola approached Deborah Oladiran, a pastor's wife and nurse-midwife who trained in London and Nigeria to become the matron of the Faith Home Training Center.[131] As such, Oladiran, an evangelist, would bring her biomedical qualifications, training, and experience to bear in the organization of the faith home, although she could not administer any medications in accordance with church tenets. Since Nigerian law permitted independent maternity practice by trained midwives, Oladiran's capability or qualifications to run the faith home would be beyond question.

The first set of students at the school enrolled in 1959. Initially, enrollment was slow. Church officials recruited women interested in becoming midwives and sent them to Ede for training. Some churches sponsored their pastor's wives for training while others sponsored respected elder women who could dedicate their time to prayers and the service of midwifery.[132] For most candidates, their enrollment was premised on a divine call to service. In my visits from one faith home midwife to the other, I asked the same question: "How did you decide to become a midwife?" The answers were very similar: "I heard the call from God that I should go for the training of midwifery," one said.[133] Another explained, "It wasn't my opinion to go for the course, but God made it compulsory for me. I was in the North doing my trading business then. I did not want to answer [the call] because my husband was already late and my children were enrolled in school. But when tribulations arose in my trading business, then I came back from the North to go and do the course at Ede."[134] In addition to those who expressed their agency to become midwives through religious calls, members of the church who had hospital training as nurse-midwives or auxiliary midwives also joined the faith home for training as faith home midwives.[135] Others became assistants to faith home midwives while awaiting their own training and posting.[136] This was how the faith home's second matron, Lydia Ajayi, joined the services of the faith home. Ajayi, who was certified by the Nursing and Midwife Board of Nigeria, had first started as an assistant to the first matron, Oladiran, and replaced Oladiran as matron in 1987.[137]

Training in the early 1960s lasted for three to six months and included personalized training by the home's matron on how to safely deliver babies. This training also emphasized the spiritual nature of the job and focused extensively on the use of prayers and psalms, as established by Babalola in the 1930s, to protect pregnancies from evil machinations or other unknown benign forces. This spiritual component of the training was partly provided by the matron but mostly by the prophetess who oversaw the women's Bible College, also situated in Ede. This prophetess and evangelist ensured that the students understood how to preach effectively, lead in their capacity as midwives, provide counseling, and utilize prayer effectively to support the goal of safe delivery.[138] One midwife's expression captured this focus on prayers and the spiritual: "Generally in this part of the world, anyone who is pregnant believes in prayer and must pray because of different forces that may want to attack the pregnancy or the mother, so you have to give yourself to prayers."[139]

The matron, on the other hand, ensured that trainees understood the processes of pregnancy and delivery as well as behaviors that could aid or deter safe delivery. In my conversation with retired midwife Comfort Aluko, she explained that some of the risky behaviors that they were instructed to dissuade in expecting mothers included taking long walks during the hottest part of the days because "the heat gets so much, which could lead to dizziness of the mother, and we don't want the heat to affect the unborn child."[140] When walking on a hot day was unavoidable, they were taught to instruct women to take cool baths when they returned home. This pattern of avoiding walks in the middle of the day had always been present in Babalola's teachings on prenatal care, but where he justified it in terms of the spiritual and a belief that *Abiku* spirits could possess a fetus at that time, the faith home midwives in the post-1960s era interpreted it in terms of an expecting mother's physical reaction to heat. High heels and tight clothes, especially during the advanced stages of pregnancy, were also discouraged.[141] In line with Babalola's earlier teachings, the training emphasized practical and natural solutions and highlighted the importance of nutrition and exercise.

During my visit to Ibadan and Lagos, the emphasis on nutrition was clear. Most faith homes had explanatory posters on the various classes of food and their nutritional values, and discussions about diet were frequent. The rationale behind this emphasis on nutrition, as Aluko explained, was because "since we don't give medications, we made prescriptions of different kinds of fruits and nutritious foods that the pregnant women should eat; we advise them and they take those things and everything would be normal."[142] Adeleye also explained that an overweight baby could cause complications during delivery, and so it was important for women to eat appropriate nutrition that was not heavy on carbohydrates and sugar.

As the number of candidates for training as faith home midwives increased in the late 1960s, training was extended to one year. It ceased to be personalized one-on-one training; instead, admission occurred yearly to enable the provision of uniform training for students and the efficient utilization of training staff. An admissions committee scrutinized applications for admissions and required successful candidates to undergo a period of fasting and prayer, a spiritual exercise that underscored for these applicants the prayer-based nature of their mission as midwives. It also prepared them for what was considered important spiritual work. As midwives, they were expected to undertake normal deliveries but also cases that defied medical intervention and could only be dealt with through prayer.[143] Admitted students resided in a dormitory that was built and maintained by the CAC Good Women, and their curriculum included subjects on basic literacy, such as reading comprehension and parts of speech. Other parts of the curriculum

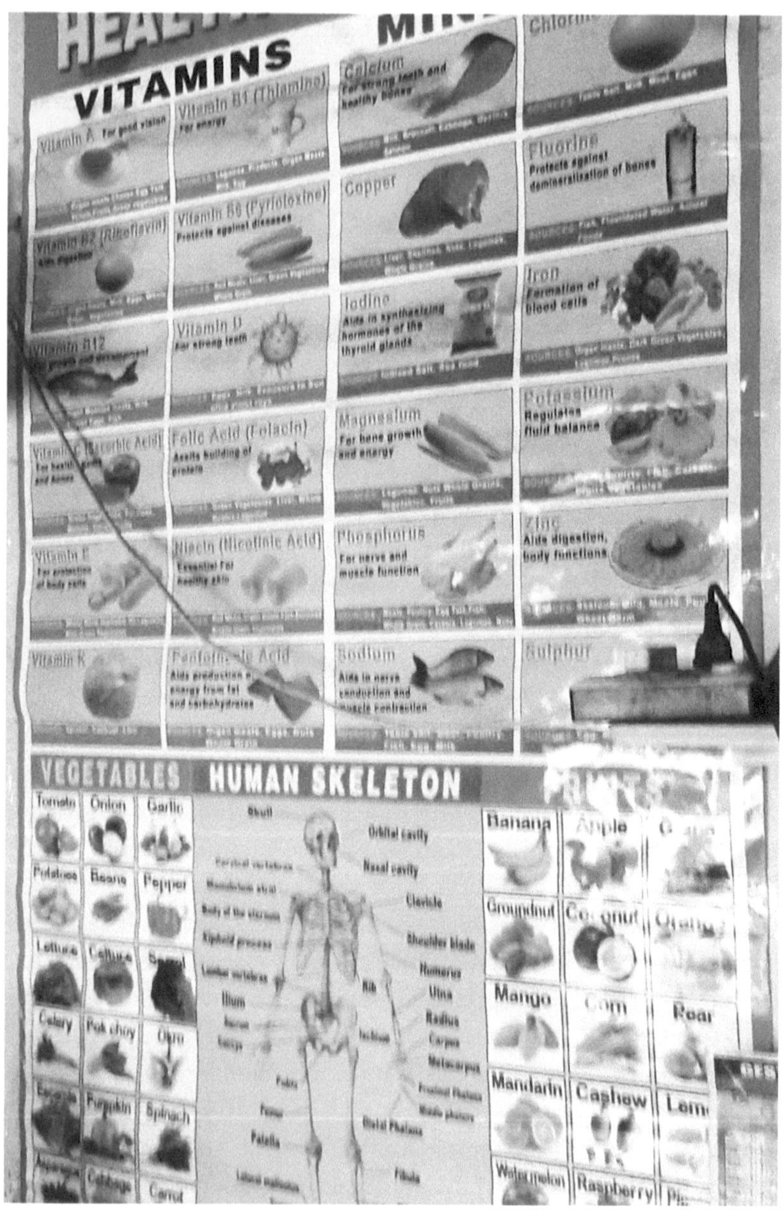

Nutrition poster on a faith home wall, common in CAC faith homes

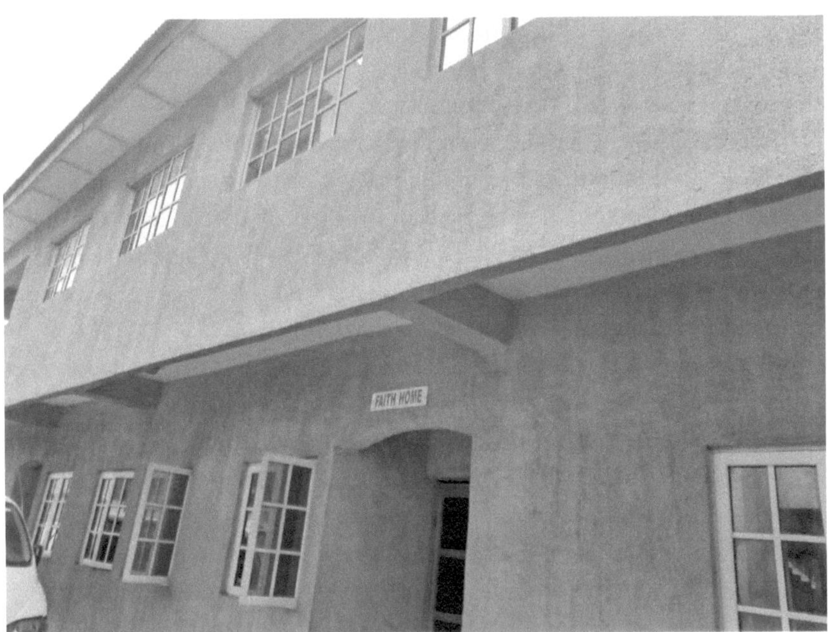

Exterior of a faith home in a Lagos CAC church

included courses on basic anatomy, basic health education, and nutrition. These lessons were provided by the matron and some visiting lecturers that included medical doctors, nurses, and professors who were largely members of the CAC.

As more trainees graduated in the 1960s, the faith home transformed from its pre-1959 format as merely a house of prayer that tended to pregnant women and all who were sick or had other types of affliction to an institution that catered specifically to pregnant women. Successful graduates were dispatched to various CAC congregations that could establish and sustain a faith home, a building that was distinct from the church structure and dedicated to the services of pregnant women. Church-sponsored candidates returned to their sponsoring institution to take on service as midwives. Throughout the 1960s and beyond, it became the norm for medium- to large-sized CAC congregations to have a faith home with one trained midwife and one or two assistants.

As CAC faith homes multiplied in the 1970s, graduating midwives spent two weeks in residence at one faith home, where they practiced under supervision to the satisfaction of designated observers and examiners. Upon the successful completion of their residency, the new midwives received more permanent postings to various branches of the CAC across Nigeria. All of these midwives were under the leadership and administration of the faith home matron in Ede and provided annual reports to Ede. In Lagos, the faith homes were divided into three districts, Lagos 1, 2, and 3, under the respective oversight of three leaders. These leaders convened monthly district meetings where midwives prayed collectively and received instructions and updates on acceptable practices.[144]

At their various faith homes, CAC midwives required expecting mothers to register with the faith home within the first three to five months of the pregnancy. Women who wished to register with a faith home beyond the fifth or sixth month of gestation were routinely turned away due to the emphasis on identifying and addressing any spiritual or physical hindrances to safe delivery through proper prayers and timely consultations. In Esther Oluwafemi's faith home, women could register with the faith home no later than the fifth month of pregnancy. As a rule, expecting mothers had to attend a minimum of four months of prayer and prenatal sessions to deliver in the faith home.[145] After registration, expecting mothers attended weekly prayer meetings presided over by the midwife. These sessions aimed to address every potential spiritual obstacle to safe delivery, including those that had been foreseen through prophecy.[146]

Such a scene played out before me at the CAC faith home in Odi Olowo. The church was filled with about thirty women who had begun arriving by 9 a.m. on a Thursday morning. Shortly afterward, the midwife began a service that ended with an extended prayer session in which the attendees prayed against stillbirth, cesarean sections, infertility, ill health, and evil eyes or other spiritual forces. Cesarean section was particularly highlighted not only because it was an expensive undertaking but because it defeated the biblical promise, "You shall deliver like the Hebrew women," and cast aspersion on cultural expectations that women should be capable of delivering babies naturally.[147] Even more important was the fear that cesarean sections produced postpartum complications and frequently led to a mother's demise during the procedure. For these praying women, therefore, a cesarean section was akin to a death sentence and had to be listed alongside other negative conditions or outcomes in women's reproduction. One could easily replace cesarean section on this list with "death." At the end of the meeting at Odi Olowo,

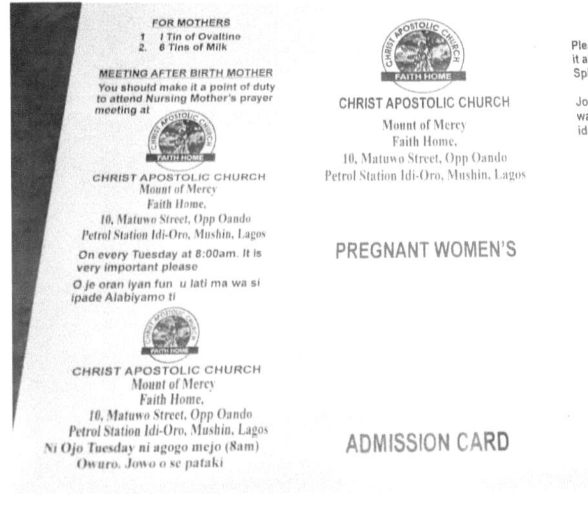

FOR MOTHERS
1. I Tin of Ovaltine
2. 6 Tins of Milk

MEETING AFTER BIRTH MOTHER
You should make it a point of duty to attend Nursing Mother's prayer meeting at

CHRIST APOSTOLIC CHURCH
Mount of Mercy
Faith Home,
10, Matuwo Street, Opp Oando
Petrol Station Idi-Oro, Mushin, Lagos

On every Tuesday at 8:00am. It is very important please

O je oran iyan fun u lati ma wa si ipade Alabiyamo ti

CHRIST APOSTOLIC CHURCH
Mount of Mercy
Faith Home,
10, Matuwo Street, Opp Oando
Petrol Station Idi-Oro, Mushin, Lagos
Ni Ojo Tuesday ni agogo mejo (8am)
Owuro. Jowo o se pataki

CHRIST APOSTOLIC CHURCH
Mount of Mercy
Faith Home,
10, Matuwo Street, Opp Oando
Petrol Station Idi-Oro, Mushin, Lagos

PREGNANT WOMEN'S

ADMISSION CARD

NOTICE

Please keep this Card clean and bring it along with you to the Faith Home for Spiritual and Prayerful care

Jowo se itoju kadi yi dada ki o ma mu wa si ipade Alabiyamo fun adura ati fun idari Emi ko si gbodo doti

CHRIST APOSTOLIC CHURCH
Mount of Mercy
Faith Home,
10, Matuwo Street, Opp Oando
Petrol Station Idi-Oro, Mushin, Lagos

NOTE

Please always bring this Card to every Tuesday Meeting.

AKIYESI

Jowo mu kadi yi dani ti o ba mbo wa si ipade

ADMISSION

THE BEARER

Mrs ____________________

Is a member of
CHRIST APOSTOLIC CHURCH

____
Assembly

Please admit her to the Pregnant Mother's Prayer Meeting.

THANKS

____
Assembly Pastor or Evangelist

Date ____________________

MEETING ATTENDED
DATE, MARK & MIDWIFE'S SIGNATURE

AWON OHUN ELO FUN OMO TITUN

1. Cotton wool
2. 4 Sunlight Soaps
3. Baby Sponge
4. 2 Towels (Big & Small)
5. Flannel
6. Gauze Bandage
7. 3 Pads
8. Flask
9. 4 Medium Blue Omo
10. Napkin & Nappy
11. Oil (1 Litre)
12. Raid
13. 5 Poly Bags

Awon ohun elo wonyi je ohun ti o ni lati ra, ki akoko ati bimo yin to to

Midwife in charge

Registration card (front and back) tracking women's attendance to weekly prayer and prenatal sessions

the women lifted bottles of water into the air, and these were blessed by the midwife and taken home for drinking and for infusion into baths. As in the early days of the Aladura movement, this blessed water was believed to confer divine protection. Beyond the prayer meeting, women attended a prenatal session on a different day when the midwife checked mother and

Requirement for Delivery & Baby Needs

1. Small Towel and 1 Shawl, Socks, Cap.
2. Disposable Nappies
3. 1 Vaseline and Cotton Buds
4. 1 Goya Oil 1 Flit (Mointeen)
5. 2 baby soap and sponge
6. 1 Medium Dettol / 1 pair long glove
7. 1 Dele cotton wool / Mothers Pampers
8. 6 Brown Paper, 6 Toilet rolls
9. Gloves 3 surgical, 1 pack Test gloves
10. Izal and Jik
11. Airfreshner (tin)
12. Markintouch (2)
13. 1 Oma or Lemon Bonux 1kg
14. Baby Oil and Spirit
15. Baby Dress
16. Cord clamp & 1 mucus Extractor
17. Comb, Cup, Spoon
18. 1 packet of Blade
19. 1 Face Towel / 2 Poly Bags

For Mother

1. Tea, Milk, Glucose D
2. 2 Comfit pads, Pants and Culteter
3. Wrappers, Slippers, Cup, Spoon and Plate

List of items required for delivery at a faith home in Ibadan

baby to ensure good health and provided advice on proper nutrition, self-care, and emotional well-being.

The deliveries at the faith home remained free during the 1960s and 1970s, an attribute that kept it appealing to the general public. Expecting mothers were required to pay for a registration card, a token fee. At the end of childbirth, they could offer monetary or other gifts, or nothing at all, to their midwives, in accordance with local cultural practices of midwifery. They were also responsible for providing the items essential for delivery. At the seventh month of pregnancy, they presented these items, which included soap, towels, disinfectants, blankets, and baby clothes, to the midwife. At the onset of labor, women arrived at the faith home for birth, after which they spent a twenty-four-hour observatory period to rule out any complications for the mother or baby. Throughout the 1970s, the faith homes operated in this manner until changes in the next decade, to which we will turn in subsequent chapters, forced them to adapt their approach to maternity care to accommodate women whose complications needed biomedical intervention.

Conclusion

Aladura intervention in the reproductive health field highlights how local actors inserted themselves in an evolving maternal health care arena by providing local solutions to maternal health challenges that the colonial government largely ignored in the first quarter of the twentieth century. Babalola's focus on maternity services, which also occurred at a time when birth and motherhood were central to European missionaries' "civilizing mission," was an attempt to address mortality and birth complications stemming from what Babalola considered mismanagement or the work of evil forces. The CAC's approach to this problem differed from government's in that CAC believed that maternal health could be optimized through prayers, good nutrition, cleanliness/godliness, sexual morality, and exercise, without the use of biomedical services. This view put the CAC at odds with European missionary groups and the colonial government and launched the CAC into colonial Nigeria's politics of birth.

Babalola's intervention in reproductive health care prompted letters by missionaries in Nigeria to their supporters in the United Kingdom about the need to increase medical personnel in the western region. As local converts left churches and hospitals in large numbers and flocked to Aladura rallies in search of healing, missionaries reasoned that a good counter to Aladura faith-healing was the expansion of medical services in the area, especially because medical personnel were severely depleted from the beginning of World War I into the 1930s. The movement's momentum was depicted as the missions' failure to provide adequate medical services among local communities. To this effect, missionaries in the western provinces issued a call: "We want a doctor, and we want another doctor, or nurse, to give instruction quite simply to the African woman . . . , midwives in the villages, a central hospital for the difficult cases. God has emphasized the need."[148] The calls for more medical workers and infrastructure were partly heeded when the colonial government became more involved in developing medical facilities and expanding infrastructure for maternal and infant welfare in the post–World War II era. However, the inadequacies of maternity services persisted, compelling women to utilize other options for birth, such as homebirths and faith homes.

By the late 1950s, at a time when private medical practice was expanding and midwifery was becoming a popular career option for Nigerian women, the CAC's venture in childbirth evolved into a more permanent institution with its own midwifery school and dedicated birthing centers. The decision to create a midwifery training institution and an exclusive class of midwives was mostly a response to government opposition against the Aladura and criticisms that they meddled in public health affairs. These oppositions, which ranged from denying children of Aladura members admission into mission schools to withholding death certificates to families of individuals known to use Aladura services during ill health, stimulated the CAC to develop a more reputable and respectable framework.[149] In the realm of childbirth, the church created an organized system that was headed by biomedically trained nurse-midwives and included a central curriculum, a system of administration, standardized practices, and a dedicated staff of career midwives.

The move to establish a professional cadre of midwives was also an economic one. In a 1950s era in which the field of midwifery both expanded and became less accessible to women who lacked advanced colonial education, the faith home school of midwifery offered CAC women a means to earn a living as midwives. Religious women who trained as auxiliary midwives in the biomedical setting who had difficulties securing positions in government facilities due to more stringent educational requirements embraced the faith homes as alternative avenues to maintain their own practice as midwives. Between its early years and the 1970s, enrollment into the CAC's school of midwifery was not based on Western academic qualifications but on candidates' spirituality and commitment to faith-based work. As such, the school provided adult education and a means of training and employment to CAC women and members of other charismatic or Pentecostal churches in Nigeria who could not read or write adequately. Thus, for midwives, the faith homes provided alternative career paths that the colonial government had largely closed off. For patients, they provided access and control over the contested terrain of their own bodies, families, and childbirth experience that was based on their own religious and cultural interpretations of birth and birth risks.

The faith homes gained popularity because of their attentiveness to cultural issues and taboos surrounding pregnancy—notably the belief that health outcomes could be shaped by natural, spiritual, psychosocial, and physical factors—but also because they were affordable, compared to hospital services. Aluko's reflection aptly illustrates this: "We deliver them free of charge and they put to bed without any health issues; that's the reason why they will always come and have their babies here. . . . For some, it is their problems that lead them here."[150] Faith homes drew their funding not from patients' bills but from church dues and donations as well as funding from the CAC Good Women Association worldwide, who were largely responsible for maintaining the midwifery school, the matron's house at Ede, and the faith home dormitories. While expecting mothers were charged a token fee for registration cards and required to provide the personal items needed by mother and baby during delivery, local CAC churches provided these personal items for indigent community members who could not afford them. At the end of birth, some families offered the midwife gifts in appreciation of her work, but no service bills were charged.

Beginning in the 1980s, the faith homes began to consolidate their position as a primary maternity care provider in Nigeria and evolved their practices to suit changing social, cultural, and economic circumstances of the era. These changes and the pressures to adapt occurred within an emerging landscape of birth politics that featured the strong presence of international nongovernment institutions and their politics of birth control. It is to these new actors and the changes that they wrought in the reproductive landscape that we now turn.

4

"Birth Control Under Whatever Name"

The International Population Control Movement and a New Reproductive Politics in Nigeria

We are introducing health services; we are likely to introduce general prosperity. . . . It is, so far as I can see, essential that Birth Control (under whatever name!), shall not merely be available, but offered, and urged.

Dr. Julian Huxley, *Birth Control West Africa*, 1943

Every possible way of making children expensive should be considered.

Summary Report, *Conference on Population Problems*, 1952

Introduction

In July 1943, Julian Huxley, an English biologist and eugenicist, wrote to Britain's colonial secretary of state about the need to initiate preemptive population control measures in West Africa, considering the expansion of colonial health services and the increase in life expectancy that Western biomedicine would bring. Huxley's letter read in part: "We are introducing health services; we are likely to introduce general prosperity. This means that the population will start shooting up . . . and shooting up just when all the white peoples (except the U.S.S.R) will be starting to go down. It is, so far as I can see, essential that Birth Control (under whatever name!), shall not merely be available, but offered, and urged, at whatever health centers and maternity and infant welfare places are set up."[1] Huxley's letter reflected both the growing influence of a eugenics movement that had become rooted in Britain and elsewhere and rising concerns during the World War II era about global population growth.[2] Supporters of eugenics like Huxley, who was the vice president of the British Eugenics Society at the time of his letter, believed that it was crucial to control reproduction to eliminate unwanted elements, including the poor, sick, and disabled, from the society.[3] Huxley's letter to the colonial office about the "population problem" brought these growing questions on population control to British colonies in West Africa and to Nigeria.[4] As chapter 2 demonstrates, Huxley's letter arrived during the decade when the colonial government in Nigeria was expanding maternal health care infrastructure to improve women's reproductive health, win local support, and maintain a robust labor supply. Thus, reducing the colony's population was not in the government's agenda at the time.

One concern among eugenicists in Britain, as expressed in Huxley's letter, was that the population growth rate in most of Europe was beginning to stall or decline while that of nonwhite peoples was on the rise, a result, in part, of improved medical services in these territories. Huxley pointed out emphatically that "the death-rate is almost double ours and the infant mortality is 5 to 10 times over!," which in turn meant that improving health conditions for British West Africa could result in the survival of these individuals who would have perished otherwise.[5] For eugenicists, this trend signaled that the Black population in many African countries would be on track to outnumber the population in many white nations, which would mean a new world order in which Blacks outnumbered whites.[6]

In response to Huxley's inquiries, the colonial office declined to take on matters of birth control. Britain's official attitude at the time was to avoid any government-supported birth control agenda in its African colonies. Colonial officers reiterated that "it would be too easy for colonial peoples to believe that birth control was a trick of the white races to destroy the colored peoples."[7] This conclusion was drawn from the controversies and backlash surrounding birth control campaigns in the West Indies.[8] It also reflected the conflicts around the racial framework of the eugenics movement up to the 1940s and 1950s when birth or population control was overtly espoused in terms of race and class, in which Black bodies were considered degenerate and Black reproduction inherently diseased.[9]

Although the British colonial office refused Huxley's request for an "investigation into the population problems," his letter reflected the centrality of population control and world demographics in discourses on the world scene, particularly within governmental and nongovernmental organizations in Europe and the United States. According to Matthew Connelly, groups such as the Colonial Advisory Medical Committee in Britain were indeed concerned by 1948 that advances in public health programs might lead to the rise of "overpopulated and impoverished nations."[10] In the British Empire, the US-based Carnegie Corporation and UK-based Population Investigation Committee (PIC) co-funded and arranged to publish a major work examining the population demographics in British colonies, titled *Demographic Survey of the British Colonial Empire* by Robert Kuczynski, a German who spent parts of his life in the United States and Britain.[11] The colonial office itself was becoming more sympathetic toward the PIC, awarding it 500 pounds in 1943 toward the completion of Kuczynski's project.[12] The colonial office sought to catch up on global population trends by establishing a Demographics Group through the Colonial Research Committee to study "vital statistics questions."[13] Kuczinsky, the architect of the *Demographic Survey of the British Colonial Empire*, was part of this group. Nonetheless, government focus during the 1940s was not set on birth or population control policies but on issues of labor supply and the poor state of (maternal) health care infrastructure in its West African colonies, including Nigeria.

Elsewhere in the world, particularly in the United States, concerns about population growth in non-Western societies heightened in the 1950s, as colony after colony in Africa gained independence. In June 1952, the Office of John D. Rockefeller III convened a "Conference on Population Problems" to address this subject.[14] Afterward, conference participants recommended that the conference become a permanent annual assembly of experts on fertility, demographics, and other themes related to global population balance between developed nations and developing ones. Central to the agenda of major US philanthropic organizations, particularly the Rockefeller Foundation and Ford Foundation, was to "deal with population problems in the underdeveloped countries,"[15] with particular attention to "population planning with respect to the world as a whole and particular societies within it."[16] The goal, as stated in a memorandum to Rockefeller III, was to control "both the quality and quantity of human fertility to assure a population . . . that does not impose an excessive strain on the world's other resources."[17] This focus drew attention to Nigeria, West Africa's largest colony by size, resources, and population, and marked an era of a reproductive politics that was centered on birth control and dominated by international aid, philanthropic organizations, and US Cold War politics.

The researchers and political strategists involved in these population control efforts recognized that newly emergent nations were wary of foreign interference in their affairs, especially an intimate one like reproduction. Educated elites in Nigeria, some of whom studied in the United States, were familiar with and influenced by Black people's assertions in the United States and the Caribbean that birth control was simply another form of imperialism or a tool of racial purge. The various stakeholders in global population control tackled these concerns by working through local partners to establish birth control and reproductive health programs that were perceived as locally driven and adapted to local economic, social, and cultural circumstances. These birth control campaigns borrowed from traditional ideologies of birth control to promote rapid buy-in across local communities.

The international community brought a new intensity to birth control advocacy in Nigeria, but it was not the catalyst for this movement. Before this international involvement in the population control scene in Nigeria, various groups within Nigeria sought to promote birth control measures in an industrializing country where large swaths of the population retained their desire for large families that was typical of their agrarian past. The greatest of these efforts were championed by a coalition of women's rights organizations across Nigeria called the National Coalition of Women's Societies (NCWS). In 1964, NCWS founded the Family Planning Council of Nigeria and supported the creation of the Planned Parenthood Federation of Nigeria, two organizations that sponsored family planning clinics and birth control work in Nigeria's major cities. The NCWS's need for funds to expand their work beyond the cities merged with the international organizations' determination to penetrate the country with their population control ideologies, leading to a partnership that resulted in the coalescing of the population control agenda. In exchange for the funds that the NCWS needed to continue its work by and for Nigerian women, the sponsoring organizations could use the NCWS programming as a vehicle to implant their own state and institutional programming to control Nigeria's population in communities across the nation—all made to appear as though they were local health and socioeconomic measures.

This period in the 1960s and 1970s was marked by public debates about family planning and expanding links between family planning and maternal health. Advancing these family planning programs in a country whose attitudes toward family planning were deeply rooted in local views of morality and religious beliefs would not be easy. Therefore, the international organizations implemented their family planning initiatives through local organizations like the NCWS, alliances with universities due to their connections with the younger segment of society, health institutions to whom women of reproductive age were bound to consult for maternity services, and outreaches to men whose consent was required to dispense contraceptives. Throughout the 1960s and 1970s, policies surrounding birth and reproduction shifted away from maternal mortality issues, which had become a key problem for Nigeria's colonial medical service in the late 1940s and 1950s, to birth control, the new preoccupation of the international community.

However, efforts in Nigeria and elsewhere to make the birth control movement more acceptable to local communities led to a shift away from the eugenicist precepts that shaped the population control movement and the amplification of family welfare, women's empowerment, and children's health in the birth control rhetoric. This shift was not unanticipated by the main actors of the population control movement, however. Back in 1952, when plans for regulating population growth in underdeveloping countries were put in place, its architects speculated that "birth control programs could be put across better as maternal health measures than as a means of population control."[18] This approach gave rise to a fairly robust family planning climate in Nigeria by the late 1970s in which various segments of the society, including members of conservative religious groups like the Aladura, began to articulate and rearticulate their perspectives on contraceptives and how the subject intersected with the goals of maternal welfare.

This chapter signals a shift in the political and social climate—from maximizing birth and infant survival to birth control politics—that influenced Nigeria's *birthscape* toward the end of the colonial period and in the postcolonial era. Tracing the rhetoric of birth control in Nigeria from the 1940s through the 1970s highlights the new directions of reproductive health policy between the end of the colonial period and the height of the Cold War. The colonial government's birth control policies closely aligned with their efforts throughout the 1940s until the eve of independence in 1960 to boost maternal health and sustain higher birth and infant survival rates. As other international actors, especially from the United States, became more vested in events in colonized territories, notably Nigeria, which was portrayed as

Africa's economic giant, maternal health targets shifted from the British goals of boosting successful reproduction to the independence era goals by international institutions of curtailing it.

In this chapter, I trace British colonial approach to the global "population problem" and other birth and population control issues in Nigeria, as well as how the transition to independence brought new actors to the scene and re-oriented the colonial-era goals of boosting population growth to a Cold War–era goal of curtailing it. Local partners and cultural ideas of fertility and reproduction became crucial for the success of these initiatives, leading to the indigenization of the birth control movement for Nigeria and ultimately the creation of a more vigorous family planning campaign in the country. As the subsequent chapter demonstrates, these new shifts in priority and in actors shaped the politics of birth in postindependence Nigeria and developments within the biomedical, faith-healing, and traditional midwifery realms.

British and Local Approaches to Birth Control and Population Issues Before the 1950s

When Huxley submitted his multiple requests to the colonial office for preemptive action to reduce the African population in the 1940s, the official response was that "there is room for an increase of population on the African continent."[19] Up to the time of Huxley's writings, issues surrounding birth control were subjects that the colonial government did not care to engage. For instance, a 1936 letter from the Joint Council of Midwifery (JCM), a volunteer organization based in Britain, to the Colonial Office seeking information on birth control, including abortion, in Nigeria and other British territories elicited the stern response from government officials that "we had better not give much encouragement to the colonial aspect of this inquiry."[20] Birth control was, at the time, a volatile subject understood among non-Western nations as part of a racist and eugenicist ideology. Thus, Britain was conscious of maintaining a good image within the colony, especially in the interwar and World War II years due to growing nationalist sentiments among its subjects and an international outlook, especially in the United Nations, that was more sensitive to the conditions of colonized territories.[21]

Thus, in response to JCM's inquiry about birth control, the colonial office stated, "There is little exact information available for this country. . . . It would I think be difficult or impossible to obtain information of any value."[22] Kuczinsky, author of the *Demographic Survey* and member of the colonial government's Demographics Group, wrote that "to appraise fertility, morbidity, mortality, and migration is about as difficult in most African Dependencies as to appraise the frequency of adultery in this country [UK]."[23] As such, even if the government had wished to enact population control measures before the 1940s, it did not possess the information to justify such interventions. Censuses, which occurred every ten years in Nigeria from 1911 until the census of 1931, were based on guesses drawn from faulty data from earlier years.[24] No census was conducted in 1941 due to the ongoing World War II, and so current data on which to judge population growth or birth and death rates did not exist. The census officer, S. J. Jacobs, responsible for the 1931 census, remarked that any data ensuing from previous censuses, including that of 1931, "must be viewed with considerable caution" due to omissions, inconsistencies, and wild extrapolations.[25]

Apart from Lagos, where medical statistics had been collected since the nineteenth century and mandatory birth and death registrations were enforced, very limited data on fertility and mortality existed up to the end of the 1940s because the government lacked any significant interest on the subject.[26] The 1931 annual report effectively summarizes the state of the data: "The Registration of vital statistics is extremely sparse and the only knowledge approaching accuracy of longevity, and of birth and death-rates in Nigeria, is provided by Lagos Urban area. . . . A number of Emirates in the North make returns of births and deaths but in most cases their accuracy is doubtful."[27] As established in chapter 2, government involvement in women's health-related issues before the 1940s was of limited scale. When it finally became more active in women's health care during the 1940s, its focus was on improving maternal and infant welfare and addressing maternal and infant mortality rather than deterring reproduction. Its discussions on population did not center on birth control but on the high infant mortality rates caused by malnutrition, malaria, and other tropical conditions in Nigeria, which ensured that women had multiple pregnancies to increase the odds that one or more children would make it beyond infancy.[28] These concerns around women's health were tied to securing a future labor supply in Nigeria. As one colonial official put it in the earlier decades of the 1920s, "Her [Africa] great obligation is and will continue to be to meet an ever increasing world demand for her agricultural products."[29] Yet another wrote of government interventions around the same time in Lagos to reduce infant death and improve childhood survival, "Children are one of the greatest assets a country can have."[30]

When the Colonial Research Group published Kuczinsky's survey in 1948, some of its findings, especially for the Southern Province, which included the Trusteeship Mandate territory of the Cameroons Provinces, showed that despite the incompleteness of available data, "the Medical Censuses afford no evidence that fertility on the whole was high."[31] Given that interventions in the 1940s did not, therefore, prioritize any restrictions on population growth, it is no wonder that Huxley's letter got the reception that it did. Efforts were instead directed at decongesting existing congested areas and relocating labor from these areas to parts of the colony where labor was direly sought. This remained a core part of Britain's population strategy in Nigeria until the end of colonial rule.

Population control per se thus never featured prominently on health education campaigns during the 1940s and 1950s. Government focus was instead on the diseases that ravaged existing populations and the colony's current and future labor supply. Dr. Samuel Manuwa, the first Nigerian director of medical services in 1951, described these conditions: "The infant mortality and sickness rates are still unnecessarily high. Malaria, dysentery, infantile diarrhoea, and other diseases which can be prevented still produce a large number of needless deaths and suffering; and the overcrowding and slum conditions which are still all too prevalent in Lagos today make the problem of pulmonary tuberculosis more serious than ever and than it need be."[32] If anything, government tackled its population problem—overcrowding—in a way that solidified its connection between labor and population density in Nigeria.

In the aftermath of Kuczinsky's demographic survey, the colonial government adopted population resettlement plans whereby populations in overcrowded or densely populated areas would be resettled in more sparsely populated regions of Nigeria. One part of Nigeria that attracted government attention in this case was the area of Igboland in the Southeast, which was densely populated per square mile, notably by farmers. An earlier report in 1945 viewed Igboland, the lauded gem of missionary maternity work in the early twentieth century, as "the most thickly populated area in all tropical Africa" and stated that population density in some areas was about 200 to 400 people per square mile, whereas the average density per square mile for the entire colony was estimated to be 55 persons per square miles.[33] The problem with this density, as government interpreted it, was that the land in these territories became overcultivated with no fallow periods, to the extent that "it is now not uncommon for some land to fail to give back the seed which it was planted with."[34]

In 1948, government approved plans to resettle people from densely populated areas to sparsely populated areas in the same region. Its goals were largely economic as the resettlement territories were tasked with producing palm oil, an important cash crop for Britain and a crucial raw material for European industries. The territories also acted as trial grounds for novel "ideas of composting, night soil disposal, cultivation and planting of fallow crops, sanitary and health measures on a small scale before applying them, if successful, to the larger area."[35] Going into the 1950s, these kinds of interventions in population redistribution and boosting the infant survival rate shaped the colonial government's programs regarding population. Interest in any form of birth control campaigns at the government level in Nigeria during this period was sparse.

Nonetheless, birth control thrived among the locals, although, as one woman put it, "Family planning wasn't a talk of the town then [an open conversation in the public sphere], unlike now when modernity is everywhere."[36] Among married couples in various communities, it was an unspoken taboo because great importance was attached to the number of children that a nuclear family could produce, as these offspring guaranteed the economic productivity and social relevance of their families.[37] The importance of birth was such that many Nigerian cultures celebrated the birth, by individual women, of an abundance of children. Among the Igbo, *Ewu Ukwu* was offered during a celebration in honor of wives who had produced up to twelve offspring.[38] Notwithstanding, birth control measures were in place within these communities, even if conversations around them were removed from the public domain and inaccessible to the colonial government.

Polygamy, still practiced for its social and economic benefits, also continued to provide new mothers with a system of birth control. Mrs. Adedeji, an independent midwife, described how men and women in polygamous households arranged intercourse: "In our mother's days, the husband may have more than one wife . . . and there is a way that they rotate it to meet together as husband and wife. The one with more than one wife would always shuffle the women based on who is pregnant or just gave birth."[39] It was the norm in these cases for men and their wives to abstain from intercourse until the new mother ceased breastfeeding or the infant took their first steps due to beliefs that the semen ruined breast milk and could result in malnutrition for the baby.[40]

In such polygamous households, breastfeeding became a major form of birth control. Due to the understanding on the part of women that it deterred menstruation, some women, including those in monogamous and polygamous marriages, quietly used it to control child spacing and reproduction.[41] Mrs. Balogun aptly describes how she utilized breastfeeding for birth control during her reproductive years in a monogamous marriage:

> When I just deliver a baby, I won't see my period until I stop breastfeeding and that is the reason why I didn't usually stop breastfeeding on time. I breastfed my children until they were three years old. My lastborn was three years and two months before I stopped breastfeeding. Even when my neighbors started telling me to stop breastfeeding at that age so as not to spoil such child, I told them not to worry and that I loved it like that. Such neighbor or friend did not know that I was using that system to prevent myself from getting pregnant.[42]

Mrs. Adedeji remarked too that this method of breastfeeding as a tool of contraception was not uncommon during the 1940s and 1950s as "these our mothers understood their bodies and recognized that they ceased to menstruate during breastfeeding."[43]

Among married and unmarried women, herbs and incisions were also common. A traditional doctor, Dr. Alalaye explained that ingesting *aseje*, a kind of herbal mixture, was "how our mothers in those days prevented pregnancy."[44] This practice was common in the colonial era and only became less preferable in later decades due to the possible complications associated with it. It was very important for the correct antidote to be applied to reverse the effects of the herbs that were ingested to stop ovulation and the accompanying menstruation, or infertility was bound to follow.[45] "The best [birth control] is the one our fathers do in those days—the herbs," another women recalled.[46] "I know the ingredients but I won't suggest it for my daughter or daughter in-law. If my father was still alive, well, I could take them to him to prepare it for them."[47]

Incisions, waist beads, and rings were also common throughout Nigeria during the colonial era. Among the Yoruba, Igbo, and Hausa, incisions were sometimes combined with the beads to achieve birth control. As described in the first chapter, such waist beads were taken off a woman's waist on the day of her marriage ceremony to facilitate pregnancy. These beads were worn by sexually active unmarried women or by married women when they wished to avoid pregnancy. Fortified rings worked in similar fashion as the beads and were worn during intercourse to fend off pregnancy. Some of the taboos associated with the rings and beads, according to an herb seller who specialized in reproductive herbs, was that the beads should neither cut nor touch the ground to be effective.[48] The rings must also be taken off during the menstrual period.[49]

In conservative Christian settings, notably among members of the Aladura faith who are the subject of chapter 3, the use of traditional contraceptives in the 1930s and especially in the 1940s clashed with church doctrine on faith healing and abstention from the use of any kind of medicine. Among the Christ Apostolic Church (CAC), pastors and faith home midwives encouraged methods of birth control, including prayers, withdrawal method during intercourse, and the isolation of sexual activity to women's safe periods. According to several members of the church, the CAC taught the principle of prayerful commandment and encouraged couples to join in prayers to God—the giver of children—to declare that they did not want children at any given period.[50] Mrs. Adeyemi gave a sample of the prayer that was passed down by CAC pastors and midwives: "God you are the one who owns the womb. I don't want to have any child again. The grace that you have given me to have children, I want you to pass it across to my children and let them also have as much as they want when they are grown and get married."[51] Such prayers, when said by a couple in faith and agreement, were believed to work just as healing through prayers was the bedrock of the CAC. "Once we attach faith to the teachings they [pastors] gave us on commanding our wombs in prayers, and how to do it effectively, then it will work," Mrs. Adeyemi finished.[52] As demonstrated later, these CAC approaches changed in the postcolonial era as other economic, social, and political changes overtook the country. These natural methods were not exclusive to CAC churches or other Aladura but also widely practiced in secular settings.

As Nigerian women negotiated the practices and policies of birth control from the grassroots, the global population control movement was growing stronger in Britain, the United States, and elsewhere. The major actors in this movement, most of them emerging from the United States, the newly anointed world police and global superpower at the end of World War II, were giving ever greater attention to African nations on the verge of independence.[53] Nigeria, with its size, growing urban population, and projections for future population growth, was a key focal point. The population movement's expanding interest in Nigeria began to draw local attention away from the focus on maternal and infant health infrastructure spun by Britain and its Nigerian colonial officers toward a population control rhetoric that shaped foreign interventions into reproductive matters and local attitudes to limiting their family size.

Nigeria and the Global Birth Control Movement

A lot of the efforts at the preemptive control of Nigeria's population began in the 1950s when some of the world's wealthy philanthropists, especially from the United States, got involved in the population control movement. On February 1, 1952, a memorandum titled "The Population Problem. A Tentative Analysis" and addressed to John D. Rockefeller III analyzed the "population problem" and offered some proposals to remedy what some in the eugenics, demography, and population studies circles considered an emergency.[54] The paper surmised the action to be taken on population growth. Thus, "we must therefore devise and apply widely simple and effective contraceptive measures, look more closely at the possibilities of sterilization, and otherwise do everything we can as quickly as possible to reduce human fertility. Failing this, it may be a mistake in the long run to pursue measures, particularly in the undeveloped areas, which result in the lowering of the death rate without a corresponding decline in the birth rate."[55] During the "Conference on Population Problems" in the same year, which assembled individuals and stakeholders, notably from the United Kingdom and the United States, to discuss this issue, participants proposed to set up a permanent organization and a group of experts whose primary goal would be the "control of fertility, especially in light of the economic and health infrastructure developments that were leading to greater life expectancy in non-western countries."[56] One of their primary goals for these non-Western countries was to craft their offers of birth control in ways that local communities would readily accept because, as the conference report put it, "the people in underdeveloped countries were likely to be suspicious of outsiders meddling with matters which intimately touched the value systems and the structure of their society."[57] As such, the conference sought ways to present population reduction schemes as local rather than Western so as not to be interpreted as American or Western attempts to interfere in other nation's affairs.[58] The 1952 conference led to the formation of the Population Council (PC), a nongovernmental organization with financial backing from the Rockefeller Brothers Fund and whose goal was to address issues of global population problems as well as "population planning" in specific societies.[59]

In the late 1950s, the Population Council and other nongovernmental and US government organizations began to develop population control programs that targeted Nigeria due to its size. US government involvement in Nigeria was also important for a different reason—the Cold War. A US country review of Nigeria conducted by the Program Development Task Force in 1961 explained this Cold War context: "With about 35 million people, Nigeria is at present one large country in Africa with significant world power potential. . . . Nigeria has a special importance to the U.S. as one large African country where the U.S may be able to conduct a major effort in economic assistance to help demonstrate that the way for newly independent Africans to achieve their economic and political aspirations lies in cooperation with the Free World."[60] As such, Nigeria became the focus of attention from the United States Agency for International Development (USAID), the US-based Population Council, and other organizations like Ford Foundation and Planned Parenthood Federation in the contests over whether, when, and how babies were born.[61]

This expanding US interest in Nigeria moved rhetoric on women's reproduction in the late 1950s and early 1960s from the British colonial focus on expanding maternal and infant health infrastructure to a population control rhetoric that shaped foreign demographic interventions in the country. Although Britain was wary of growing US influence in Nigeria, the imperial ruler did not wield as much direct control in Nigeria as it did in the 1940s or early 1950s because many key positions in the social service sector were transitioning or had been transitioned to Nigerians during the Nigerianization policies of the 1950s. In the political realm, Nigerians had also increasingly taken over political appointments in preparation for self-government, which was ultimately achieved on October 1, 1960. With these developments, a lot of the British staff took on more advisory roles as Nigerian officials paid heed to both UK and US advisors and leveraged the resources and other support that they could get from either nation or their representatives before making decisions.[62]

In the foreground of the Cold War, the United States embarked on economic and educational projects in Nigeria through USAID, an organization that provided nonmilitary foreign aid and development assistance. USAID was also involved in the health care sector, although it shied away from direct involvement in birth control interventions or other potentially controversial matters that may be offensive to the government of Nigeria or perceived as US meddling. In 1973, for instance, the US government, through USAID and its embassy in Nigeria, approved a population research and demographic data collection project proposed by an American university but refused to be associated with the project itself out of concern that certain (mis)perceptions might arise over US government backing of such a project in Nigeria.[63]

In the initial decades after independence, USAID and embassy officials were keen to accommodate the Nigerian government's preferences and requests in order to keep Nigeria pro-West in the course of the Cold War. On its part, a recently independent Nigeria was sensitive to potential public uproar that certain foreign policies might cause in the country due to the country's not-too-distant colonial history. Nevertheless, USAID sponsored and approved numerous birth control projects and demographic-related programming that were executed through nongovernmental US institutions, notable of which were the Population Council, Ford Foundation, International Planned Parenthood Federation (IPPF), and Pathfinder Fund.[64] It also provided logistical and financial support to universities and academic groups that were directly involved in population control work. In the 1960s and 1970s, for example, USAID provided part of IPPF's funding for its work in Nigeria and proposed to cover more than 40% of the organization's budget if IPPF expanded its sterilization program in the country, a program that offered sterilization as a form of birth control to women who were adjudged by Nigerian representatives of IPPF to benefit from it.[65] Nongovernmental organizations like Population Council expanded their research on Nigeria's existing birth control programs, finding natural partners in local family planning programs that had been instituted in the country in the 1960s.

Family planning measures existed in Nigeria in the early 1960s, before the large-scale involvement of international agencies in the country's demographic matters, but did not gain a lot of traction. In his survey of family planning acceptors in Lagos, Steven Morgan, a research fellow at the University of Lagos, summarized the challenges of locally groomed family planning programs at this time: "lack of funds and of governmental support, the inadequacy of available contraceptive techniques, the widespread faith of the Nigerian public in traditional contraceptive techniques, including the use of charms, abortifacients, and the traditional period of abstinence from sexual relations during lactation, and the cultural value placed in many African societies on large families."[66] These existing family planning measures were put in place by some of the country's medical practitioners whose motives were not to save the world from impending overpopulation doom but rather to curb the unchecked reproduction that sometimes endangered women's lives and saddled families with children that they could not support, especially as the economy continued to shift from an almost exclusively agrarian to an urban industrial one.

These local movements for birth control began to gain a little traction in 1964 when the National Council for Women's Societies, a women's coalition and pressure group founded in 1959 to advocate for better policies for Nigerian women, created an advisory council on family planning that then assumed the name Family Planning Council of Nigeria (FPCN).[67] With the inauguration of the FPCN and the sponsorship that it received from the mother organization, the FPCN opened several family planning clinics of a limited scale in Lagos, its headquarters.[68] These clinics were operated one evening a week and were staffed by one or two doctors, but attendance remained low due to people's attachment to some of the traditional contraceptive methods already discussed earlier as well as the lingering practice of raising large families.

In the ranks of the Nigerian government, apathy continued to exist about the controversial subject of global population control and the invasive issue of meddling in family size, so very little support for family planning programs came from this direction. In fact, the same reasoning behind Britain's reluctance to promote birth control in Nigeria or elsewhere in West Africa was still present as sentiments persisted among the Nigerian public that birth control was a means by well-to-do countries in the West to maintain control over decolonizing countries in Africa. According to O. Ojo, who instituted a family planning clinic in 1965 at Nigeria's first university hospital, the University College Hospital Ibadan (UCH), there was opposition and unsavory rumors among UCH personnel about the clinic, including assertions that it served an imperial agenda of depopulation and went against local culture.[69] To overcome these setbacks, the various foreign sponsors of demographics control, notably Ford, Population Council, and Pathfinder Fund, partnered with the FPCN and began to frame birth control around improving the quality of women's health through adequate child spacing and providing families with the ability to deliberately determine their family sizes. Their efforts to gain public acceptance also emphasized the importance of family planning in eliminating a cycle of poverty in Nigeria in which families could neither own property nor maintain savings due to an abundance of dependents.[70] In his pitch to the Nigerian public on the need for family planning, the chief research officer of the Economic Research Bureau in Ibadan aptly framed children as economic burdens instead of blessings: "In a situation where a man can only support three to four children but bring into the world eight to 10 children and in addition has married extra young and productive wives, he will be creating for himself complex socio-economic problems which he may never be able to solve before he dies."[71] Family planning was also framed around parents' ability to give their children a good education. According to a US country report on Nigeria, "There is a great popular demand for education, which is generally seen as the key to economic and social betterment."[72] Families only positively considered family planning in economic and health-related terms in which a planned and limited number of children meant better education and better chances for the children to advance socially and in turn care for their parents in their old age. Such arguments resonated more with many Nigerians than abstract population projections.

Throughout the 1960s and 1970s, the birth control rhetoric continued to shift from the need for a global population strategy to concerns about a looming global population crisis. In Nigeria, arguments about birth control centered on the economics of family size. The director of Food and Agriculture Association of Nigeria, in an exchange in which he encouraged the Nigerian government to ban family planning, warned that reducing the nation's birth rate could cause food shortage, perhaps because he was associating any reduction in family size to a reduction in agricultural labor. Another correspondent countered his argument by stating that family planning "is not based

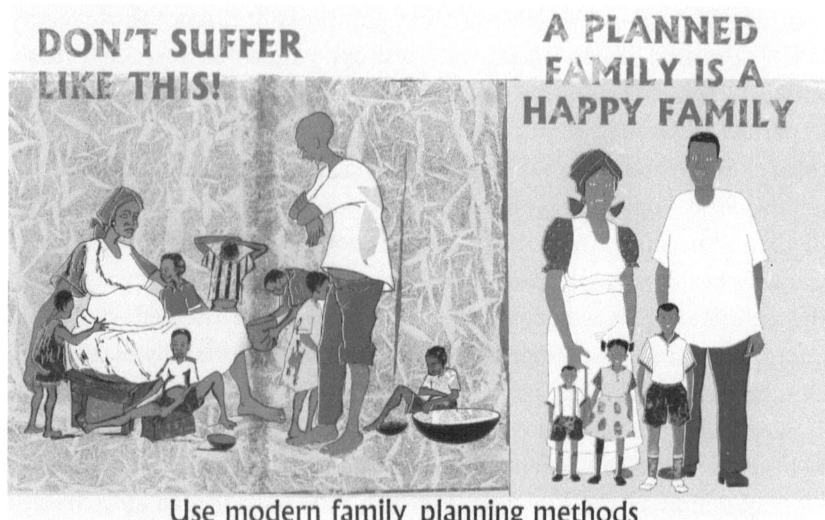

Flyer portraying the need for birth control in economic terms. *Source*: Wellcome Collection.

on the fear of over-population but aimed at curbing the bearing of 'unwanted children'—who suffer as a result of poor upbringing."[73]

This exchange of economic arguments was not unique. In another instance, an information/education officer argued that family planning was not limited to birth control but involved the provision of assistance to couples who could not conceive or who wanted more children but could not. This officer tied arguments for family planning closely to the family's economic well-being and the mother's health. He emphasized that family planning was part of maternal health care and ensured that women would not become anemic and die due to unspaced consecutive pregnancies.[74] Another expert who made the case for some population growth measures viewed the problem not in terms of a global population crisis but of welfare and economic growth. In his view, a rapidly expanding population was not necessarily a problem. Rather, it becomes a problem when "the productive capacity of a nation VIZ a VIZ food and natural resources is not sufficient to meet increased demand."[75] In these cases, any population problem or the need for family planning was articulated in economic terms of increasing education, jobs, and technical skills to improve the lifestyle and decision-making of the existing population.

Birth control became all the more hotly contested as Nigerian nationalist figures brought their warnings about the ulterior motives behind this Western agenda into the public arena. The nationalist and activist Ken Tsaro-Wiwa publicly argued that birth control was an attempt to reduce the African population and, as such, sabotage a potential military struggle against Portuguese-ruled African territories, white-ruled Rhodesia, and the apartheid regime along with its system of oppression in the southern African region.[76] Other nationalist leaders were similarly wary of what one *Daily Times* correspondent referred to as "pill peddlers—the Euro-Americans."[77] The public divide on birth control was such that major Nigerian newspapers dedicated columns for debates on the subject.[78] *Daily Times* had a column titled "Birth Control Row" while the *Nigerian Observer* had "Birth Control Controversy" featuring several articles for and against family planning.

Official Nigerian policy, as espoused by the Nigerian minister of health to representatives of the IPPF in 1968, stated that "it was somewhat too premature to establish a policy on the question of family planning. Nigeria had not had a nation-wide study of the problem which raises very sensitive issues of social, economic, moral and religious questions."[79] At this point, the country was not concerned about a global population explosion and an impending global population crisis in ways that international organizations framed it. While Nigeria was industrializing at this time, many parts of the country still relied on agriculture, and the correlations between family size and agricultural labor supply still existed. It was in light of these arguments that popular Nigerian nationalist Chief Obafemi Awolowo, then vice president of the Federal Executive Council, stated, "Nigeria need not exercise unnecessary fear over the question of population explosion. . . . It might be possible for Nigeria to produce more than what she is producing now if she could cultivate only one 6th of her land very well."[80] Other Nigerians were mindful of the same sentiment about population distribution between Blacks and whites that had first driven eugenicists like Huxley to advocate for preemptive population control measures in Nigeria. This class of people argued that the world was in the age of majority domination and the "minority hardly has the chance of obtaining its rights."[81] One opinion stated, "The continent of Africa is scantily populated and so it is out of season for the aborigines to practice birth control. The result of such uncalled for practice in the future may be that some of those prolific nations of the world would spread to Africa so that what happened in North America and Australia would repeat itself in Africa. What happened in those places was that the aborigines who were very small in number were driven from their soil by the teeming strangers."[82] These kinds of sentiments shaped Nigeria's official stance on avoiding the divisive sentiments about population or birth control.

When Nigeria finally adopted an official population policy in 1970 as part of its National Development Plan, it was wary of pushing a population control agenda and instead opted to establish a National Population Council that would serve as a clearinghouse for Nigeria-based and international family planning programs and their activities across the country.[83] The council came into being in 1975 but was criticized two years later as "yet to formulate meaningful and comprehensive population policies."[84] The bulk of fertility control and family planning activities remained orchestrated by international agencies and their local allies in Nigeria.

The Birth Control Movement's Customization for Nigeria

As debates about birth control raged in public and private domains, the various foreign stakeholders sought ways to customize their programs for a Nigerian audience. Along with the Ford Foundation, the Population Council determined that an effective birth control movement in Nigeria must target key groups in the Nigerian society who directly influenced attitudes and decisions on reproductive health and could shape attitudes of the Nigerian public on birth control. Their primary target groups were medical and paramedical personnel.[85] To rapidly harness the influence of this group, most birth control efforts in the 1960s and 1970s were concentrated in the western region of Nigeria, notably Lagos and Ibadan, because this region was the center of colonial and postcolonial governance and a stronghold of European missionaries since the mid-nineteenth century. As such, health measures and medical institutions were most concentrated in this region and had been present for an extended period relative to other parts of Nigeria. Thus, there was a general understanding by international organizations that this area would be most open to new measures related to birth control, especially those measures presented as health interventions.[86]

One of the goals was to closely tie birth control to maternal health care. In 1967, the Population Council and Ford Foundation identified Lagos Island

Maternity Hospital, which they considered the largest maternity hospital in Africa, as a prime candidate for the Population Council's Postpartum Program, a program that was set up in various countries to offer contraceptives to women under the auspices of postpartum care.[87] This program also provided an avenue for data collection on birth control, fertility, and related subjects. The Lagos Island Maternity Hospital was considered well suited for this program not only because of its large number of maternity patients, about 20,000 annually, but because a hospital of that size "was doing relatively nothing in the way of birth control."[88] Lagos was also well suited for such a program because the FPCN first launched in the state and had an established presence in the area since 1964. Planned Parenthood Federation of Nigeria also began its activities in Lagos during the same year.

The Postpartum Program at the Lagos Island Maternity Hospital took off in 1969 with a mandate to offer birth control services and access to short- and long-term contraceptive devices to regular postpartum patients in the family planning clinic. In 1970, one year after the postpartum program's takeoff, the Population Council and Ford Foundation sent a representative to observe the family planning clinic and the postpartum program in the Lagos Island hospital. This representative painted a grim picture: "Getting patient education in this clinic is near impossible. . . . Group discussions are impossible due to the lack of space and the tremendous amount of noise. There is no evidence of posters and patients are not given any literature on discharge from the hospital."[89] In addition to the problems identified above by this representative, the Lagos Island Maternity Hospital limited its postpartum clinic to patients with difficult deliveries and cesarean sections only, which translated to about 10% of annual deliveries or 50 patients a week and around 2,000 patients annually out of an average of 20,000 maternity patients.[90] This arrangement meant that most women did not return for a postpartum visit and, therefore, did not receive any information about contraceptives.

An additional setback was a requirement by the Nigerian government that hospitals and family planning clinics must obtain a husband's signature before dispensing contraceptives of any kind. Men who were suspicious of birth control methods withheld their signatures from the consent forms and threatened clinics or their wives with police and civil action should they proceed to administer or obtain contraceptives without the men's consent.[91] Women, on the other hand, resorted to signature forgery to procure their contraceptives. According to FPCN officials, "Some have paid professional letter writers to forge their husband's signature on the consent forms and some even sign them themselves."[92]

Historically, in many Nigerian communities, women mostly controlled the space of childbirth but had little direct control over their reproductive bodies—bodies that were routinely viewed both by colonial agents and local communities as objects for measuring and enforcing communal morality.[93] The family unit was also a patriarchal space in which men were the primary decision-makers. As such, attempts at regulating reproduction were interpreted in terms of gendered power, patriarchy, and family dynamics. Discourses about birth control through family planning, therefore, resulted in expressions of discomfort in a patriarchal society over women's potential ability to regulate their reproduction at a significantly larger scale and what changes in power dynamics that this might bring to the home. For some men, their wives' ability to access birth control meant increased opportunity for economic empowerment that would be absent if there were chances of conception and pregnancy. One woman rendered an example on this matter:

> Let's say a woman had given birth to four children and the husband deliberately doesn't want her to work so that he can always control her, he'd say he wants more children, to which the wife refuses. The husband may decide to withhold feeding allowance and out of the ensuing hunger, the woman yields to her husband's request. But when you have your job or business as a woman and can take care of yourself, if your husbands refuses to perform certain functions at home, you as the wife can do them and in fact the husband will see that such a woman cannot be intimidated.[94]

As such, the oppositions by some men and the embracing of birth control by women were as much a matter of power and economic control as they were about women's health.

Concerns about women's bodies and public morality remained a significant part of the public debate. Many Nigerians feared that allowing women access to the more discreet "modern contraceptives" would constitute a license for their promiscuity and render the society incapable of monitoring women's sexual relations.[95] To those who shared this view, eliminating the consequences of sex—the possibility of pregnancy—through contraceptives would hide the evidence necessary to identify and judge promiscuity or unsanctioned sexual relations. This would in turn encourage women to engage in illicit sexual acts. As one Nigerian put it, "Even spinsters, school girls and promiscuous housewives who indulge in premarital sex will capitalize on it to indulge themselves with reckless living."[96] This sentiment was so far-reached that one of FPCN's objectives for their programming in 1972 was to "help allay the fears of some men that family planning leads to promiscuity."[97] Other opponents of contraception believed that it caused infertility and would render women incapable of bearing children. In fact, the prophet of a Pentecostal church was quoted in a major Nigerian newspaper as declaring, "If women take to family planning, they will be permanently barren."[98] Late in the twentieth century, these beliefs that contraceptives "spoils the womb" persisted.[99]

To address some of these obstacles and advance their agenda, the Population Council and Ford Foundation advised the Postpartum Program to expand the reach of the family planning clinic by blurring the lines between the clinic and other postpartum services. One excerpt from a review of the Postpartum Program read, "Routine postpartum programs should be conducted in the family planning clinic at all times and such examinations should be made available to all postpartum and postabortion patients regardless of whether they desire family planning or not."[100] Postpartum visits, which were initially reserved for difficult labors, were now extended to all deliveries. Nurses and physicians encouraged mothers to schedule a postpartum visit within six weeks of birth or up to three months afterward.[101] Prior to this time, nurses and midwives advised mothers that they could return within two months of delivery or not at all. The new approach meant that women who were unable to return within six weeks to three months could return anytime without being turned back.

The nurse-midwives who ran the postpartum and family planning clinic became charged with the responsibility of providing birth control care, such as inserting the intrauterine device or administering other contraceptives options, while the position of a designated inserter was eliminated.[102] This move was aimed at routinizing family planning and encouraging the outlook that it was part of regular maternity care. It also dealt with issues of staff shortages that had always been present in Nigeria's health sector. The streamlined process reduced the need for additional staff and funding for the staff and instead utilized the nurses and midwives who already operated in a hospital's maternity ward to cover needs for contraceptives services. This arrangement also meant that family planning work did not have to be restricted to one or two nights a week, as was the case with the FPCN clinics in the early 1960s, but could operate as part of a hospital's daily work.

The Population Council and Ford Foundation recognized that administering birth control without the consent of husbands could render the act illegal, according to Nigerian laws; therefore, they emphasized the importance of including men in conversations and campaigns about birth control. Motivators, tasked with recruiting women in the prenatal clinics and labor wards for birth control, were instructed to contact "as many husbands as possible at the time of visiting hours."[103] During the hospital's daily visitation periods for newly delivered mothers and postabortion patients who typically stayed in the clinic for twenty-four hours, these motivators introduced themselves to the patient's male partners and provided them with information about birth control. This approach was not adequate, however, as it was premised on reaching the men who visited their partners in the clinics but not others outside the clinics.

Postpartum staff, including midwives, whose responsibilities were to visit patients who did not return for scheduled postpartum visits, were now required to discuss birth control programs with the male members of the patients' families at the patients' homes. The Population Council recognized, however, that many motivators were young women, and so conversations with men about conception and birth control might prove awkward. To address this challenge, it proposed the recruitment of male fieldworkers whose responsibilities were to conduct community outreaches and educate men on contraceptives. Prior to this development, women were the exclusive target of the Postpartum/Family Planning Clinic and the Family Planning Council of Nigeria.[104]

A public education campaign was also launched in urban areas targeting low- and middle-income families that may not otherwise know about family planning or understand prevalent literature on the subject. The first campaign was funded by the Ford Foundation and executed through the FPCN. It lasted for four months in 1972 and included mass communications programs through cinema, radio, billboards, and printed materials. A second campaign was proposed to specifically target men for education and information dissemination on birth control by positioning materials specific to the male audience in male-centered spaces. Billboards with messaging about contraception were located in stadiums, and contraceptive-themed clips ran in commercial cinemas, as the movies were considered "a medium for young men."[105] This male-oriented campaign also sought to promote condom use among men as a method of birth control. According to William Sweeney, a Ford Foundation agent who evaluated these projects, "Few programs in the world, to date, have focused on the male. None have undertaken a program as broad in scope."[106] Sweeney hoped that Nigeria's programming for men could provide a model for other West African countries.[107]

The proliferation of information on birth control and responsible sexual relations over Nigeria's print media, radio, television, and cinema became such a normal part of daily life that by the 1970s and 1980s, Nigerian newspapers were emboldened to publish numerous debates on birth control that it might not have in prior decades. A look at *Daily Times*, a major Nigerian newspaper, showed that younger people, educated audiences, political activists, women leaders, and medical practitioners created and debated emerging narratives of birth control in Nigeria. This use of mass communication to advance birth control agenda yielded some of the most popular birth control and sex education music videos of the twentieth century in Nigeria—*Choices* and *Wait for Me*—which were performed by two popular Nigerian musicians, Onyeka Onwenu and King Sunny Ade. The videos were funded by Johns Hopkins Population Communication Services and became a subject of public and private conversations in the 1980s.[108]

Beyond a focus on men and popular media, birth control sponsors sought to win over educated elites, including medical personnel, who could be instrumental in shaping societal trends. Davidson Gwatkin, program advisor for the Ford Foundation in Nigeria, argued, "Nigeria will be able to mount aggressive, effective family planning programs only where the large numbers of educated people who will be responsible for policy decisions and program development and administration fully understand the consequences of uncontrolled population growth."[109] To this end, the FPCN and its foreign partners targeted educated elites in Nigeria's higher institutions, including doctors, nurse-midwives, and social workers in teaching hospitals, under the premise that these academics were routinely in contact with a significant amount of Nigeria's younger generation. They were, therefore, positioned well to shape public opinion in favor of birth control. Thus, the Ford Foundation and similar organizations directed resources at promoting family planning initiatives among this category of people. In 1972, for instance, Ford organized a six- to eight-week family planning training program at the University of Ibadan that prioritized doctors, nurses, midwives, and social workers. The training was free and included need-based allowances, especially for out-of-state residents, for the duration of the program.[110] Academic departments that had any broad connections to health education, demographics, or social services also received funding to promote birth control initiatives.

A lot of the population control and family planning messaging in Nigerian academic institutions was championed by various universities in the United States that were themselves hosts to population studies and demographics projects. In 1973, for instance, the International Program of Laboratories for Population Statistics (POPLAB), based in the University of North Carolina, Chapel Hill, proposed to establish a POPLAB at the University of Ife in Nigeria, although this did not materialize that year because the US government "was willing to have a POPLAB in Nigeria but in effect wished to have nothing to do with the POPLAB itself."[111] POPLAB was geared toward constructing a global demographic data collection method and registry. In the same year, the American Home Economics Association (AHEA) and the International Family Planning Project in the United States hosted an international conference to promote the role of home economists in family planning. This conference, held in Chapel Hill, included participants from Nigeria. Afterward, members of the US association reached out to the Ministry of Education in Nigeria to coordinate with Nigerian home economists on promoting and incorporating family planning initiatives in their work.[112]

This focus on home economists reflected the broader logic that partnerships with influential groups who had access to less influential members of the community could advance family planning. In this case, home economists were chosen as a focal point because they were mostly women who tended to work with female groups. As Dr. Doris Hansen, director of AHEA, put it, "The home economist would be concerned with the women in the village, in the poverty area, and other isolated settings. . . . The profession's longterm focus on the individual in the family environment provides a dimension which we believe will be useful in finding solutions to this vital problem which involves people everywhere as well as in the less developed countries. . . . A large number of women from the lesser developed countries have received home economics degrees."[113] Home economics was already a well-established field in Nigeria in the 1970s because missionary education for most of the colonial period centered on domestic sciences and home economics training.[114] The population control and family planning movement tapped into this group of educated women to advance its birth control narratives. Similar to missionary logic for focusing on women to advance its agenda of converting families and communities, home economists were believed to have access to other women, girls, and families in difficult-to-reach rural areas.[115] As educators, they also had access to young people in primary and secondary schools and universities.[116]

In the late 1970s, these outreaches and aids extended to religious institutions, although a religious-based opposition against contraceptives stalled progress, especially from Pentecostal denominations and the Catholic Church. In addition to the widely held belief that contraceptives promoted promiscuity and moral laxity, a view also held strongly by charismatic churches and evangelical groups in Nigeria, the Catholic Church believed that it was an attack against the family. Pope John Paul II, who became pope in 1978, vigorously campaigned against the use of contraceptives and, when he visited Nigeria four years later, admonished all Nigerian Catholics to defend the family against "the modern enemies of the family, the disturbing degradation of more fundamental values" by vices like "divorce, contraception, and abortion."[117] Protestant denominations, however, were more open to the idea of birth control. The few inroads made by family planning groups among religious institutions occurred within this Protestant circle, albeit with resistance among some groups.

In 1978, for example, Family Planning International Assistance (FPIA), the international wing of Planned Parenthood Federation of America, provided funding to the Church of Christ in Nigeria (COCIN), a successor of the colonial-era British missionary group, Sudan United Mission, for a "Birth Spacing Project." This project was intended to distribute contraceptives and educational materials on family planning to approximately 20,000 people in the COCIN's catchment area of about 1,380,000 people in Plateau State, northern Nigeria.[118] Because this catchment area included twenty dispensaries and five maternities within the church's district as well as an existing COCIN Rural Health Program founded in 1976, the FPIA believed that the COCIN would be influential not only in distributing contraceptives but in cultivating positive attitudes toward it.[119] According to the FPIA, "COCIN is the only agency in the area prepared to provide family planning information and services."[120] Medical development in the northern region of Nigeria was slow throughout the colonial era due to colonial policies that limited missionary advancement in the region, which created a dichotomy in the pace of educational and health services development between northern and southern Nigeria.[121] In 1979, the FPIA reported similar problems as in the colonial era, stating that many newly constructed rural health centers in the area were not operational. As such, the FPIA had to advance its program through a missionary body whose parent organization had been active in Nigeria since 1904 and had an established health network.

The birth control work with the COCIN was not without opposition. Eight influential church leaders from various COCIN congregations in one district, the Daffo District, opposed the birth control measures as alien to their culture and against Christian tenets of purity. The view that the use of contraceptives, including condoms, corrupted the minds of young people was after all widespread across Nigeria, irrespective of religious affiliations. As a result, these COCIN congregations were wary of welcoming such teachings about contraceptives among their ranks. To convince this group of leaders, birth control was explained merely as an attempt to restore the local custom of three-year birth spacing in between births, except that this would now be achieved not through extended breastfeeding and abstinence among married couples but with modern contraceptives methods.[122] The primary audience for these birth control efforts was identified as married couples rather than the unmarried. These explanations were satisfactory to the local church leaders and calmed the opposition, which, thereafter, allowed distribution of pamphlets and discussions of family planning in the churches.

In another religious setting, that of CAC faith homes and midwifery school, midwives continued to embrace and teach prayers of commandment and abstinence during a woman's fertile period. According to CAC midwife Mrs. Omotosho, these two methods of contraception were taught to prospective CAC midwives due to the foundations of faith healing that Joseph Babalola, the CAC's most prominent figure, laid. These midwives-in-training were also empowered to teach the withdrawal method in which a husband avoided ejaculation inside his wife during intercourse.[123] Those who could not observe the withdrawal method were encouraged to monitor their menstrual flow and only engage in intercourse during the safe periods before and after the menstrual cycle.

Notwithstanding, opposition to contraceptives gradually waned among the CAC not because of any government intervention but due to the economic and social realities of the time. As the stance on total reliance on faith healing softened in some circles due to increased educated membership

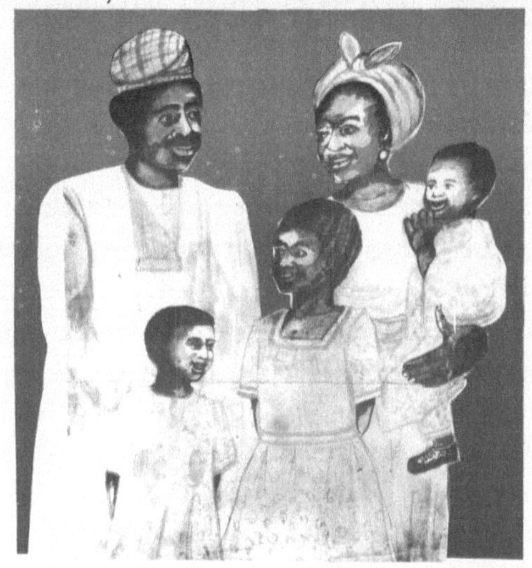

A family planning promotional material explaining birth control as local cultural practice. *Source*: Wellcome Collection.

and the harsh economic conditions, which meant that families were less able to support large unchecked family sizes, the scripture, "be fruitful and multiply, and subdue the earth," often interpreted as a biblical sanction for unchecked reproduction, became subject to reinterpretation. Many people in the CAC and other Aladura churches argued that this biblical injunction was not just about reproduction. "'Subduing' has to do with control," Mrs. Adedeji, a CAC midwife and an active member of several associations on childbirth, argued.[124] "Of what use is plenty of children and not being able to take care of them and having them loitering the streets and under bridges. That is not control."[125]

Those who argued for family planning of some kind, based on family's preferences, emphasized that it was not a new concept. According to the midwife Adedeji, "Even God had a natural way of which he has helped every woman to plan childbirth, because there is a safe period and unsafe period in every woman's cycle. There was a pastor that I first worked with in the 1980s. He told me he never did family planning in the hospital or used contraceptives with his wife, but there was an agreement between him and his wife to only meet sexually when the wife was in her safe period, and that was how they planned their pregnancies until they gave birth to all their children."[126] Increasingly in the 1980s, the CAC's approach became that of letting individual families make their own decisions about family planning. "CAC still believes and maintains faith healing and birth control through prayers, but now that we have modernization, CAC did not ban any member from doing family planning or using contraceptives. Anyone who likes it can go for it," midwife Olaoba stated.[127] Another CAC midwife emphasized, "We can't say categorically that CAC supports the use of contraceptive or goes against it per se."[128] Yet another agreed, "The way Babalola laid the foundation of the church and how we were trained as midwives is healing without medications, injections, or drips. . . . CAC does not advocate contraceptives, but when they [members] go and do it, we don't discourage them."[129]

As contraceptive use became more widespread and a part of public discussions throughout the 1970s, people also became more aware of the limitations of traditional methods of birth control. As a result, more people were willing to try Western biomedical methods. The reservation with the traditional methods was that it could go wrong if the right antidote was not found.[130] Mrs. Olaoba recounted that a family had secured an *aseje* for their daughter to prevent unwanted pregnancy until childbirth. However, the antidote was neither disclosed nor given to the family. When the girl got married years later, the herbalist who had prepared this particular mixture had died and the antidote to her medicine was unknown and undisclosed. Since the birth control could not be reversed, the woman remained childless. According to Dr. Alalaye, knowledge of the antidote to counteract such birth control was of absolute importance, and it was standard practice for herbalists and traditional doctors to disclose or give this antidote to the woman seeking birth control or to a close family member in the case of a dependent. The incisions were also viewed by many as unreliable when conception was desired. It had the tendency to work rather too well, in which case it became irreversible when conception was sought.[131]

Biomedical contraceptives were not without their own challenges, ensuring that the traditional methods remained widespread. The debates about their disadvantages played out publicly in the pages of Nigerian newspapers. One commentary, titled "Beware of the Pill," argued that birth control pills caused a decrease in libido and were unreliable in preventing pregnancy when compared to natural methods.[132] The writer argued, "Between thirty and fifty per cent of women who start on the pill abandon it inside one year."[133] Another article in the *Sunday Tide* in 1981 also associated pills in particular to loss of libido and vaginal health challenges within four to six months of use.[134]

The concerns that played out in the newspapers were corroborated by several interviewees who pointed out that they or many women that they knew abandoned the pill and other artificial contraceptives at different points due to undesirable side effects like nausea, unchecked weight gain, irregular menstrual cycles that could last up to fifteen days, and, in some cases, sudden weight loss.[135] One of these women recounted, "There was a time I did it; that was after my third child, when my husband said he did not want any additional children. So I went for the three month injection, and suddenly I saw that many things nauseated me, including my own soup."[136] In this woman's case, the injection failed to prevent pregnancy since she became pregnant one month later. Mrs. Adeyemi summarized these hesitations about modern contraceptives: "Even though family planning is free at every government health center, some still prefer not to take it; some will substitute it with a ring that won't allow them to get pregnant. Some will go for it, but often the complaint about how the contraceptives injection react on some of the women is what makes some not to go for it. Some say it makes them shrink and some that it makes them fatter."[137] In her observations, another woman, a chemist who was familiar with what she described as "artificial contraceptives and dispensed pills," recounted similar side effects and stated that women in her circle who used the injections, intrauterine insertions, or arm implants felt generally unwell within six months of adopting these methods until they returned to the health centers to remove the implants.[138] These concerns and complaints influenced the number of acceptors who continued to use the pills, injections, and implants in the long term.

By the end of the 1970s, birth control and family planning was a well-established topic in Nigeria's public realm. In a 1977 news article, one writer surmised, "In the olden days a man's importance was judged by the number of wives and children he had. That was when all the requirements of the family came mostly from the farms and these children and wives were employed on the farm. This is not the position these days. Every family now must cut its coat according to its size and the only way is to practice family planning. . . . So anybody still wallowing in the sentiments of following his grandfather's footsteps may suffer the pains of incongruous predicaments."[139] This remark aptly summarizes the economic changes that were rapidly shaping rural and urban Nigerian landscape. It also characterized the postindependence attitudes toward family planning that had taken roots in the country. As these public debates raged about contraceptives, the Federal Government of Nigeria quietly began to provide subventions to the National Council of Women's Societies and the Planned Parenthood Federation of Nigeria, the Nigerian wing of the IPPF, in 1975.[140] By the 1980s, and as a result of the economic depression that befell Nigeria following its oil boom in the 1970s, even the Federal Military Government of Nigeria waded directly, albeit unsuccessfully, into a field that it had largely left to international actors, launching the country's first national population program in 1988. This program was funded by USAID and most remembered for a failed attempt to institute a limit of four children per family and restrict the minimum age of marriage to eighteen for women and twenty-four for men.[141]

Conclusion

As the colonial era approached its final decade in Nigeria, interests in expanding maternal health care infrastructure were overtaken by the desire to regulate global population. From the 1960s, maternal health policies became dominated largely by concerns about demographics and a growing population. However, this population control rhetoric was championed by external institutions in their quest to change attitudes toward fertility and reproduction. These agents found allies among women's organizations and medical actors who were keen on providing resources for families to regulate their family sizes, largely for economic and health reasons. By the early 1970s, the foreign interests and local agendas meshed to create rigorous public debates about birth control and family planning throughout that decade. Although the knowledge of family planning was increasingly widespread at this time, the embrace of family planning was not sudden as many still believed in the importance of large families, despite growing narratives that family size should correspond with the family's economic capability.

The transition from a population control rhetoric controlled by the state and international organizations to a family planning rhetoric that was based on individual buy-in and voluntary participation was gradual. In Nigeria as in many developing and newly independent nations, the population control rhetoric was blunted by the colonial and racial history of its chief advocators, and so these countries were, in many cases, outrightly hostile to such sentiments. Their concerns lay instead with the challenges that confronted their maternal health sector. In colonial Nigeria since the 1940s, this attention had been mostly tailored to the improvement of maternal health care and skilled birth attendance.

In the independence era, the population control and maternal health sectors allied with each other to advance work in maternal health, on the one hand, and birth control, on the other. The latter had always been in dire need of funds to build this sector and improve maternal health infrastructure while the other party had the money but could not advance into the society because of distrust that the population control rhetoric had garnered throughout the twentieth century. At a meeting in 1971, sponsored largely by USAID in conjunction with Ford and Rockefeller, for instance, the International Council of Midwives (ICM) insisted to USAID that "working parties must concentrate on midwifery training with emphasis on the importance of involving midwives in family planning."[142] It also insisted that its "interest is in the improvement of maternity services," which in its account also meant work in family planning.[143] Thus, while the ICM was deliberate to advocate maternity services, it also made itself relevant by arguing that midwives were the natural partners to advance the work of family planning. At the end, the joint coalition of family planning and population control advocates agreed that family planning would become a part of midwives training and a part of the routine work that midwives undertook.[144]

With this new coalition, interests in demographics and population control became increasingly framed as an effort to improve women's health, promote children's quality of life, and save parents from persistent cycles of poverty. These family health rhetoric and mass media campaigns, advanced by international foundations and their local collaborators, inserted family planning into Nigeria's public health narrative. The engagement of nurses and midwives in family planning work in the country increased the number of known acceptors and spread family planning services to rural and urban health facilities. Between 1972 and 1979, that number of acceptors had grown from 13,320 to 105,369, a statistic given by the national director of the Planned Parenthood Federation of Nigeria on a national TV broadcast in 1980.[145] Into the 1980s, even the World Health Organization made direct connections between family planning and safe motherhood, arguing that the former was essential to achieving the latter.[146]

This era, which was also characterized by continued personnel shortage in Nigeria's health sector and increased international interest and focus on maternal health care, as well as the economic shortage that plagued Nigeria in the 1980s, created heightened interests in utilizing skilled and unskilled traditional midwives and birth attendants to augment the services provided by biomedical personnel and improve safe motherhood. It birthed an era of partnerships, changes, and adaptations among various local childbirth actors, and it is to these evolutions that we now turn.

5

Reinventing Themselves

"Decolonized" Hospitals, Tradomedical Maternities, and Legitimate Faith Homes

For too long Africans had accepted definitions of being civilized that did not arise from their own cultures but which had been imposed on them. The present medical system is a colonial legacy which is unsuitable for the Africans, and my suggestion is that we should create a forum where medical and tradomedical doctors can meet . . . to decide what will be the pattern of medical system whose universality will not be prejudiced. The view I take is that Africans can master modern and western technology without abandoning their cultural heritage.

J. O. Mume, *Tradomedicalism: What Is It?*, 1974

Introduction

In Ibadan in 2015, I came upon a one-story building that served as a health care facility. The sign on the building read "Abimbola Hospital," followed by "Traditional Gynaecologist." The word *hospital* was written over an erased description that probably represented sentiments from a prior century. This hospital catered to general ailments but was notable for childbirth and other gynecological issues. Abimbola Durodola, the practitioner who owned this hospital, prided himself in handling complicated births, ectopic pregnancies, fertility issues, and fibroids during pregnancy. He had learned his skills as a traditional doctor from a renowned practitioner in what is now Ogun State in Nigeria.[1]

In 2022, a new signboard in front of a renovated Abimbola Hospital site read, "Abimbola Hospital Ultrasound Diagnostics and Medical Laboratory Services." These name changes reflected broader shifts that had occurred within this tradomedical hospital and other facilities like it, where the

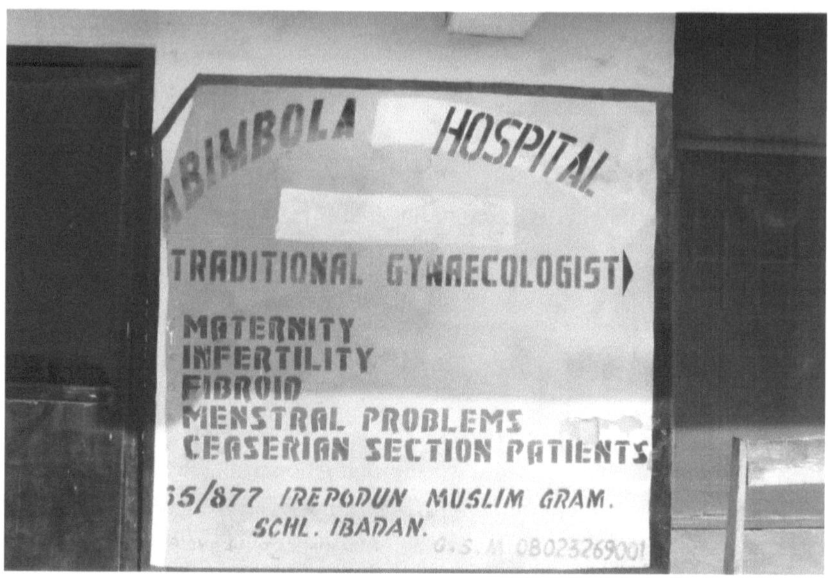

A tradomedical hospital in Ibadan

colonial-era hardlines between traditional medicine and biomedical technologies had begun to blur in the former's bid to stay relevant and competitive. In fact, the term *tradomedicalism* became common among some traditional doctors in the 1980s for addressing traditional medical practice and signaling its shifts in response to internal political and economic forces. The term was specifically adopted to defy the negative stereotypes that the words *native* and *traditional* had come to signify in colonial labels as stamps of condemnation. Durodola explained the changes in his hospital by first producing his certificate of registration as a traditional doctor recognized and certified by his state government to practice traditional medicine. Next, he displayed the hospital's medical certificate, a federally recognized document that granted his hospital the right to function as a primary care hospital that was subject to federal standards of care for such facilities. The federal document was followed by a certificate from Nigeria's Corporate Affairs Commission that recognized the hospital as a legitimate facility authorized to operate within set parameters.

Within the hospital itself, the workers demonstrated the bridge that Durodola had strategically built between his traditional medical practice and

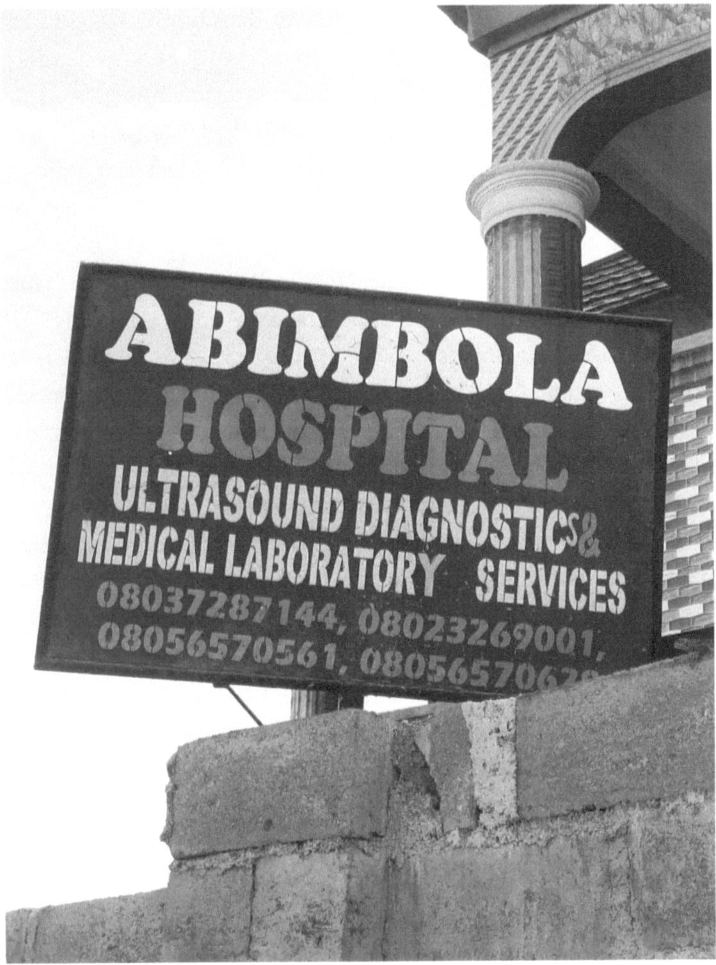

Signboard of the newly renovated Abimbola Hospital

Western medicine. One of the most active staff in his facility, his son Saheed, began training in traditional medicine when he was eight but also became a nurse with a graduate-level degree. Saheed also possessed medical certifications in several health fields and utilized his biomedical training in his father's hospital. In addition, the hospital employed the services of doctors and lab scientists in its provision of health care, including gynecological services, to the public.

These kinds of intersections of multiple medical traditions, as in Durodola's hospital, were not always possible, especially in Nigeria's colonial era, in which missionaries and the colonial administration interpreted medical traditions that were rooted in African cultures of health and healing as backward and undesirable, to support the Euro-supremacist logic of early imperialism. As an independent Nigerian government took over governance and the continued "Nigerianization" of the civil and public service, including the medical sector, brought Nigerians en masse into the workforce to replace foreigners, these institutions became more tolerant of cultural and religious-based ideologies.

In the medical realm, what resulted from these more tolerant views of health and health care was an atmosphere of competition, reinventions, and intersections between traditional practitioners, their biomedical counterparts, and faith healers in order to remain relevant. This chapter explores those intersections and co-constitutions that were created between traditional, biomedical, and religious birthing institutions, as well as the adaptations that they made to remain relevant and be considered legitimate. I consider the changes that Nigeria's major maternal health care actors—faith homes, biomedical hospitals, and traditional medicine practitioners—implemented as they scrambled to adjust their practices in a period of economic depression and global shift from population control to the maternal mortality statistics that heralded the Safe Motherhood era. This narrative of readaptations begins with changes within the biomedical setting in the 1940s, followed by corresponding reactions in the ranks of traditional midwives and other traditional experts and efforts by faith homes to receive official recognition as legitimate purveyors of maternity care. The intersections that ensue are set within broader economic, political, and international contexts that compelled all the major actors in this *birthscape* to evolve in the face of societal changes and growing rivalry.

Following Nigeria's independence, various postcolonial governments did not approach traditional medicine with the outright dismissal that it received in the colonial era. This was partly because they understood the longevity of this medical tradition and the practical necessity of allowing it to thrive. In 1980, J. O. Mume, a respected traditional doctor who had doctoral degrees in natural therapeutics and was an influential member of the Nigerian Association of Traditional Medical Practitioners, expressed this necessity thus:

There are at present about 8,000 registered medical doctors in the country whose practices are concentrated in the big cities whereas there are about half a million traditional doctors scattered throughout the country in both urban and rural areas. . . . The services of the tradomedical physician is the highest contribution of medical service to the Nation's health, compared with the limited healthcare which only 8,000 medical doctors have to offer the 80 million inhabitants of this country. And if by misadventure, the half a million tradomedical doctors are deprived of rendering this essential service to the public, the result can be catastrophic to the nation.[2]

Thus, in the absence of a biomedical service that could provide health care to the millions of people in Nigeria, the nation's government was in no position to adopt a hostile zero tolerance for traditional medical care.

Despite the postindependence government's position on other non-Western medical traditions, the decades of colonial criminalization and stereotyping that were perpetuated through missionary schools and churches had created an urban educated population that frequently looked down on traditional institutions. As such, areas that embraced Western education also treated Western forms of medical care as a status symbol. The location of birth became a matter of not only faith but also class and prestige. Those who subscribed to the "old" ways were looked down upon as underprivileged and inferior, while many educated families preferred hospital birth or delivery in facilities run by biomedical midwives.[3]

As the location of childbirth progressively shifted to hospitals in an increasingly urban and educated Nigeria, changing interpretations of proper birth compelled traditional medicine specialists and their faith-healing counterparts to alter their "traditions" and identities in line with the changing environment and economy. These changes manifested itself in various ways. On the part of traditional gynecologists and midwives, the adaptations occurred in terms of the use of certificates and certification to legitimize themselves. Abimbola explained this need for layers of certifications in terms of the government's capability to "play fast on people and switch up their stance on traditional medicine at anytime."[4] Other changes involved apprenticeships by traditional midwives with their biomedical counterparts as well as the employment of nurses, doctors, and laboratory technicians as partners in traditional health care facilities. This fusion, as exemplified in Abimbola hospital, resulted in what some traditional doctors have described as tradowestern maternities or tradomedical hospitals.

A new category of traditional midwives—Traditional Birth Attendants (TBAs)—also came into existence in the late 1980s during a period of economic, political, and social crisis in which the Nigerian economy could not support an already embattled health care system. This somewhat new category in the maternal health arena was the brainchild of the World Health Organization and other international actors whose interests had shifted from the population control rhetoric that dominated the 1960s and 1970s in Nigeria to a maternal health crisis that had become undeniable. Similar to a failed 1930 effort to train what was considered "lower-grade tribal midwives" to undertake the work of delivery in the rural areas and fill the shortages of biomedically trained midwives in Nigeria, the creation of TBAs was an effort to improve the number of skilled attendants at birth.[5] They served as the equivalent of the traditional midwife but with basic training in biomedical methods and sometimes without the traditional midwife's knowledge of herbs and depth of experience in delivery work. Their practice was premised on collaborations with biomedical doctors, but it also became a site for the blending of traditions as some of those who trained as TBAs were also traditional midwives who had knowledge of herbs and the indigenous modes of attending deliveries. Stacey Langwick, who wrote extensively on this phenomenon in Tanzania, points out that this was a common trend in developing countries that lacked sufficient professionally trained biomedical staff.[6]

Before this postcolonial introduction of the TBAs, the colonial government had made attempts to mimic the services of the traditional midwife. In the late 1950s, the government had begun to recognize the need to create a cadre of nurse-midwives that tended to women in their preferred spaces of birth. This development was brought about by local women's continued preference, for various reasons, to give birth in their homes and with their midwives rather than in the hospitals. The proposed solution to this problem and to the shortage of personnel and biomedical facilities in various parts of the country was to create community nurses and domiciliary midwives who undertook work in the community and women's homes.

Further changes that occurred in the hospital setting were a direct result of the increase in Nigerian personnel within the medical service, which created an atmosphere in which Nigerian health workers were more willing to accommodate cultural beliefs about health. This development opened the door for faith healers and traditional medicine specialists to feature in biomedical spaces as part of patients' search for healing and well-being. Patients and their families brought their traditional beliefs about the reproductive body and the disposal of items like the placenta and umbilical cord into the hospital setting. Some biomedical workers, on the other hand, recognized the skills that were possessed by their traditional counterparts. Nurse-midwives in training consulted with traditional midwives to learn some of their techniques, while the latter, in return, sought information on current biomedical techniques that may improve birthing outcomes. Some hospitals ventured to invite notable traditional experts to administer care to patients and sometimes manage certain complications within the hospital setting under close observation.

Akin to changes in traditional medicine in which members sought to professionalize their services to remain relevant, the faith homes of the Aladura church, Christ Apostolic Church (CAC), embraced an institutionalization process to protect their midwives from government or nongovernmental persecution. CAC faith homes began to adjust their anti-biomedicine stance and implement partnerships with hospitals to improve outcomes and avoid narratives of illegality. They also adopted the structural and training patterns of their biomedical counterparts to remain relevant and overcome any persecution from their rivals who accused them of endangering women's lives. The bulk of these changes occurred during the economic depression of the 1980s, in which access to maternal health facilities became more problematic and too expensive for many. It also coincided with the heightened global attention on maternal deaths and the era of "safe motherhood."[7] This increased attention on maternal deaths fueled the dual-pronged issue of providing more accessible and affordable health care to Nigeria's extensive population but also regulating the non-biomedical spaces that had become undeniable sources of maternal health care. These developments, in turn, broadened intersections and collaborations that culminated in a plural approach to maternal health care.

Biomedical Maternities and Adjustments to Non-Western Birthing Traditions

Adjustments within the biomedical framework were present before independence, especially in the 1940s and 1950s. One recurrent complaint in annual medical reports in the late 1940s about maternal health, which became the center of the plural medical practices adopted by expecting parents and the changes implemented by the colonial government, was that although more women embraced prenatal services, most of these women chose homebirths for delivery.[8] This issue was rooted in not only cultural preference but also the problem of inadequate maternity centers. Despite the colonial government's ten-year development plan in 1946 that pledged to expand hospital and maternity services throughout the country by 1956, it could establish only a limited number of maternities. This was mostly due to a shortage of trained midwives, inadequate training centers, and the overstretching of personnel, materials, and equipment in the administration's Works Department.[9] In Brass (Rivers Province), where a hospital was not scheduled to be built until 1955/1956, the lack of maternal and infant welfare services grew so dire that the government approved a mobile unit that would transit through communities and health facilities to provide services, including maternity care.[10] In communities across the country, advances in infant and maternity welfare could not be made due to staff shortages. These challenges in the colonial medical service created an environment in which growing and unmet demands for maternity care created room for hybrid birthing institutions but also stimulated change within the biomedical system.

The government's initial approach to the challenges of inadequate maternity centers and personnel shortage was the conversion of dispensaries into health centers. These centers provided prenatal and postnatal care to women. However, in many cases, they had no maternity wards and compelled women, including many who attended prenatal sessions, to deliver at home. Families that could not afford the rising prices of hospital birth retained the assistance of traditional midwives or experienced relatives whose services were repaid with gifts or minimal monetary payment.[11] For instance, in Udi Division, known for their late embrace of Western institutions, a growing number of women attended prenatal clinics to receive biomedical attention, vitamins, and other clinical examinations around the 1950s. However, they still retained their traditional midwife's services during labor and delivery.[12] Such examples of need and indispensability of non-biomedical actors existed in other parts of the country and fueled some of the intersections between hospitals and their traditional or faith-healing counterparts.

The Nigeria Medical Service also created a new kind of midwife, the community nurse, also known as the domiciliary midwife, whose services closely reflected that of the traditional midwife in terms of home-based care. This was targeted at addressing personnel shortages in maternity centers.

These types of nurse-midwives became common in the late 1950s and were primarily drawn from the lower cadre of midwives—the Grade II midwife— who then received additional training in nursing and other aspects of health education. The training lasted for a year and a half and involved a six-month refresher course on general nursing and midwifery. This was followed by a one-year training on public health, with emphasis on "domiciliary midwifery, home visiting, and child welfare."[13]

At the end of the training, candidates wrote examinations conducted by the Nursing Council. Preferences for candidate selection were given to local governments with health centers or plans to establish one, especially because these health centers were ideal locations for the community nurse.[14] Although many health centers did not have maternity wards, the community nurse became a mobile maternity service provider that coordinated maternal and child welfare services in the center and attended to labor and delivery in women's homes.[15] Since community nurses served as domiciliary midwives who visited homes to administer their services, they became popular among local governments, which typically had health centers rather than hospitals in their jurisdictions. According to Dr. E. M. Poulton, a medical officer in the eastern region, these community nurses and domiciliary midwives were "trained to help the mothers in childbirth, to cut and dress the umbilical cord of the new-born and to advice on the upbringing of children."[16] They visited homes on a schedule, and when pregnant women could not come to the clinic during labor and childbirth, they readily conducted deliveries in the women's homes.[17]

For the rest of the 1950s and beyond, local governments sponsored candidates who applied for such training in exchange for the candidate's services upon graduation. In some instances, they wrote to Grade II midwives expressing interest in sponsoring them for community nurse training.[18] In Lagos, domiciliary midwifery was set up by the Lagos Town Council and served a large proportion of the population. The nurse-midwives adapted their care to the conditions of the homes, which, according to the council's medical officer, "vary according to the people."[19] Patients who were booked for this service paid a registration fee that covered the cost of the domiciliary birth and were required to obtain a chest X-ray at the beginning of their prenatal care.[20]

In many ways, the influence of the community nurse was set up to rival that of the traditional midwife, who, in her role as a birth attendant, influenced community opinions on maternal and child health. In Poulton's reflection on the community nurse's position, he speculated, "She becomes in her district a person of great influence, the adviser of chiefs and coun-sellor, as well as of the poorest farmer; for she has assisted their wives and children. . . . She can herself see the health needs of the village, and after discussing their remedy . . . she can assist by going to the right people who can take the agreed action. The community nurse also has a great opportu-nity of building a healthy public opinion through her weekly talks to ante-natal mothers, and her mothercraft classes."[21] Responses to them varied from one community to another, however.

In Lagos and elsewhere, community nurses improved public knowledge and utilization of child welfare, but progress in maternity care varied. In Nsukka Division in 1960, for example, one community nurse reported that many mothers still delivered at home under the care of traditional midwives, although they attended the child welfare clinics in greater numbers.[22] An-other community nurse in Nanka, Awka Division, reported that between January and September 1960, her center recorded fifty-seven deliveries, 1,049 prenatal visits, and 1,914 child visits in the child welfare department, as opposed to what she described as lower figures from the previous year.[23] This signified an uptick in prenatal and child welfare services utilization but not much progress in domiciliary home birth attendance as no home deliv-eries were recorded by domiciliary midwives in the period covered by the report.[24] In the urban center of Lagos, on the other hand, the number of supervised domiciliary births was 883 in 1958, as opposed to 615 in the previ-ous year. Home visits by midwives also expanded.[25]

Further shifts had occurred in biomedical hospitals since the 1950s as more Nigerians took charge of these facilities and more local workforce oc-cupied these spaces. In the Federal Medical Service, Lagos, in 1958, 96.1% of the nursing and superintendent staff were Nigerians as opposed to lower numbers in the previous five years.[26] Around this time also, the Federal Min-istry of Health significantly increased the already expanding number of trained Nigerian registered nurses.[27] The result was that these health work-ers became more tolerant of local beliefs about health and healing in clinics and hospitals. As they generally shared the same sentiments and ideologies about the roots of illnesses in spiritual as well as natural causes, they increas-ingly accommodated the manifestation of these local beliefs within the hos-pital setting, laying foundations that have persisted in Nigeria's health care system.

Roseline Ezekwem's account of her last pregnancy exemplified how this interweaving of cultural sentiments about pregnancy and delivery within the hospital setting created complexities in accessing care. As her pregnancy progressed past the ninth month into the eleventh and she trekked to the nearest hospital, located a reasonable distance in a neighboring town, an alarmed nurse who had attended to her during prenatal visits immediately sent her to the labor ward but made sure she carried a note that authorized entrance into the ward. Nurses in this hospital believed, as did the broader Igbo society of which Roseline was part, that pregnant women risked miscarriage if they ventured into the presence of a woman who had just given birth. When Roseline got to the entrance of the labor unit, another nurse refused entry, querying, "You are pregnant. Are you due for delivery that you are trying to enter the delivery room? You should not be here or you could miscarry."[28] Roseline tendered the note she had been given, which stated that it was urgent that she be delivered today and should, therefore, be allowed into the labor unit. These nurses as well as their patients acknowledged and were guided in their care by some traditional taboos surrounding childbirth, irrespective of the location of care.

Another aspect of this symbiosis played out in the disposal of the placenta and umbilical cord. As pointed out in chapter 1, these items were cared for in particular ways and had rituals associated with them designed to tie the newborn to the land and ensure their access to its resources. In the colonial era, when hospitals were largely staffed by missionaries and European personnel, these traditional preferences for disposing of the placenta or the umbilical cord were not acknowledged or respected, a factor that discouraged some families from utilizing hospitals and maternity centers for birth. Key members of the extended family, whose responsibility it was to police the observance of the traditional practices associated with birth, were often not allowed in missionary spaces and so could not influence practices and outcomes. In the late 1950s, however, the increased presence of local staff with shared acknowledgment of local customs facilitated such cultural observances. It became common for nurses to save the placenta immediately after birth and hand it over to new parents. In private hospitals especially, where patients had more say on care and outcomes than in government facilities, the disposal of the placenta and umbilical cords followed local rules. Families received children's cords for proper burial in the babies' natal homes.

Similarly, some Nigerian doctors became more amenable to the adoption of traditional and religious modes of healing within their hospitals, especially in difficult circumstances. Those patients who believed in the healing power of God but also the importance of biomedicine could, for instance, invite their priests, prophets, or faith healers to intervene with prayers and other spiritual ministrations in the hospital setting. One woman explained this kind of occurrence in her testimony about the delivery of her babies: "I had been seeking the fruit of the womb for many years since I got married. When I finally got pregnant with twins, I had a difficult and prolonged labor in the hospital. As it became clear that I may not have a normal natural delivery, I asked my husband to call my pastor's wife. She was allowed into the labor room and placed her hand on my belly and prayed for some time while the nurses did their work. Shortly after her intercession, I had my babies."[29] Stories like hers abound in both cases of childbirth and other health interventions. One traditional doctor explained how some biomedical doctors discreetly sought the skills of traditional practitioners in dire cases, even if they would not acknowledge such collaboration publicly because of the stigma associated with traditional medicine and the rivalry between traditionalists and their biomedical counterparts.[30] Banire Alalaye, a traditional doctor in Ibadan, argued that some doctors invited their renowned traditional counterparts during complex deliveries that were not attributed to a narrow pelvis and of which the imminent last resort was a potentially risky and expensive cesarean section.[31] In many cases, these traditional doctors were successful in stimulating delivery. Where they failed, the cesarean section was performed.

Nurses and midwives, in fact, recognized the skills of their traditional counterparts like Onyeugwu Nwa Ogwo and Mary Ugwuanyi, who insisted I must be a student of midwifery when I interviewed them for this study. Knowing that acquiring these skills in traditional midwifery of midwives like Onyeugwu and Mary could give the nurses an advantage in their own private practices, biomedical nurses and midwives sought out renowned and well-respected traditional midwives for training on useful traditional skills that could aid labor and delivery. The prevalence of this practice and the traditional midwives' recognition of their worth in this regard explains the confusion that arose in my interactions with many of the elderly traditional midwives that I interviewed for this study. Mary, who had retired from midwifery, insisted that I must pay her training fee before she could grant me audience. Imagining I could only be engaging her for training in traditional midwifery, she explained that it was standard practice for nurses from the major hospital and training school in town to visit her for training.[32]

Chizoba, the traditional midwife described in the introduction and whose name resounded across her community and in rural health centers for her skills as a midwife and her knowledge of herbs, similarly gave examples of intersections between traditional medicine and hospital birth, as exemplified in Onyeugwu's experience. She had been invited to a major colonial-era Catholic hospital, where she was asked to apply her skills to difficult deliveries. After one such successful session, Chizoba was asked to bring her herbs to the hospital, a request that she refused. When asked to sign a paper, she declined and explained her reasoning thus: "I am uneducated; I cannot even spell my name. How do I know what they are asking me to sign? They are not looking to protect me. I must protect myself. That place is for educated people. I did not have anybody to look out for my interest. I help them with some cases, but I refuse to deal with them or sign any paper for them. There are people who are jealous of my success and have accused me of different things."[33] The same hospital that Chizoba visited often invited and partnered with well-known traditional midwives in the hospital's maternity wards. Here, doctors, nurse-midwives, and matrons watched their traditional counterparts manage complex cases like breech pregnancies or cord entanglements. Some of the nursing and midwifery students who came seeking training from Mary came from this hospital.

Mary also had an encounter similar to Chizoba. When Mary's pregnant daughter was close to her due date and Mary visited her home in faraway Abuja only to learn that her daughter had been in labor for two days, Mary immediately asked to be taken to her. When she got to the hospital, she inserted a medicine in her daughter's anus, and delivery happened shortly afterward. She was instrumental in managing her daughter's needs during and after delivery such that the fascinated doctor inquired into her background and promptly offered her a job. Mary declined this offer because she had other younger children at the time and was unwilling to uproot her entire family, including her husband, to a faraway city for a position as a midwife in a hospital. She also displayed the same distrust as Chizoba and expressed that she had worked with hospitals in the past but received insults and little pay in the process because of practitioners who looked down on her as a traditional practitioner.

Many of the shifts that occurred in the biomedical space were largely stimulated by the shortage of nurses and midwives that was prevalent in the Nigerian medical system during the colonial and postcolonial eras. The staff shortage was so pronounced that it became standard practice for patients' relatives to move into hospital premises or lodge with friends or relatives close to the hospital to tend to the daily needs of the inpatients and provide meals daily for such patients. Those who stayed in the hospital sometimes slept on the floor in the patients' ward or on the corridors outside the hospital unit, but they became essential caregivers for the patients, providing baths, personal care, nourishment, and company. A delegation of Kalabari people complained to the director of medical services about relatives' forced predicaments as hospital caregivers as early as 1947, arguing that relatives had no choice but to provide such care to hospitalized family members due to a lack of personnel.[34] Such occurrences facilitated outcomes in which local beliefs and practices shaped the nature of hospital care and brought some local sentiments into the hospital space.

In the realm of childbirth, these relatives incorporated local dishes believed to aid delivery and postpartum healing into hospital care. In many cases, women combined hospital medicine with herbal mixtures as part of their medical therapy. The fallout in this kind of care, as the Kalabari group pointed out, was that these caregivers did not often abide by prescribed food and dietary restrictions due to their own beliefs that varied foods and drinks would aid recovery. The group stated that "if the number of nurses is increased, their duties will be distributed evenly and all patients will come under the exclusive care of and supervision of nurses who will observe all medical rules and prescriptions."[35]

Tradomedicalism and Biomedical Maternities: Intersections

Changes in traditional medicine were forced by the hostile attitude that its practitioners historically received from missionaries and government officials. As such, traditional practitioners began to look for ways to maintain their appeal to society but also legitimize themselves in the eyes of the government. One of the avenues that they adopted in this push to be viewed as efficient and respectable was triggered by the widespread emergence of private maternities established by their biomedical counterparts. In efforts to address the shortage of nursing and midwifery personnel in the 1940s and 1950s, the Medical Service began to certify auxiliary nurses and midwives whose qualifications were generally lower than that of the higher-tier Grade I midwives. When government loosened restrictions that originally required midwives to practice only in the community in which they trained, these auxiliary midwives established private maternity homes across the country. These types of private practice were permitted by the government because they offered a way to fill the void in the nation's maternal health care infrastructure. A typical maternity home comprised four beds, the government-recommended number of beds per midwife.[36] Some midwives built larger maternity homes and employed other midwives.

As private birthing homes expanded, an apprenticeship system emerged in which traditional midwives attached themselves to hospital-trained midwives to learn and combine important components of biomedical birthing methods in their own practices. Traditional midwives who completed apprenticeships with their hospital-trained counterparts established their own birthing centers and adopted beds in place of traditional birthing postures or an itinerant practice. Conditions in many urban and rural areas no longer permitted birthing in open backyards, as previously practiced, and so traditional midwives shifted their own birthing locations to fixed sites equipped with the necessary items for maternity care.

From their biomedical counterparts, these midwives learned contemporary ways of dealing with complications like hemorrhage, new techniques for palpations, and basic vitamins for managing pregnancy. In the colonial and postcolonial medical landscape where injections, tablets, and syringes had become symbols of efficient medical therapy to locals, these elements became coopted by traditional practitioners as part of their repositioning. One missionary, for example, associated some of the increased attendance at her clinic to people's desire to obtain a tablet or bottle of medicine with the belief that the power of the tablet could subdue any illness.[37] Such associations of syringes and tablets to a speedy or credible cure continued into the postindependence era and shaped the rivalry between traditional practitioners and their hospital counterparts, such that doctors sometimes objected to the former's use of medical equipment like blood pressure machines, stethoscopes, and sugar test strips.[38] These apparatuses had become symbols of contests for legitimacy. As such, biomedical doctors claimed these machines as the exclusive symbols of biomedicine, while their traditional counterparts claimed that "they [biomedical doctors] are not the only ones that should be in possession of these machines."[39]

Many traditional midwives attached themselves to nurse-midwives to learn the use of general monitoring tools like blood pressure machines, blood sugar tests, and other diagnostic techniques. Others like Ngozi Ikwueze fortified their traditional knowledge with emerging biomedical trends. Ngozi, a certified nurse who also studied community health in the 1970s, was knowledgeable in the use and administration of herbs. When she retired from government employment, she opened a private maternity clinic where she utilized her biomedical training and herbal knowledge gained from an herbalist and her grandfather, a traditional doctor.[40] Unless patients expressly indicated that they did not want herbal treatment, she utilized traditional therapeutics at particular stages of pregnancy where she believed traditional rather than Western therapeutics were most effective.

On the other end of the spectrum, younger traditional midwives bolstered their standing and economic opportunities by attaching themselves to hospitals and maternity homes to train as auxiliary midwives. Equipped with the new knowledge that the modern methods bestowed on them, they provided services that integrated knowledge from both medical traditions. Felicia, a midwife, was a product of this new cultural synthesis. She gained her knowledge of indigenous medicine from her mother, a traditional midwife who practiced between the 1940s and 1980s. She served as her mother's apprentice, a natural successor to her position. With the discrediting of traditional midwives under colonial rule, however, Felicia was sent to a midwifery training center to acquire knowledge about hospital births. In this way, she created a practice that combined traditional and Western knowledge.[41] In the earlier stages of pregnancy, she applied biomedical therapies. Between the fourth and eighth months, however, she administered local roots and herbs that she picked out biweekly from the forests of a neighboring town.

Other traditional midwives, such as Mary, affiliated with nurses specifically to secure licensing and, therefore, operate a birthing center that could not be victimized by law enforcement or other government offices for operating as a noncertified midwife. Like Felicia, Mary learned her herbal and midwifery skills from her mother but apprenticed with a nurse in the early 1970s to secure a license that would protect her from arrest or detention. Of this decision to train with a nurse, Mary stated, "I got license from the person I apprenticed with for six months. I went because of the license, not that I do not know the work of midwifery or was not knowledgeable with what I was doing."[42]

Mary also registered with the Nigerian Union of Medical Herbal Practitioners, an organization formed to stave off bullying by the government and the police, as well as make traditional medicine more legitimate. When the police showed up on her doorstep because of complaints that she was practicing without any license or recognition, Mary simply tendered her certificate and was promptly left alone by the police. Organizations like Mary's provided a united front for dealing with federal, state, and local governments, as well as for protecting members. They had specific laws that included conferring membership only on those whose skills had been ascertained by older members.[43] Organizations that showed the most promise and expansive membership were routinely coopted into state ministries of health in the 1980s and 1990s, a symbol of recognition and legitimacy.

These kinds of intersections between traditional medicine and biomedicine increased tremendously in the 1970s and 1980s, as symbolized by newspaper dialogues in these decades highlighting the crucial role of traditional

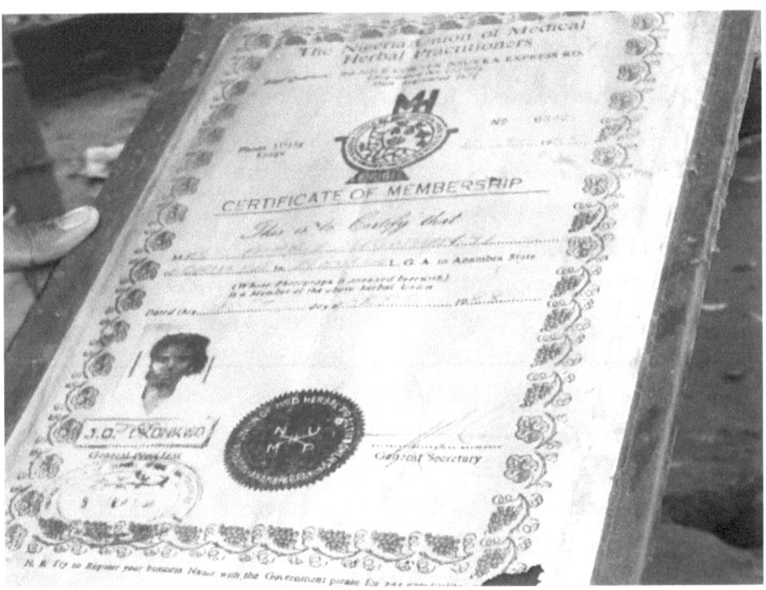

Mary's Certificate of Membership for Nigerian Union of Medical Herbal Practitioners

medicine in addressing the inadequate infrastructure and personnel that continued to assail Nigeria's medical services. Many Nigerians touted traditional medicine as a solution to this bottleneck in biomedical care. One commentator invoked the support that traditional medicine had received from some biomedical doctors like Oguntola Sapara, who had conducted research into traditional medicine throughout his career until his death in 1935, and T. Lambo, who revolutionized the use of traditional medicine and psychosomatic techniques to advance treatment of mental health in Nigeria.[44] The efficacy of traditional medicine, as demonstrated by these Western-trained trailblazers, this *Daily Times* writer argued, should be the basis for why "traditional medicine should be improved and not condemned."[45] It was, after all, a proven method of addressing issues like "family planning/birth control."[46]

As a result of these growing interests and public dialogues on traditional medicine, it received a boost in public, especially because it was often the only viable alternative for some people who needed care. Olikoye Ransome-Kuti, the minister of health from 1983 to 1992, admitted in 1991, "As at now many communities have only traditional healers to look after them. Traditional medicine thrives where scientific medicine has not established itself."[47] Of the renewed interest in traditional medicine, J. O. Mume, a respected traditional physician with a PhD in natural therapeutics, wrote, "For almost a whole century, traditional medicine has suffered innumerable setbacks and degradation under colonial tutelage," and the moment had now arrived for practitioners to begin "a vigorous fight for the emancipation of traditional medicine in Nigeria."[48]

Independence-era governments gradually recognized the important role that traditional medicine played in society, although widespread stereotypes from the colonial era remained.[49] Under the health minister Ransome-Kuti's leadership, the Medical and Dental Practitioners Decree No. 23 of 1988 formally recognized traditional medical practitioners, stating that "any person recognized by his or her community as having been trained in the system of therapeutic medicine traditionally in use in the community is automatically qualified to practice."[50] Various state governments also launched efforts to harness the capabilities of traditional medicine in health care. One such example was Lagos State, where the state government introduced a Traditional Medicine Board under the Ministry of Health with ten hectares of land for a botanical garden to aid research.[51]

This general interest and support of traditional medicine led to the development or adoption of what traditional practitioners have called tradomedical and tradowestern hospitals. As Mume explained in his writing on tradomedicalism in 1980, the adoption of this word became necessary in the efforts by traditional medicine practitioners to disassociate themselves from the connections of the word *traditional* to primitiveness or backwardness.[52] The use of *tradomedical* signified instead that, far from being obsolete, traditional medicine had therapeutic use that was based on empirical knowledge, a long tradition, and an established philosophy of health care.[53] Traditional practitioners who employed the word and its counterpart, *tradowestern*, also sought to convey that they combined elements of traditional medicine and biomedical techniques. The message was that they were not steeped in superstitions and religious rituals but rather on administering a broad range of medicinal therapeutics to effect cure. In his letter to his colleagues in the Nigerian Association of Traditional Medical Practitioners advocating the adoption of tradomedicalism, Mume wrote, "Fellow practitioners, I feel we have reached a stage where it has become necessary and compulsory for us to adopt a new name for ourselves and our profession."[54]

Throughout the 1980s, as the endorsement of traditional medicine intensified, hospital-style facilities like Abimbola Hospital, run by traditional medicine experts and specializing in gynecological issues, began to proliferate. In addition to the birthing centers built by midwives, those traditional doctors who specialized in gynecology and intervened in traditional midwifery during difficult deliveries or problems with conception began to set up hospital-style facilities. Similar intersections that featured in the midwives birthing center also became obvious here. Abimbola Durodola's son, Saheed, provides a good example of a medical personnel who strategically situated themselves in the world of traditional medicine and biomedical training in order to get the most benefit from the medical services that he provided. When Saheed enrolled in nursing school at the bachelor's and master's level to augment what he had learned from his father and grandfather as traditional gynecologists, his goal was to figure out "what are we doing right traditionally that I need to improve on? What are we doing wrong that I need to correct? What are we doing effectively and where or how can we combine techniques?"[55] Saheed was confident that figuring out these questions "has helped me to combine both the medical and the traditional methods of healing together. Those cases that require medical [biomedical intervention] at the hospital [Abimbola Hospital] are attended to medically and those that require combination of traditional and medical are combined equally."[56]

At Abimbola Hospital, where the traditional doctor worked alongside biomedical personnel, cases such as breech positioning of the baby, which could not be addressed except by a cesarean section in many hospitals, were treated with herbs. Such herbal applications were believed to initiate a repositioning of the baby within a twenty-four-hour period. Cases of placenta previa, in which a low-lying placenta obstructed the cervix, were also addressed with herbal treatment if the baby had not reached maturity and the pregnancy was under thirty-two weeks. If the pregnancy was more advanced, then the biomedical team handled this situation due to the presence of vaginal bleeding at this stage. In the case of threatened miscarriage, which was typically handled in the biomedical scenario by prescribing bedrest, herbs were applied to secure the pregnancy and prevent involuntary abortion. These were some of the points of convergencies between tradomedical and biomedical therapy. In general, difficult births that could not be resolved by biomedical practitioners were frequently referred informally through friends and relatives to traditional practitioners. Those who defied the tradomedical experts were referred to hospitals.

These kinds of synthesis between traditional and biomedical therapeutics were not new but were visible in the colonial era despite opposition by the colonial administration. Prior to Nigeria's independence, the government was skeptical of such an admixture of traditional and Western medicine that officials arrested traditional physicians whose former or current patients died suspiciously. Traditional practitioners sought to cultivate government support for herbal interventions by requiring members to obtain statements from patients indicating that they were not currently receiving treatment from an "English doctor."[57]

Some regional organizations had rules regarding medical practices surrounding women and maternities. The Yoruba Native Doctors of the House of Shangodeyi required traditional medical practitioners dealing with difficult deliveries to summon other practitioners for help or face expulsion from the group.[58] Maiyedum Otu Dibia, founded in Onitsha in 1938, had similar rules. The latter organization imposed fines on practitioners who failed to assist other doctors, herbalists, and midwives in need.[59] These traditional doctors failed to receive colonial government backing, irrespective of the steps that they took to obtain it. At most, the government adopted a deliberate policy of neither endorsing nor condemning such organizations as their existence made it easy to track these practitioners or gain access to their medicinal plants for biomedical research in Europe.

Postindependence governments addressed this potential problem of contraindication by ruling that traditional and biomedicine could not be used within six hours of one another. At Abimbola Hospital, for instance, one course of treatment had to be completely stopped and results assessed before an alternative could be introduced. Dosages were enforced with every herbal medicine, and a mandatory six to eight-hour interval was observed between the administration of traditional and biomedical techniques.[60] This dosing requirement seemed to have been put in place by traditional doctors in the 1980s as they sought to address concerns over the complications surrounding the mixing of herbal medicines and synthetic drugs. In cases where pregnant women exclusively required biomedical intervention or the traditional one, these were utilized. Abimbola also partnered with hospitals in the area, such as old names like the University College Hospital and Adeoyo Hospital, both colonial-era government facilities, for ailments that required an advanced level of management. These traditional medicine facilities also could not store human blood or possess human body parts, a rule put in place to curb any abuses.[61] Abimbola was, in this case, an exception because it was registered as a tradomedical facility but also qualified as a hospital under the Federal Ministry of Health.

In the broader landscape of international interventions in reproduction and a global recognition of the crisis in maternal health care, made possible in the 1980s by decades of data that had been collected through the birth control movement, a new category of practitioner, the Traditional Birth Attendant (TBA), was created. In 1987, the World Health Organization (WHO) launched the Safe Motherhood program during an international meeting in Kenya.[62] From then onward, various nongovernmental health organizations and national governments adopted the initiative to help curb maternal deaths in their countries. This program was adopted in Nigeria following a national conference on maternal health care in 1990 and became implemented by local women's groups across the country.[63] These Safe Motherhood networks worked toward improving community health education and training programs for midwives. They were largely funded by international organizations like Pathfinder and the United Kingdom's Department For

International Development (DFID)-directed programming and trainings. One of their major focus throughout the 1990s was the promotion of skilled attendance at birth through TBA trainings, especially considering the shortage of personnel and medical resources in various parts of the country.

In many papers assessing TBA roles in birth, it is common to see TBAs categorized as "the custodians of traditional practices," as one paper put it.[64] In this case, TBAs and traditional midwives frequently got classified as the same. The reality, however, was that since the TBA category became popular in the late 1980s, following WHO's adoption of the Safe Motherhood program, traditional midwives distinguished themselves from TBAs as a category. A nurse at the Enugu Ministry of Health pointed out this difference, arguing that all traditional midwives did not see themselves as TBAs, and all TBAs were not considered traditional midwives.[65] Traditional midwives, such as Chizoba and Mary, did not consider themselves TBAs as they did not possess the certification that classified them as such but also because their practice was based on herbal knowledge and the traditional methods of managing pregnancy learned from their mothers. Thus, the difference between the two categories lay in "the custodians of traditional practices" labels implied for both groups.

The most obvious symbol of a TBA was their possession of certificates that they obtained from training in Safe Motherhood programs. Some traditional midwives, in efforts to bolster their standing as midwives, registered and received training as TBAs. Those traditional midwives seeking to improve their skills through apprenticeship seized this moment for training and certification. When Saheed Durodola registered for such TBA training before he had commenced his bachelor's degree in nursing, it was to further protect his practice as a traditional specialist and an aspiring nurse. Others, especially well-established traditional medicine practitioners, neither participated in this way nor considered themselves in the category of TBAs. They were frequently knowledgeable of the herbs and other cultural methods of managing pregnancy. The other category of TBAs were auxiliary nurses or others who saw the training as an opportunity to advance their economic standing. Acquiring this title of TBA and the certificates that came with it also became a strategic way to avoid bullying by law enforcement.

This thread of persecution, featured in the narratives of various traditional midwives about rivalries with biomedical health personnel, shaped decisions by many traditional practitioners to seek training and certification as TBAs. Chizoba recounted how she was arrested on trumped-up charges by rivals that she performed surgery illegally at home. Mary Ugwuanyi, from the same area as Chizoba in the southeastern town of Nsukka, also received similar visits from law enforcement under accusations initiated by a medical staff that she practiced illegally without a license. In the western city of Ibadan, a nurse and wife of a traditional doctor had her birthing center shutdown by the police due to reports that she operated illegally as a TBA. These cases were all dropped once the women provided proof, including registration documents and certifications, that validated their rights to practice. Chizoba, who practiced as a traditional midwife rather than a registered TBA, was released once police verified her credibility in her community and ascertained that the charges against her were false. In rural communities, the work of midwives like Chizoba was often so essential that they were less subject to abuse by law enforcement unless a proven case of abuse had been filed against them.

Faith Delivery Homes and Efforts at Modernization

Aladura faith homes were not exempt from the changes during this era. From their inception, they were subjected to derisions from European administrators for their rejection of biomedicine, which was the central part of Aladura doctrine during the 1930s. In CAC, changes occurred to address long-running sentiments from government and biomedical circles that CAC structures were mediocre. The hardline in the early days of the Aladura movement between faith healing and biomedicine began to soften, especially in a postcolonial atmosphere of urbanization, expanding education, and increased opposition from biomedical practitioners. According to midwives like Adeleye and Ajayi, who trained or practiced in CAC faith homes during the 1970s and early 1980s, and mothers like Comfort Aluko and Folashade Akande, who had kids in the faith home during the same period, barely any change in CAC's exclusive emphasis on prayers and divine healing in maternity care occurred.[66]

By the 1980s, however, shifts in CAC members' attitudes toward the use of medicine and medical technologies began to occur due to developments in the economic and social arena. CAC members who worked in the civil service and other government or institutional positions at the time required paperwork from government hospitals to secure sick or maternity leave. This unavoidable circumstance required the use of hospitals, even briefly. Grace

Abiala, who used the faith home for the birth of her children, recalled how she registered her pregnancy at a government hospital and attended their prenatal clinic at various intervals to secure a medical certificate and other relevant paperwork for her maternity leave.[67] For Isaac, a CAC pastor whose wife had their first child at the University College Hospital, Ibadan, in the early 1990s, his employer, an international nonprofit institution, required employees to commit to utilizing hospitals for birth.[68] Changes were thus inevitable in a church whose membership cut across social strata and included educated people and members of the public service.

The 1980s also coincided with the "Safe Motherhood" era in which global attention was drawn to maternal mortality in Africa, specifically Nigeria, where about 75,000 women died annually from birth-related complications.[69] The heightened attention by local biomedical doctors and international supporters of the WHO's Safe Motherhood initiative on traditional midwives extended to and contributed to adjustments within faith homes. Doctors argued that institutions like faith homes facilitated maternal deaths due to their approach to maternity care and opposition to the use of medicine. One newspaper that headlined "Aladuras" captured the sentiments of the time: thus, "it is criminal to carry a patient dying from severe bleeding, obstructed labor . . . to a prayer house instead of a hospital."[70] Such scrutiny compelled faith home leaders, including the matrons who were professional nurses and midwives and were attuned to conversations in the biomedical world, to make changes in faith homes' approach to maternity services.

To overcome the increased scrutiny, the Faith Home Midwifery Training School, discussed earlier in chapter 3, sought partnerships with the biomedical sector. Between 1983 and 1986, its leaders created a referral system with nearby hospitals for the faith homes. This partnership was targeted at addressing doctors' criticisms that faith homes exceeded their limits by refusing or failing to refer critical cases to the hospital in a timely fashion.[71] Dr. Ajuwon, whose hospital served as a referral location for the faith home beginning in 1983, when this referral system was adopted, expressed such criticism while simultaneously pointing out that "most of them [CAC midwives] are well trained and qualified midwives."[72] Prior to this formal arrangement of a referral network, some medical doctors and nurses of CAC background provided assistance or counsel in faith homes on an ad hoc and voluntary basis. However, the need to address the criticism that they endangered lives made this relationship with biomedical staff more permanent.

As former matron Lydia Ajayi pointed out, "At any station our students find themselves, it is compulsory that they have a professional doctor that they can refer their patients to because we don't want anybody to die or tarnish the image of our maternity."[73]

In 1988, the Faith Home Midwifery Training School expanded the scope and duration of its training from one year to two years to conform with practices in the biomedical sector. They implemented annual refresher courses in which health representatives observed and participated in students' workshops. Medical doctors and nurses, including CAC members, were involved in providing training at these workshops.[74] The session's goal was to reinforce earlier instructions, introduce midwives to new techniques, and provide opportunities for networking with visiting physicians and health workers. It was also a time for spiritual reinforcement in which the midwives dedicated themselves to prayers, fasting, and admonition.[75] These increased interactions with biomedical personnel created a better understanding of complications during pregnancy and the importance of early referral. CAC midwife Adeleye explained, "During our weeklong program, the government will usually come and train us on what to do and otherwise. We know these things. . . . We don't wait till our patient is weak; we follow protocol. . . . When we see that the patient is not okay and there is complication, we quickly transfer. We have gynecologists who will come and lecture us, and we buy handouts [books or course packets]."[76] Faith home patronage increased significantly during the 1980s and 1990s. It was a reliable alternative for many who could not afford rising hospital bills. As the faith homes did not depend on revenue from patients for their operation but were largely sustained by monetary contributions from the CAC Good Women worldwide as well as grants from the CAC, it was possible at this time for faith home services to be rendered free to the public. According to former matron Alabi, "Some families willingly might hand out compensation to the matron, but there was no admission fee and discharge fee from the Faith Home's inception until I retired in 2012. . . . In fact we did give our patients gifts after delivery."[77] This was further incentive for those who could not afford hospital bills.

By the 1990s, CAC faith homes had to confront the tensions between medical science/technology and their belief in divine intervention.[78] As noted earlier, the CAC's membership, especially in the postcolonial era, included doctors, nurses, midwives, government workers, and employees in higher education. It had an expanding educated youth population who grew up in

Christ Apostolic Church

Mount of Mercy
Faith Home,
10, Mutuwo Street, Opp Oando
Petrol Station Idi-Oro, Mushin, Lagos

DECLARATION FORM

I Mr...

Of (your denomination)..

....Living at No..............................

....Hereby declared as follows:

I,...That my wife, Mrs...................

Should attend all prayer meeting of pregnant women throughout the period of her Pregnancy.

That she should deliver in this Church/Faith Home

May God help us. Amen.

....
Husband Signature   **Date**

....
Midwife Signature   **Date**

....
Pastor-in-charge   **Date**

Form signed by husbands of prospective faith home participants, especially of non-Christian background, to avoid clashes or misunderstandings over a woman's attendance

a different environment than 1920s and 1930s Nigeria. This younger generation increasingly pushed for a loosening of the church's rules against the use of medicine, which was strictly imposed in the 1940s. Joshua Alokan and E. Olorunwa described them as a new generation of the church who came up under different technological and developmental circumstances than the church's first generation.[79] As discussed in chapter 3, Babalola's condemnation of biomedicine in the 1920s was premised on its inadequacies and inability to protect from illness and death. Moses Olowe explained the ease of nonreliance on biomedicine during the colonial period in terms of access and availability: "In the village and even in Ibadan around 1949 when my mother was pregnant and my father was sick, how many hospitals do we have then? At times we have just one or two government hospitals, because we were still in the colonial era that time. My mother was taken to a prophet and she was delivered; no doctor, no injection, no paracetamol, just prayer."[80] By the 1990s, however, biomedical institutions were more widespread and more advanced, and the CAC had to adjust its stance on the use of biomedicine to remain relevant and competitive.

Increasingly, the faith homes began to view some medical procedures, such as medical tests, lab work, ultrasound, and fetal monitors, to ensure positive pregnancy outcomes. Under the guidance of the faith home matrons at the midwifery school and CAC member-physicians, especially after 1993, when a new evangelist-matron who had been in the medical field since the 1960s assumed office, these medical procedures became routine in faith homes' prenatal care. Patients were required to complete basic lab work, such as PCV, genotype, and blood tests, and if a Rhesus factor injection was necessary, this was administered in the hospital by the partnering doctor or another doctor chosen by the patient.[81] To ensure that these medical exams were conducted, matron Alabi explained, "We took our time to monitor their cards regularly."[82]

At the annual refresher courses in the 1990s, midwives were encouraged by doctors to administer vitamins, such as folic acid, B-complex, calcium, and iron, to augment easier pregnancy and delivery. However, the dispensing of these vitamins was subject to an individual midwife's interpretation of faith healing and views on the acceptability of such vitamins. Many midwives abided by Babalola's original teachings on maintaining good nutrition and balanced diet as the best way to ensure the necessary balance of nutrients required to sustain a pregnancy. A lot of the weekly or biweekly prenatal instructions provided to pregnant women focused on these. Explaining these changes, the bulk of which occurred in her tenure as matron, Alabi mused, "CAC did not believe in drugs. But over time we found out that Babalola did not forbid the use of medically proven drugs. It was concoction and other uncertified substance that he advised us against. The use of ring against dizziness during pregnancy or making of sacrifices for free delivery was some of the things that Babalola preached against."[83] The prophecy that Babalola received in 1928 did indeed specifically condemn the use of herbal medicine and other concoctions from traditional doctors and herbalists, but

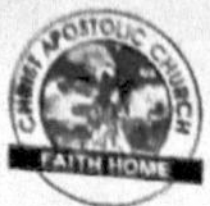

Christ Apostolic Church

Mount of Mercy
Faith Home,
10, Matuwo Street, Opp Oando Petrol Station Idi-Oro, Mushin, Lagos

ANTE NATAL RECORDS

NAME (ORUKO)			
DATE OF BOOKING OJO IFI ORUKO SILE		**L M P**	**EDD**
ADDRESS			
AGE OJO ORI	**RELIGION** IJO	**GSM**	
OCCUPATION ISE OWO			
HUSBAND'S NAME ORUKO OKO			**HUSBAND'S OCCUPATION** ISE OWO OKO
HUSBAND'S RELIGION IJO OKO		**GSM**	
MEDICAL / SPIRITUAL HISTORY IRU AWON ISORO TI O NI			
PREVIOUS PREGNANCIES OYUN MELO LO TI NI	**PARA**	**NO OF LIVING CHILDREN** OMO MELO LO WA LAIYE	

DATE OF BIRTH OJO IBI	DURATION OF PREGNANCY OSU TI OYUN LO	PREGNANCY LABOUR CONDITION ISELE NINU OYUN ATI IROBI	BABY ALIVE/DEAD OMO WA LAYE/OKU

ANTE NATAL VISITS

DATE OJO	HEIGHT OF FIYNDUS BI OYUN SE GA TO	PERSON TATION ORI/IGE	FOETAL HEART MIMU OMO	B.P. IFUNPA	WEIGHT IWON	OEDEMA SE ESE WU	REMARKS KINI ENI LATI SO

Form tracking data and vital statistics of faith home attendees

PROGRESS OF LABOUR
ILOSIWAJU NINU IROBI

DATE OF LABOUR OJO IROBI	TIME ASIKO	OBSERVATION AKIYESI	DURATION OF LABOUR ASIKO TI IROBI NGBA
ONSET OF LABOUR IGBATI IROBI BERE			1st Stage Igbese Kini
MEMBRANES RUPTURE OMI ARA DA			2nd Stage Igbese Keji
CERVIX FULLY DILATED ORUN ILE OMO LA PATAPATA			3rd Stage Igbese Keta
CHILD BORN OMO WAIYE			Total Hours Gbogbo Asiko Ti ogba
PLANCENTA EXPELLED EKEJI OMO (OLOBI JADE)			

PRAISE THE LORD!
EYIN OLUWA!

3RD STAGE	TIME FOR DELIVERY OF PLACENTA	PROGRESS OF LABOUR	
IGBESE KETA	ASIKO IROBI TI OLOBI NUADE		
CONDITIONS OF PLACENTA BAWO NI OLOBI SE RI			

FOURTH STAGE WAKA TI KINI LEHIN IROBI

DATE (OJO) ______________________________

TIME (ASIKO) ______________________________

TEMPERATURE ______________________________

PULSE STATE ______________________________

BLOOD PRESSURE (IFUNPA) ______________________________

URINE PASSED (SE OTI TO?) ______________________________

CONDITION OF MOTHER
(BAWO NI IYA SE NSESI?)

CONDITION OF BABY
(BAWO NI OMO SE NSESI?)

BIRTH WEIGHT (IWON OMO)

Another example of data collection and tracking during labor and delivery the application of this prophetic injunction was extended to biomedicine due to early church leaders' belief that the failure of biomedicine would drive members to traditional doctors and, therefore, idolatry.[84]

Although the Faith Home Midwifery Training School had an increasingly cordial relationship with government physicians by the 1990s, some doctors argued that faith homes had overtaken hospitals' roles in maternity care.[85] To protect itself from fallouts from these types of arguments, the Faith Home Governing Board, a cross section of pastors, nurses, members of the CAC Good Women, doctors, and faith home alumni, formally ratified the office of a Doctor-in-Charge in 1996.[86] This positioned the faith home to argue that it observed the necessary protocols required in women's primary health care. Matron Alabi made exactly this argument in 1996 following a meeting with local government doctors who had witnessed a decline in hospital attendance by expecting mothers and hoped that the matron could redirect pregnant women to their facilities.[87] The first medical doctor who acted in this role as doctor-in-charge was J. K. Fagbo, a CAC member and respected physician. The doctor-in-charge was not domiciled in the faith home but served in an advisory capacity and participated in student training and curriculum development. This official also served on the Faith Home Governing Board, a cross section of CAC members who made decisions on the faith home's development.[88]

Like their tradomedical counterparts, CAC faith homes sought to protect themselves from accusations of illegal existence by registering with government bodies and health agencies. The faith home training center in Ede registered itself with the Osun State Ministry of Health—its home state—receiving authorization from the state to offer maternity and child welfare services.[89] However, because its subsidiary faith homes were scattered throughout other states where Osun State's jurisdiction did not extend, these became subject to visits from local government agents, especially in Lagos, where faith homes were randomly searched and accused of practicing illegally because "all our certificates, everything we have is under this school that is only registered with Osun state."[90] The three matrons, Alabi, Ajayi, and Awoyungbo, emphasized that these searches and accusations were not all authorized by the local government but were frequently the work of agents acting independently in their capacity as real or fake state employees to extort money from birthing centers.

The solution to these harassments became the registration of all CAC faith homes in Nigeria under a health agency that was duly registered by the country's Corporate Affairs Commission. Some faith homes independently registered with the Federal Ministry of Health as providers of primary maternity services. This approach of embracing registration as an avenue for securing their practices and gaining legitimacy in the government and professional setting was a tactic that became common among the two major providers of maternity care in their efforts to compete favorably with their biomedical counterparts. The competition between the trio, as well as the society's assigning of value to each category of care providers, sustained the impetus for these changes.

Conclusion

The attempts at building a more modern appeal and outlook in the realm of childbirth created new layers of contests and collaborations in which members of the different birthing traditions sought alliances to promote their practices and stay competitive. These changes were especially magnified in the 1980s and 1990s, despite heightened scrutiny of non-hospital-based spaces of birth by government agencies and international health organizations. These decades were fraught with shrinking wages, price hikes, rising unemployment, and wage freezes for workers, making it difficult for people to afford necessities, including health care.[91] Capturing the situation at the time, popular Nigerian politician Chukwuemeka Ojukwu stated, "In the past you needed a pocketful of naira to bring home a basketful of goods. Now you seem to need a basketful of naira in order to bring back a pocketful of goods."[92]

The federal government's restructuring of the Nigerian economy through its Structural Adjustment Program (SAP) cut spending on the public sector and escalated issues in a health sector that was already fraught with challenges. A medical doctor in Lagos commented on the situation: "Things have never been this bad for health services. Even the general hospital which was supposed to be the last hope of the common man now charge fees in most cases."[93] The doctor considered this a terrible development, "particularly now that most people are jobless."[94] Newspapers in the late 1980s and early 1990s were riddled with tales of strikes by nurses, midwives, and doctors.[95] Others recounted stories of mistreatment and shortage of medical personnel at government hospitals.[96]

The effects of these challenges were severely felt in maternal health care, where lack of personnel and poor infrastructure escalated a crisis in maternal deaths. In a presentation given in 1991 by Grace Nwabuisi, senior midwifery tutor at the Lagos State University Teaching Hospital, a hospital whose history dated back to 1955, maternal deaths in Lagos Island had gone from 4.7% to 7.8% per 1,000 live births between the 1960s and 1970s to 36.4% per 1,000 births in 1986 and 1987.[97] These numbers, Nwabuisi emphasized, were representative of trends in other locations across Nigeria.[98]

As a result of the growing inadequacies in biomedical maternity care as well as the affordability of alternative modes of health care delivery, many individuals resorted to the use of alternatives beyond the hospital for childbirth. An Ede woman, Lydia Ajala, explained the treatment she and others had experienced at hospitals as well as their preference for faith homes: "The attitude of the officials at the government hospitals is nasty towards pregnant women. Sometimes, they pester, yell, and demoralize pregnant women. But, at FH [Faith Home], the attitude differs such that they ensure that one receives adequate care."[99] Ajala continued, "When a woman enters labor and is brought at FH, the very first thing is to ascertain if such woman has appetite and has eaten. . . . In addition, after delivery, the care is different [than the hospital]."[100] These general views of hospital care and personnel as inadequate fueled the popularity of faith homes and their tradomedical counterparts, as well as the rivalry between the competing health care traditions.

In the tradomedical realm, professionalization efforts went beyond adaptations in midwifery to broader conversations in traditional medicine. In the bid to gain footing alongside biomedicine as an officially recognized network for health care, tradomedical practitioners began deliberate efforts to create a distinction between their medical practices and the more religious rituals associated with traditional religion. Educated traditional doctors like J. O. Mume and Banire Alalaye were examples of the general attitude in which some traditional practitioners sought to eliminate one of the biggest stereotypes and obstacles to tradomedicalism: its association with paganism, cultism, and witchcraft.

When Banire Alalaye completed his doctoral training and joined a tradomedical association in Ibadan, he made a push within the association to separate traditional religious performances and tradomedical events. On the association's anniversary, for instance, which was attended by government and biomedical representatives as well as community members, Banire did not support the incorporation of very visible and sometimes exclusive elements of Yoruba traditional religion, arguing that it alienated those who did not share similar belief systems and diverted attention from the association's medical work. Similar conversations occurred elsewhere in which national traditional medicine associations, such as Mume's National Union of Medical Herbal Practitioners and Alalaye's Organization of Competent Divine Therapists, sought to publicly promote their tradomedical work as separate from their sometimes ethnic-based African traditional religions. This, in turn, opened membership to people of different religious and cultural backgrounds who wanted to be affiliated with such organizations.

In the field of midwifery, adaptations entailed becoming stewards of nurse-midwives in order to combine biomedical and traditional therapies and, in some cases, obtaining certificates that qualified them to practice. Traditional midwives themselves were also sought out as instructors by nursing and midwifery students who wished to improve their own portfolio by familiarizing themselves with traditional techniques for managing pregnancy. For the traditional midwife Gloria Ozoani, this involved a trade-off with these nursing and midwifery students in which she learned new techniques from them in exchange for her knowledge of traditional treatments. For Mary Ugwuanyi, this new mobility opened a new source of income. She could charge fees to the stream of students who showed up at her doorsteps in exchange for the tradomedical training that she provided. Both the biomedical and the tradomedical camps increasingly recognized the relevance, at least to the public, of their various approaches to childbirth and sought to maximize these opportunities.

Among rural residents, the stigma that developed against traditional midwifery throughout the colonial era and beyond as associated with paganism and poverty was less pronounced because of the scarcity of medical facilities. Where biomedical services existed, rural residents found ways of integrating traditional and biomedical birthing methods in ways that best suited them. Elements of indigenous cultural practices that fulfilled some social purposes were retained. The biomedical system was itself infiltrated by indigenous ideas of healing and care. Nigerians infused their belief systems within the hospital setting, especially as these biomedical spaces had become increasingly occupied by locals since the 1950s. Hospital midwives and nurses also attempted to stay competitive by trading their knowledge of biomedical techniques for traditional ones, especially in rural settings, where value was placed on traditional medicine. Even the faith-based CAC ultimately desisted from its total rejection of biomedicine to incorporate components that suited their goals of securing legitimation. However, CAC faith homes controlled this interaction with biomedicine to reflect and respect their own core concepts of faith healing. By the end of the twentieth century, each birthing actor had become involved in a maze of co-constitutions that were shaped by the intricate and frequently overlapping values allotted by various segments of the society on them.

Coda

An Ongoing Era of Medical Pluralism

in the Realm of Birth

The past is still with us. You ask me about childbirth in the olden days as though these things no longer exist. If you go to the interiors of my natal home, Ibagwa, you will see these practices still in play.

Chizoba, interview, 2016

The strategy to achieve this goal [maternal health plan] . . . rests on the foundation . . . which is context-specific, systems-oriented and people-centric.

Dayo Adeyanju, *Vanguard*, 2015

Contested Spaces of Birth: Cause and Effect

When Mary Ugwuanyi and Onyeugwu nwa Ogwo insisted in 2013 and 2016, respectively, that I was a midwifery student at a school of midwifery seeking knowledge of traditional methods to improve my public marketability, they were signaling the outcome of a century-long struggle over the control of childbirth in Nigeria. These two elderly midwives had become accustomed to operating in a new *birthscape* that was a product of rivalries, competition, and adaptations that followed the economic, sociocultural, and political contest that childbirth had become in the colonial era. Mary's insistence that I pay the fee that she stipulated for training biomedical midwives was the new way in which she demonstrated her agency and assigned value to her knowledge in a field dominated by biomedical institutions.

While part of Mary's gain in this exchange—the provision of training— was economic, the other part symbolized a continued relevance of her skill as a traditional midwife, a skill that she considered both valued and devalued by her biomedical counterparts. From her own experiences of partnerships with doctors and hospitals, her skills as a traditional midwife were appreciated and coveted by medical personnel while she simultaneously experienced disrespect and disregard due to her status as a traditional practitioner. For Mary, therefore, compelling monetary compensation was also a claim to power and a forced acknowledgment of value for her skills. This reflection on Mary raises broader questions: what were the outcomes of this contest for Nigeria's maternal health sector?

The marginalization of women in the colonial economy had direct consequences on maternal health care services and the nature of infrastructure in this sector. In a colonial-era environment in which British administrators viewed women as invisible citizens whose primary responsibility was domestic service rather than the economic and political activities that characterized the lives of many precolonial women, women's health care infrastructure barely received any attention from the government even as health care facilities for locals were concentrated in urban areas. With few exceptions, women were not active parts of the colonial machinery; the education system, therefore, focused on Nigerian males. By the time the colonial government began to revisit women's education in the 1930s and 1940s and sought to build maternity care structures, the realization became apparent that few women had the standard of education required to enroll in the schools of nursing, midwifery, and medicine that were being established by the government. Nigeria, therefore, entered the postcolonial era with a gap in personnel that affected the entire health care sector but particularly impacted the largely female field of nursing and midwifery.

The shortcomings in women's health care and the underdeveloped nature of biomedicine throughout the colonial era boosted the pluralistic environment and the endurance of faith homes, traditional midwives, and other auxiliary medical practitioners that characterized the history of birth in Nigeria. Throughout the colonial and postcolonial eras, urban-sited government hospitals were prioritized in terms of staffing and funding over rural health centers, dispensaries, and maternity homes. The situation became even more dire in a postcolonial environment in which health service personnel who tended to rural areas prior to the 1970s, such as dispensers and public health assistants (sanitary inspectors), were phased out. Both state and federal governments failed to fill the gap left by the colonial government in advancing maternal and infant health services. This government lapse throughout the twentieth century can be tied to the country's economic woes from the late 1970s but is also partly connected to Nigeria's political climate after independence, in which the country fell to a series of military dictatorships within six years of independence and only had its first consistent democratic rule from 1996. The logic here is not that democracy is somehow tied to good health care. Rather, it is that political stability enables the sustenance of health care policies.

The problem of access to hospital-based care was evident throughout the course of my fieldwork. As I navigated various rural communities without consistent means of public transportation, I pondered over the fate of birthing women who went into labor without means to get to the "nearest" hospital. What if a complication arose with a home birth? How could the women get to a hospital in time? According to a midwife, such women were ferried in stretchers by runners until a means of transportation was secured, or a community member who owned an automobile was located to transport such women to a hospital. Moses, an Ibadan resident, painted a clear picture of what happens in such scenarios: "When my mother was pregnant . . . how many hospitals do we have then? At times we have just one or two government hospitals. . . . My mother was taken to a prophet and she was delivered; no doctor, no injection, no paracetamol, just prayer."[1] Another woman who lived in Lagos but could not reach a hospital in time due to unrest and hospital closures in the 1990s had her fifth and final baby in a nearby accessible faith home.[2]

Amid the atmosphere of gaps and inefficiencies in maternal health and the desire to overcome them, the multiplicity of maternity actors vying for influence created an interconnected atmosphere of competition that pushed the various providers of maternity services—CAC faith homes, hospitals, traditional practitioners—to adapt. Throughout the postcolonial era in the twentieth century, CAC faith homes constantly adjusted their beliefs and practices to withstand the increasing scrutiny, intensified by the proliferation of maternity-focused nongovernmental organizations in the 1980s, about maternal deaths. Chief among the criticism of their services was their inability to deal with medical emergencies, including conditions requiring surgery or involving hemorrhage, a common source of maternal death. The precautions that CAC faith homes took to address these views that they exceeded their limits and jeopardized women's health included maintaining referral networks with biomedical doctors in the case of emergencies while remaining steadfast to their own principles of healing through faith, prayers, nutrition, and hygiene. The utilization of biomedical technologies, such as blood pressure monitors and ultrasound equipment, to monitor health indicators also became part of this adaptation.

The reality of these adaptations played out in front of me at a CAC branch in Lagos. An expecting mother who had visited this CAC faith home for their weekly prayer session during the previous day had a high blood pressure reading. Blood pressure monitoring was part of the faith home's care but was not scheduled to occur until the prenatal session the following week. The midwife, however, took this blood pressure reading at the prayer session because the woman was reported to be involved in an intense altercation with another woman in the community. Following this high reading, the midwife instructed her to return the next day, and when the blood pressure measurement remained dangerously high, she immediately accompanied the woman, now full term, straight to a hospital within her referral network. Accompanying the woman not only ensured that she went to the hospital without delay but guaranteed that she would receive quicker attention, considering that she was a referral patient rather than the hospital's original patient.

Like faith homes, traditional midwives and gynecologists also received increased attention in the 1970s and 1980s era. However, a slightly different conversation occurred at the local level. The shortages and shortcomings of biomedical services forced a national rethinking of traditional medicine and public conversations about the need to invest in and harness the services of tradomedical hospitals as part of the nation's health care network. Akin to Mary's encounter with students of nursing and midwifery, traditional practitioners also sought ways to take advantage of this growing interest. Individuals who had backgrounds in traditional medicine, such as Ngozi Ikwueze and Saheed Durodola, sought biomedical training to boost their appeal to an audience that may be looking for traditional or biomedical therapy or a combination of both. One of the biggest concerns that they had to address was the potential side effects of this co-utilization of traditional medicine and biomedical substances in patient care. The approach that they and other experts in traditional medicine adopted involved administering both remedies at a minimum of six hours apart, at which time the medicines were considered to have waned in the bloodstream.

An Ongoing Reflection

By the last decade of the twentieth century, Nigeria's *birthscape* had assumed a well-established pattern shaped by economic, sociocultural, and religious factors. The continued popularity of the various maternal health care providers highlights the agency that locals assume in what is considered legitimate or valuable. In the case of CAC faith homes, for instance, interviewee accounts highlighted the importance that health seekers placed on the spiritual and the belief that some health situations needed spiritual solutions. In a 2016 focus group with pregnant women of non-Aladura backgrounds, including Muslim women, attending a prenatal session at a CAC faith home in Lagos, the women explained their choice of a CAC faith home in economic and religious terms.[3] Most women appreciated the faith homes' focus on the expecting mother and child's physical and spiritual welfare. In the case of the faith home headquarters in Ede, issues that defied hospital treatment were informally referred to them. Those who had experienced tragedies in hospital births or could not afford hospitals turned to the faith home not only for prenatal care but also for delivery. According to Isaac, a father of five children, "Four out of my five children were born in the faith home. The first child was born in the hospital, and that's the one I lost."[4] Other stories like Isaac's abound, including stories of circumstances for which biomedical remedies appeared useless. Traditional midwives and their Traditional Birth Attendant (TBA) colleagues similarly received patronage due to issues of access and cost. These narratives highlight the importance of sociocultural relevance in health care.

Despite the presence of this pluralistic maternity setting, challenges persist. As students at a School of Midwifery in Enugu discussed the challenges of contemporary midwifery in Nigeria in 2013, I listened with interest. One issue that was prominent in this discussion, as well as others, was that more successful interventions would be made if traditional and faith-based midwives referred emergencies and other difficult births to hospitals in a timely manner. "Some of the mortality rates we have in these hospitals are not attributable to the hospital," one student stated. "These TBAs do not refer patients until all is lost and they know that the patient will die. The patient dies upon arrival to the hospital and such demise enters the hospital records while the midwife, especially the faith-based ones, claim little or no casualty."[5] Early referral is, therefore, a major issue. Among all the faith home midwives that I interviewed, only two opened up about mortality issues in their practices. For others, this was a subject that could not be broached. One mentioned a death but emphasized that this client died in the hospital and not at the church facility. Another stated that she had referred the patient to a hospital, but she and her family refused the referral, ultimately leading to death. The midwives' unwillingness to confront mortality weakened the prospect of referrals, and it is here that local and state government efforts to bridge the gap between these birthing sectors become critical.

While an independent network of partnerships and collaborations has developed in Nigeria's *birthscape*, what has remained lacking is a deliberate nationwide policy to coordinate and support these partnerships. Regardless of Nigeria's consistent ranking among countries with the worst maternal health indices, maternal and reproductive health campaigns in the country remained largely in the hands of international and local organizations. Where government interest in maternal health has been galvanized at the local level, success has been recorded. An example of such efforts exists in Ondo State in southwestern Nigeria, where the then governor, Olusegun Mimiko, a medical doctor and former state minister of health, launched Abiye (born to survive or safe delivery) in 2009, a maternity project aimed at improving maternal and infant health outcomes.[6] The Abiye project adopted a comprehensive outlook that established basic primary and secondary facilities to address the needs of pregnant women. Its core objectives addressed the four critical delays that affected maternal health care: delay in deciding to seek care, delay in reaching care, delay in receiving appropriate care on arrival, and delay in referral.[7] By targeting each of these delays, the state government developed appropriate responses, including assigning specially trained community health auxiliary workers to monitor and act as a liaison between pregnant women and the maternity hospitals and coordinating transportation in areas with poor modes of transport.[8]

More importantly, the Abiye project paid attention to the high utilization of TBAs and faith-based birth attendants and explored these existing modes of birth to improve outcomes. Rather than criminalizing these nonbiomedical platforms that remained popular for varying reasons, the government established a task-sharing partnership in 2014 that incentivized these birth attendants to provide prenatal care but refer their patients to maternity hospitals for birth. In return, these TBAs and church-based birth attendants received cash incentives for each successful referral, access to vocational training, and start-up funds for alternative businesses.[9] To make the referral network more seamless, the Ondo government created a set of hospitals, Mother and Child Hospitals, that became the apex referral locations for all maternal health service providers in the state, offering free health care for all pregnant women and children under the age of five.[10] Not surprisingly, this comprehensive approach that was adapted to local circumstances yielded results. By 2016, Ondo State went from the state with the worst maternal health indicator in southwest Nigeria in 2008—749 per 100,000 births—to the best in Nigeria—112 per 100,000, an 84% reduction.[11]

The success recorded by this locally implemented Safe Motherhood program points to the importance of rallying local support and investments from central governments in such efforts. These strides made by the Ondo project bring to the fore the fundamental argument inherent in this work: all birthing methods in Nigeria offer one or other advantages, either because of their reach and popularity or because of the position of trust that they occupy in their communities. Maternal health, especially in rural communities, will benefit from a government-facilitated partnership that harnesses existing networks and creates a political and social climate conducive to a pluralistic birthing framework to thrive. In communities where the focus on non-biomedical providers of maternity services dwelt on harassment and marginalization rather than constructive redirection, these providers simply went underground, making it harder to regulate their services or encourage partnerships and referrals to hospitals due to fear of retribution.

The effects of such harassment manifested in the course of my encounters with midwives and other locals. Traditional midwives and other women in Ibadan communities were reluctant to speak with me about midwives or how to locate them. Some students in the neighboring university explained later that these midwives were subject to random police raids and arrests for varying charges and so distrusted outsiders whose objectives they could not ascertain. They also became elusive with referrals or invitations to hospitals because of fear of persecution or sudden arrest. On the other hand, government certification and, therefore, oversight of CAC faith homes in the same community resulted in efforts by these centers to keep their facilities in good condition and up to the set standards on which they were approved. Local birthing methods (traditional and faith-based) remain popular in various parts of the country due to their affordability, access, and flexibility. There are many prospects for partnership here, especially in the backdrop of personnel and facility shortages.

Notes

Introduction

1. Interview with Onyeugwu nwa Ogwo, Nsukka, April 6, 2016.

2. Interview with Onyeugwu nwa Ogwo, Nsukka, April 6, 2016.

3. Interview with Chizoba, Nsukka, April 9, 2016.

4. See University of Illinois (UI), *Colonial Annual Reports, No. 1030, Nigeria,* "Reports for 1918," 18; Wellcome Library (WL), *Nigeria. Southern Provinces. Annual Medical and Sanitary Report for the Year Ended 31st December 1918,* 29; UI *Colonial Annual Reports, No. 1315, Nigeria,* "Reports for 1925," 12; H. W. Turner, *A History of an African Independent Church* (Oxford: Oxford University Press, 1967), 41; O. Oduntan, "Culture and Colonial Medicine: Smallpox in Abeokuta, Western Nigeria," *Social History of Medicine* 30, no. 1 (2017): 48–70; D. C. Ohadike, "The Influenza Pandemic of 1918–19 and the Spread of Cassava Cultivation on the Lower Niger: A Study in Historical Linkages," *Journal of African History* 22, no. 3 (1981): 379–391, 383–386. See also M. Ochonu, "Conjoined to Empire: The Great Depression and Nigeria," *African Economic History* 34 (2006): 103–145.

5. For more on the *Aladura* movement, see J. D. Y. Peel, *Aladura: A Religious Movement among the Yoruba* (Oxford: Oxford University Press, 1968); Turner, *History of an African Independent Church,* 8–34; Adam Mohr, "Faith Tabernacle Congregation and the Emergence of Pentecostalism in Colonial Nigeria, 1910s–1941," *Journal of Religion in Africa* 43 (2013): 196–221.

6. Christ Apostolic Church, *The Constitution and the Order of Service* (Nigeria, n.d.), 42. A later publication by the CAC in a 1976 volume of *Ecumenical Review* identifies the date of their first constitution as 1946. See Cadbury Research Library (CRL) H7/B/42/101, CAC, "The Christ Apostolic Church, Its History, Beliefs and Organization," *Ecumenical Review* 28, no. 4 (1976): 423.

7. Hibba Abugideiri, *Gender and the Making of Modern Medicine in Colonial Egypt* (Burlington, VT: Ashgate, 2010); Megan Vaughan, *Curing Their Ills: Colonial Power and African Illness* (Stanford, CA: Stanford University Press, 1991).

8. Vaughan, *Curing Their Ills,* 23.

9. Ralph Schram, *A History of the Nigerian Health Services* (Ibadan: Ibadan University Press, 1973).

10. Deanne Van Tol, "Mothers, Babies, and the Colonial State: The Introduction of Maternal and Infant Welfare Services in Nigeria 1925–1945," *Spontaneous Generations: A Journal for the History and Philosophy of Science* 1 (2007), https://doi.org/10.4245/sponge.v1i1 .1761; Ogechukwu Williams, "A Blur Between the Spiritual and the Physical: Birthing Practices Among the Igbo of Nigeria in the Twentieth Century," in *Sacred Inception: Reclaiming the Spirituality of Birth in the Modern World,* edited by Marianne Delaporte and Morag Martins (Lanham, MD: Lexington Books, 2018), 97–112; Ogechukwu Williams, "Medical

Legitimacy: Childbirth, Pluralism, and Professionalization in Nigeria's Faith-Based Aladura Birthing Homes," *Journal of African History* 64, no. 1 (2023): 96–111; Okeke, *The Better Obstetrics in Rural Nigeria (Born) Study: An Impact Evaluation of the Nigerian Midwives Service Scheme* (Santa Monica, CA: RAND Corporation, 2015); Hadiza Galadanci and Suwaiba Sani, "Childbirth in Nigeria," in *Childbirth Across Cultures: Ideas and Practices of Pregnancy, Childbirth, and Post-Partum*, edited by Helaine Selin and Pamela Stone (New York: Springer Dordrecht Heidelberg, 2009), 212–220; Chimaraoke Izugbara and Joseph Ukwayi, "The Hospital as a Birthing Site: Narratives of Local Women in Nigeria," in *Reproduction, Childbearing, and Motherhood: A Cross-Cultural Perspective*, edited by Pranee Liamputtong (New York: Nova Science, 2007); Tola Olu Pierce, "Women's Reproductive Practices and Biomedicine: Cultural Conflicts and Transformations in Nigeria," in *Conceiving the New World Order: The Global Politics of Reproduction*, edited by Faye Ginsburgh and Rayna Rapp (Berkeley: University of California Press, 1995).

11. Kelsey A. Harrison, *Sowing the Seeds of Safe Motherhood in Sub-Saharan Africa* (London: Adonis & Abbey Publishers, 2010); Chinenye Uchenna and Banke-Thomas Aduragbemi, "There Is No Ideal Place but It Is Best to Deliver in a Hospital: Expectations and Experiences of Health Facility-Based Childbirth in Imo State Nigeria," *The Pan African Medical Journal* 36, no. 317 (2020), https://doi.org/10.11604/pamj.2020.36.317.22728; Akinrinola Bankole et al., *Barriers to Safe Motherhood in Nigeria* (New York: Guttmacher Institute, 2009); Aanuoluwapo Olajubu et al., "Mothers' Experiences with mHealth Intervention for Postnatal Care Utilisation in Nigeria: A Qualitative Study," *BMC Pregnancy and Childbirth* 22 (2022), https://doi.org/10.1186/s12884-022-05177-x; Chinedu Iwu et al., "Empowering Traditional Birth Attendants as Agents of Maternal and Neonatal Immunization Uptake in Nigeria: A Repeated Measures Design," *BMC Public Health* 21, no. 287 (2021), https://doi.org/10.1186/s12889-021-10311-z.

12. UNICEF, "Maternal and Child Health," http://www.unicef.org/nigeria/children_1926.html, accessed August 27, 2014.

13. Peel, *Aladura*; Turner, *A History of an African Independent Church.*

14. Some of these works include B. Sackey, *New Directions in Gender and Religion: The Changing Status of Women in African Independent Churches* (Lanham, MD: Lexington Books 2006); I. Mukonyora, *Wandering a Gendered Wilderness: Suffering and Healing in an African Initiated Church* (New York: Peter Lang, 2007); D. Crumbley, *Spirit, Structure, and Flesh: Gendered Experiences in African Instituted Churches among the Yoruba of Nigeria* (Madison: University of Wisconsin Press, 2008); Mohr, "Faith Tabernacle Congregation," 196–221. Crumbley briefly touches on faith homes in *Spirit, Structure, and Flesh*, 38.

15. See Williams, "A Blur Between the Spiritual and the Physical"; Jonathan Roberts, *Sharing the Burden of Sickness: A History of Healing and Medicine in Accra* (Bloomington: Indiana University Press, 2021); Ekanem and A. Asira, "Religion and Medicine in the 21st Century Nigeria," *SOPHIA* 9, no. 1 (2006): 56–61; M. Asare and S. Danquah, "The African Belief System and the Patient's Choice of Treatment from Existing Health Models: The Case of Ghana," *Acta Psychopathology* 3, no. 4 (2017): 1–4; L. Lado, C. Felicien, and J. Azetsop, "The Social Construction of the Legitimacy of Christian Healing in Abidjan," *Journal of Contemporary African Studies* 36, no. 3 (2018): 334–350.

16. A. I. Adanikin, U. Onwudiegwu, and A. Akintayo, "Reshaping Maternal Services in Nigeria: Any Need for Spiritual Care?" *BMC Pregnancy Childbirth* 14, no. 196 (2014),

https://doi.org/10.1186/1471-2393-14-196; A. E. Orobator, *Religion and Faith in Africa: Confessions of an Animist* (Maryknoll, NY: Orbis Books, 2018).

17. William Olsen and Carolyn Sargent, "Introduction," in *African Medical Pluralism*, edited by William Olsen and Carolyn Sargent (Bloomington: Indiana University Press, 2017), 2; J. Amzat, *Medical Sociology in Africa* (Cham, Switzerland: Springer International Publishing, 2014), 207; M. Dekker and Rijk van Dijk, *Markets of Well-Being: Navigating Health and Healing in Africa* (Leiden: Brill, 2010); Roberts, *Sharing the Burden of Sickness*; Pamela Feldman-Savelsberg, *Plundered Kitchens Empty Wombs: Threatened Reproduction and Identity in the Cameroon Grassfields* (Ann Arbor: University of Michigan Press, 1999), 135–174; Anita Acobson-Widding and David Westerlund, *Culture Experience and Pluralism: Essays on African Ideas of Illness and Healing* (Uppsala: Academiae Upsaliensis, 1989); Waltraud Ernst, *Plural Medicine Tradition and Modernity 1800–2000* (London: Routledge, 2002); Arthur Kleinman, *Patients and Healers in the Context of Culture* (Berkeley: University of California Press, 1980); R. Cooter, *Studies in the History of Alternative Medicine* (Houndsmill: Macmillan, 1988); David Arnold, *Imperial Medicine and Indigenous Societies* (Manchester: Manchester University Press, 1988).

18. Olsen and Sargent, *African Medical Pluralism*; Acobson-Widding and David Westerlund, *Culture Experience*; Dekker and van Dijk, *Markets of Wellbeing*; Jonathan Roberts, *Sharing the Burden of Sickness: A History of Healing and Medicine in Accra* (Indiana: Indiana University Press, 2021).

19. Olsen and Sargent, "Introduction," 1.

20. The subject of TBAs is discussed in more detail in chapter 5.

21. Various dimensions of this trend are discussed in Ifi Amadiume, *Male Daughters, Female Husbands: Gender and Sex in an African Society* (London: Zed Books, 1987); Gloria Chuku, *Igbo Women and Economic Transformation in Southeastern Nigeria, 1900–1960* (New York: Routledge, 2005); Nwando Achebe, *Farmers, Traders, Warriors, and Kings: Female Power and Authority in Northern Igboland, 1900–1960* Westport, CT: Praeger, 2005); Ndubueze Mbah, *Emergent Masculinities: Gendered Power and Social Change in the Biafran Atlantic Age* (Athens: Ohio University Press, 2019); K. Sacks, "An Overview of Women and Power in Africa," in *Perspectives on Power: Women in Africa, Asia, and Latin America*, edited by J. O'Barr (Durham, NC: Duke University, Center for International Studies, 1982); Oyeronke Oyewunmi, *What Gender Is Motherhood? Changing Yoruba Ideals of Power, Procreation, and Identity in the Age of Modernity* (London: Palgrave Macmillan, 2015); Oyeronke Oyewunmi, *The Invention of Women: Making an African Sense of Western Gender Discourses* (Minneapolis: University of Minnesota Press, 1997); L. Denzer, "Domestic Science Training in Colonial Yorubaland, Nigeria," in *African Encounters with Domesticity*, edited by K. T. Hansen (New Brunswick, NJ: Rutgers University Press, 1992); Iris Berger, *Women in Twentieth Century Africa* (Cambridge: Cambridge University Press, 2016).

22. Anna Davin, "Imperialism and Motherhood," *History Workshop* 5, no. 1 (1978): 10–12.

23. Davin, "Imperialism and Motherhood," 12–14.

24. Lynn Thomas, *Politics of the Womb: Women, Reproduction and the State in Kenya* (Berkeley: University of California Press, 2003); Nancy Rose Hunt, *Colonial Lexicon of Birth Ritual, Medicalization, and Mobility in the Congo* (Durham, NC: Duke University Press, 1999); Nancy Rose Hunt, "Le Bebe en Brousse: European Women, African Birth Spacing and

Colonial Intervention in Breast Feeding in the Belgian Congo," *The International Journal of African Historical Studies* 21, no. 3 (1988): 401–432; Michael Jennings, "'A Matter of Vital Importance': The Place of the Medical Mission in Maternal and Child Healthcare in Tanganyika, 1919–39," in *Healing Bodies, Saving Souls: Medical Missions in Asia and Africa*, edited by David Hardiman (New York: Editions Rodopi B.V., 2006), 227–250; Carol Summers, "Intimate Colonialisms: The Imperial Production of Reproduction in Uganda, 1907–1925," *Signs: Journal of Women in Culture and Society* 16, no. 4 (1991): 787–807; Debby Gaitskell, "'Getting Close to the Hearts of Mothers': Medical Missionaries among African Women and Children in Johannesburg between the Wars," in *Women and Children First: International Maternal and Infant Welfare 1870–1945*, edited by Valerie Fildes, Lara Marks, and Hilary Marland (New York: Routledge Revivals, 1992); Barbara Cooper, *Countless Blessings: A History of Childbirth and Reproduction in the Sahel* (Bloomington: Indiana University Press, 2019).

25. Hunt, *Colonial Lexicon of Birth Ritual*; Summers, "Intimate Colonialisms"; Jean Allman, "Making Mothers: Missionaries, Medical Officers and Women's Work in Colonial Asante, 1924–1945," *History Workshop* 38 (1994): 23–24; Walima Kalusa, "From an Agency of Cultural Destruction to an Agency of Public Health: Transformations in Catholic Missionary Medicine in Post-Colonial Eastern Zambia, 1964–1982," *Social Sciences and Missions* 27 (2014): 219–238.

26. Thomas, *Politics of the Womb*; Amy Kaler, *Running after Pills: Politics, Gender, and Contraception in Colonial Zimbabwe* (Portsmouth: Heinemann, 2003); Beverley Chambers, *African Birth: Childbirth in Cultural Transition* (River Club, South Africa: Berev Publications CC, 1990).

27. For other examples of how this played out elsewhere on the African continent, see Jane Turrittin, "Colonizing Midwives and Modernizing Childbirth in French West Africa," in *Women in African Colonial Histories*, edited by Susan Geiger, Jean Allman, and Nakanyike Musisi (Bloomington: Indiana University Press, 2002), 72–115; Mercy Amba Oduyoye and Musimbi R. A. Kanyoro, eds., *The Will to Rise: Women, Tradition, and the Church in Africa* (New York: Orbis Books, 1992); David Arnold, ed., *Imperial Medicine and Indigenous Societies* (Manchester: Manchester University Press, 1988); E. A. Ayandele, *The Missionary Impact on Modern Nigeria 1842–1914: A Political and Social Analysis* (London: Longman, 1966); T. O. Beidelman, *Colonial Evangelism* (Bloomington: Indiana University Press, 1981).

28. Lugard's comments are recorded in Wellcome Library (WL), MEDK22987; Robert Rene Kuczynski, *Demographic Survey of the British Colonial Empire, Vol. 1 (West Africa)* (Oxford: Oxford University Press, 1948), 748.

29. Ndubueze Mbah, *Emergent Masculinities*, 3. Similar arguments are established in Ifi Amadiume, *Re-inventing Africa: Matriarchy, Religion, and Culture* (London: Zed Books, 1997), 29–51, 183–198; Gloria Chuku, "Igbo Women and Political Participation in Nigeria, 1800s–2005," *The International Journal of African Historical Studies* 42, no. 1 (2009): 81–103; Judith van Allen, "'Sitting on a Man': Colonialism and the Lost Political Institutions of Igbo Women," *Canadian Journal of African Studies/Revue Canadienne Des Études Africaines* 6, no. 2 (1972): 165–181; Barbara Bush, "Gender and Empire: The Twentieth Century," in *Gender and Empire*, edited by Philippa Levine (Oxford: Oxford University Press, 2007), 77–111.

30. This subject is explored in more detail in chapters 1 and 2.

31. National Archives Enugu (NAE) MH FED 1/1, *Infant Welfare Center, Ondo Province*, 1.

32. National Archives Enugu (NAE) MH FED 1/1, *Infant Welfare Center*.

33. CRL ACC 716/F8, *Church Missionary Outlook*, vol. LIX, January 1932, 3. Saheed Aderinto discusses the extent of sexually transmitted infections as a threat to colonial propagation in *When Sex Threatened the State: Illicit Sexuality, Nationalism, and Politics in Colonial Nigeria, 1900–1958* (Champaign: University of Illinois Press, 2014).

34. Schram, *A History of the Nigerian Health Services*, 61.

35. Deidre Helen Crumbley, "Patriarchies, Prophets, and Procreation: Sources of Gender Practices in Three African Churches," *Africa* 73, no. 4 (2003): 586.

36. NAI OYO PROF 662, *The Faith Healer-Babalola and the Faith Tabernacle*; NAI OYO PROF 1/28, *Aladura Movement (Apostolic Church)*; NAI OYO PROF 661, *Cherubim & Seraphim*.

37. NAI OYO PROF 662, *The Faith Healer-Babalola*.

38. CRL CMS ACC 716 F8, "The Prophetic Movement in Ekiti and Beyond," by Archdeacon Dallimore, Lagos Diocese, *Church Missionary Outlook*, vol. LIX, 1932, 3.

39. CRL CMS ACC 716 F8, "The Prophetic Movement in Ekiti and Beyond," 2.

40. CAC faith homes are well established in these locations and have a long history there.

41. Joshua Alokan, *Christ Apostolic Church @ 90, 1918–2008* (Ile-Ife: Timade Ventures, 2010).

42. Joseph Ayo Babalola, *Thoughts of an Apostle: His Collected Works and Teachings*, compiled and translated by Moses Idowu (Lagos: Artillery Christian Ministries, 2000).

43. Some literature on the Women's War includes Matera Marc, Misty L. Bastian, and Susan Kingsley Kent, *The Women's War of 1929: Gender and Violence in Colonial Nigeria* (Basingstoke: Palgrave Macmillan, 2011); Toyin Falola and Adam Paddock, *The Women's War of 1929: A History of Anti-Colonial Resistance in Eastern Nigeria* (Durham, NC: Carolina Academic Press, 2011); Gloria Chuku, *Igbo Women and Economic Transformation in Southeastern Nigeria 1900–1960* (New York: Routledge, 2005).

44. C. K. Meek, *Law and Authority in a Nigerian Tribe* (Oxford: Oxford University Press, 1937).

45. Amaury Talbot, *Woman's Mystery of a Primitive People* (London: Cassell and Company, 1915).

46. The most relevant of these works include Judith Eze, *Traditional Birth Control in Iheaka, Igbo-Eze South LGA*, BA thesis, Department of History, University of Nigeria, Nsukka, 2008; Chioma Akawuba, *Traditional Midwifery and Child Care in Ebenator Ekwe Isu LGA Imo State, 1900–2005*, BA thesis, Department of History, University of Nigeria, Nsukka, 2011.

47. CRL CMS M/Y/A3/1 1916–1933, "In Nigeria. Dated Achimota, 28 May, 1927," 3.

Chapter 1. Local Mothercraft

1. "The Education of the African Woman (Final Article)," *Nigerian Daily Times*, November 2, 1928, 6.

2. "The Education of the African Woman (Final Article)."

3. "The Education of the African Woman," *Nigerian Daily Times*, October 31, 1928, 8.

4. "The Education of the African Woman," *Nigerian Daily Times*, October 31, 1928, 8.

5. "The Education of the African Woman," *Nigerian Daily Times*, November 1, 1928, 6.

6. "The Education of the African Woman," *Nigerian Daily Times*, November 1, 1928.

7. "The Education of the African Woman," *Nigerian Daily Times*, November 1, 1928.

8. "The Education of the African Woman (Final Article)," 6.

9. W. H. S. Curryer, "Mothercraft in Southern Nigeria," *Nigerian Daily Times*, March 4, 1927, 2.

10. Curryer, "Mothercraft in Southern Nigeria."

11. Interview with Ezechikwelu, Adazi-Enu, May 4, 2016; interview with Philip Nnatu, Enugwu-Ukwu, April 9, 2016. For more on *mkpuke*, see Ifi Amadiume, *Male Daughters, Female Husbands: Gender and Sex in an African Society* (London: Zed Books, 1987).

12. "The Education of the African Woman (Final Article)," 6.

13. Curryer, "Mothercraft in Southern Nigeria," 2.

14. "The Education of the African Woman (Final Article)," 6.

15. "The Education of the African Woman (Final Article)." See also "The Education of the African Woman," *Nigerian Daily Times*, November 1, 1928, 6.

16. "The Education of the African Woman (Final Article)."

17. Amaury Talbot, *Some Nigerian Fertility Cults* (New York: Barnes and Nobles, 1927), 2–3, 6, 64–67.

18. Interview with Mrs. Obijelu Okpalaeze, Adazi-Enu, January 29, 2009; interview with Roseline Ezekwem, Adazi-Enu, January 27, 2009; interview with Mrs. Patty Iloghalu, Umuabu, January 28, 2009; interview with Ezechikwelu.

19. For more on this subject, see Joseph Agbasiere, *Women in Igbo Life and Thought* (London: Routledge, 2000); Gloria Chuku, *Igbo Women and Economic Transformation in Southeastern Nigeria, 1900–1960* (New York: Routledge, 2005); Nwando Achebe, *Farmers, Traders, Warriors, and Kings: Female Power and Authority in Northern Igboland, 1900–1960* (Westport CT: Praeger, 2005); Amadiume, *Male Daughters, Female Husbands*.

20. See Cadbury Research Library, Birmingham (CRL) CMS, *Mercy and Truth: A Record of CMS Medical Mission Work* 9 (1903): 6–7; CRL CMS, *The Mission Hospital: A Record of Medical Missions of the CMS* XXIX (1925): 298–299; Margaret Roseveare, *High Spring: The Story of Iyi-Enu Hospital* (London: Church Missionary Society, 1946), 25–28.

21. Roseveare, *High Spring*; Amaury Talbot, *Woman's Mystery of a Primitive People* (London: Cassell and Company, 1915), 22–34; Interview with Roseline Ezekwem, March 28, 2016; Interview with Ezechikwelu.

22. National Archives Enugu (NAE) ON DIST 12/1/1244, *Human Sacrifices and Destruction of Twin Children*, "Twin Killing," 1955, 2; NAE ON DIST 12/1/1244, "Requesting Information re Twins," 1955, 2.

23. Abena Osseo-Asare and Karen Flint compellingly demonstrate throughout their respective books on traditional healing, for instance, the constructions and flexibility of "tradition" and traditional medicine. See Osseo-Asare, *Bitter Roots: The Search for Healing Plants in Africa* (Chicago: University of Chicago Press, 2014), 1–30, 165–212, and Flint, *Healing Traditions: African Medicine, Cultural Exchange, and Competition in South Africa, 1820–1948* (Athens: Ohio University Press, 2008), 1–66. In *Healing Traditions*, Flint in fact begins her book by grappling with the question, "What is 'traditional' about traditional healers and medicines?"

24. Interview with Mrs. Obijelu Okpalaeze, Adazi-Enu, January 29, 2009.

25. Interview with Mrs. Obijelu Okpalaeze.

26. Interview with Onyeugwu Nwa Ogwo, Lejja, April 6, 2015.

27. Interview with Philip Nnatu.

28. Interview with Philip Nnatu.

29. Interview with Roseline Ezekwem, 2003.

30. Interview with Roseline Ezekwem, 2003.

31. Interview with Ichie Ezedum, Ogweni Ocha, January 29, 2009.

32. Interview with Mrs. Patty Iloghalu.

33. C. K. Meek, *Law and Authority in a Nigerian Tribe* (Oxford: Oxford University Press, 1937), 285, 287.

34. Meek, *Law and Authority in a Nigerian Tribe*, 289.

35. Meek, *Law and Authority in a Nigerian Tribe*, 269.

36. See Meek, *Law and Authority in a Nigerian Tribe*, 289.

37. Meek, *Law and Authority in a Nigerian Tribe*.

38. Meek, *Law and Authority in a Nigerian Tribe*, 52, 101.

39. The traditional doctor in this case is a general term that covers the different branches of indigenous medicine. It is often used to imply an herbalist, doctor (*dibia*), and diviner. In some cases, traditional physicians are all these things at the same time. In other cases, they are a doctor, herbalist, or diviner.

40. Meek, *Law and Authority*, 51.

41. Interview with Onye Ugwu Nwa Ogwo.

42. See Misty Bastian, "The Naked and the Nude: Historically Multiple Meanings of Oto (Undress) in Southeastern Nigeria," in *Dirt, Undress, and Difference: Critical Perspectives on the Body's Surface*, edited by Adeline Masquelier (Bloomington: Indiana University Press, 2005).

43. Interview with Ogidija Ugwuole, Lejja, April 5, 2016; interview with Onyeugwu nwa Ogwo, Lejja, April 6, 2016.

44. Meek, *Law and Authority*, 58.

45. See CRL, *Medical Missions Quarterly, Nos IX to XVI*, 1895–1896 (London: Church Missionary Society, Salisbury Square, E.C., 1897), 88; CRL CMS M/C 2/1/7 (1898–1905), "Niger Missions, June 1900."

46. A. P. Stirrett, *Medical Book for the Treatment of Diseases in West Africa* (Jos: The Niger Press, 1922), 117.

47. Miss D. Jewitt, "The Opening of a Dressing Station at Ufuma," *The Mission Hospital: A Record of Medical Missions of the CMS* XXIX (1925): 298–299.

48. Interview with Onyeugwu.

49. MH (Fed) 1/1/4075, *Infant Welfare Center Ondo Province*, "Suggestions for Starting New Centers," 1942, 2.

50. MH (Fed) 1/1/4075, *Infant Welfare Center Ondo Province*.

51. Meek, *Law and Authority*, 290; interview with Nnanna Okorom, Imo State, March 2, 2011.

52. Interview with Mary Ugwuanyi, Nsukka, June 26, 2013.

53. Interview with Chizoba.

54. Interview with Chizoba.

55. Interview with Gloria, Nsukka, April 5, 2016.

56. Interview with Gloria, Nsukka.

57. Meek, *Law and Authority*, 269; interview with Onyeugwu.

58. ON PROF 7/13/97, *Trial Exposure of Twins*, "Nigeria Onitsha Province," 1926, 2.

59. Interview with Mary Ugwuanyi.

60. Interview with Onyeugwu; interview with Ogidija.

61. Interview with Ezechikwelu.

62. MH (Fed) 1/1/4075, "Training of Midwives Grade II," *Infant Welfare Center Ondo Province*, 1942, 1.

63. MH (Fed) 1/1/4075, "Training of Midwives Grade II."

64. Interview with Mary Ugwuanyi.

65. Interview with Ogidija; interview with Mary Ugwuanyi; interview with Florence Odo, Enugu, April 4, 2008; Interview with Onyeugwu.

66. Interview with Florence Odo; interview with Felicia Agu, Imo State, March 5, 2011; Basden, *Niger Ibos*.

67. Stirrett, *Medical Book*, 117–118.

68. Interview with Ogidija.

69. Interview with Amalugo, Umuabu, May 4, 2016.

70. Interview with Ngozi Ikwueze, Orloto, April 2, 2016.

71. "Ite Ola Okike," National Museum, Enugu Nigeria.

72. "Ite Ola Okike"; interview with Onyeugwu; Interview with Roseline Ezekwem, 2016.

73. Interview with Onyeugwu.

74. Interview with Chizoba.

75. Interview with Rita Ewereji, Imo State, March 5, 2011.

76. Meek, *Law and Authority*, 292.

77. Meek, *Law and Authority*.

78. Meek, *Law and Authority*, 293.

79. Meek, *Law and Authority*, 294.

80. Interview with Onyeugwu; interview with Ugwuole.

81. Interview with Onyeugwu.

82. Interview with Chizoba.

83. See Basden's account of this type of child-spacing in *Among the Ibos*, 62.

84. CRL CMS, *The Mission Hospital: A Record of Medical Missions of the CMS* XXIX (1925): 298.

85. Basden, *Among the Ibos*, 53.

86. See Basden, *Among the Ibos*, 50; Talbot, *Woman's Mystery of a Primitive People*, 22–34; Roseveare, *High Spring*, 22–27.

87. NAE ON DIST 12/1/1247, *Triplets: Queens Bounty for the Birth of Triplets*, 10.

88. Philip Peek, *Twins in African and African Diaspora Culture: Double Trouble, Twice Blessed* (Bloomington: Indiana University Press, 2011), 1.

89. Basden, *Among the Ibos*, 50.

90. NAE OP 7/13/97, *Awgu-Rex versus Unaegbu and One Other Charged with Exposure of Twins and Committed to Trial to the Resident's Court*, "Nigeria-Onitsha Province," 1926 1.

91. Interview with Ngozi Ikwueze.

92. NAE OP 7/13/97, *Awgu-Rex versus*, 1–2.

93. "Appointment of Lady Medical Officer," *Nigerian Daily Times*, March 23, 1928, 4.

94. NAE ON DIST 12/1/1244, *Human Sacrifices and Destruction of Twin Children*, "Twin Killing," 1955, 1.

95. Basden, *Among the Ibos*, 50.

96. NAE ON DIST 12/1/1244, *Human Sacrifices and Destruction of Twin Children*, "No. 1812/27, Resident's Office," 1955, 2.

97. NAE OP 7/13/97, *Awgu-Rex*, "Nigeria. Onitsha Province," 2.

98. NAE OP 7/13/97, *Awgu-Rex*.

99. NAE ON DIST 12/1/1244, *Human Sacrifices and Destruction of Twin Children*, "Requesting Information re Twins," 1955, 1.

100. CRL CMS, *Mercy and Truth: A Record of CMS Medical Mission Work* 9 (1903): 6–7.

101. Jewitt, "The Opening of a Dressing Station at Ufuma," 298–299.

102. Jewitt, "The Opening of a Dressing Station," 299.

103. CRL CMS, *Mercy and Truth*, 9:7.

104. CRL CMS, *Mercy and Truth*, 9:7; CRL CMS, "News from Onitsha," *Mercy and Truth: A Record of CMS Medical Mission Work* 12 (1908): 27.

105. CRL CMS, *Mercy and Truth*, 12:27. For more on this king's relationship with missionaries, see CRL CMS, "A Joint Journal from Onitsha," *Mercy and Truth: A Record of CMS Medical Mission Work* XIII (1909): 89–90. See also Roseveare, *High Spring*, 26–27.

106. Roseveare, *High Spring*, 26–27.

107. NAE ON DIST 12/1/1244, *Human Sacrifices and Destruction of Twin Children*, "Requesting Information re Twins," 1955, 2.

108. NAE ON DIST 12/1/1244, *Human Sacrifices and Destruction of Twin Children*, 1.

109. NAE ON DIST 12/1/1244, *Human Sacrifices and Destruction of Twin Children*, "Murder of Twins and Triplets," 2.

110. NAE ON DIST 12/1/1244, *Human Sacrifices and Destruction of Twin Children*.

111. NAE NSUDIV 12/1/38, Midwives General, "Community Nursing Report by Patricia Eze," 5.

112. Roseveare, *High Spring*, 27.

113. Interview with Roseline Ezekwem, 2016.

Chapter 2. Instruments of Propaganda

1. Cadbury Research Library (CRL) Arthur E. Clayton, "Light on the Niger," *Mercy and Truth: A Record of CMS Medical Missions*, vol. III (London: Church Missionary Society, 1899), 216–217.

2. CRL C/2/1/8 1905–1909, "Memorandum of Interview between Medical Committee and Dr. A. E. Druitt," December 6, 1907.

3. CRL C/2/1/8 1905–1909, "Memorandum of Interview."

4. See Lawrence Amadi, "Church-State Involvement in Educational Development in Nigeria, 1842–1948," *Journal of Church and State* 19, no. 3 (1977): 483–484; J. F. Ade-Ajayi, *Christian Missions in Modern Nigeria: The Making of a New Elite* (Evanston, IL: Northwestern University Press, 1965); E. A. Ayandele, *The Missionary Impact on Modern Nigeria 1842–1914: A Political and Social Analysis* (London: Longman, 1971), 4, 28–30.

5. CRL CMS ACC 716 F8, *The Church Missionary Society* LIX (January 1932): 3; CRL M/Y /A3/1 1918–1933, *Iyi-Enu Medical Mission Report. 1919*, 2–3.

6. CRL CMS ACC 716 F8, *The Church Missionary Outlook* LIX (September 1932): 184.

7. Wellcome Library (WL), *Report on the Medical and Health Department for the Year 1931* (Lagos: Government Printer, 1932), 34.

8. See WL, *Annual Medical and Sanitary Report* Nigeria, 1929 (Lagos: Government Printer, 1930), 34–35. Besides Massey Street Hospital, the colonial government formed a partnership with the Roman Catholic Mission's Sacred Heart Hospital, in which government operated from a ward in the hospital to provide maternity services. For more information, see WL, *Annual Medical and Sanitary Report* 1930 (Lagos: Government Printer, 1931), 31.

9. National Archives Ibadan (NAI) J/1/a, *Medical Policy in the Colonial Empire*, "Medical Policy in the Colonial Empire," 1943, 5.

10. See CRL C.M.S. G3/A3/0, *Henry Dobinson to R. Lang*, May 5, 1890; F. K. Ekechi, *Missionary Enterprise and Rivalry in Igboland 1857–1914* (London: Frank Cass, 1971), 75–78.

11. For the role of medicine in the late nineteenth and early twentieth centuries as an instrument of conversion, see also Felix Ekechi, "The Holy Ghost Fathers in Eastern Nigeria, 1885–1920: Observations on Missionary Strategy," *African Studies Review* 15, no. 2 (1972): 221–222; Felix Ekechi, "The Medical Factor in Christian Conversion in Africa: Observations from Southeastern Nigeria," *Missiology* 21, no. 3 (1993): 289–309.

12. CRL CMS G3/A3/0, *Annual Report of Onitsha Station for 1886.*

13. CRL CMS G3/A3/0, "Annual Report of Onitsha Station Dated 1885."

14. CRL CMS G3/A3/0, "Annual Report of Onitsha Station Dated 1885."

15. CRL CMS G3/A3/0, *Henry Dobinson to R. Lang*, May 5, 1890.

16. CRL, "Our Title," *Mercy and Truth: A Record of CMS Medical Missions*, vol. I (London: Church Missionary Society, 1897), 1–5; see also CRL CMS G3/A3/0, *Henry Dobinson to R. Lang*, 77; CRL, *The Mission Hospital: A Record of C.M.S Medical Missions* xxxiv (1930): 110.

17. CRL, "Our Title," *Mercy and Truth: A Record of CMS Medical Missions*, vol. I (London: Church Missionary Society, 1897), 1–5.

18. Curryer, "Mothercraft in Southern Nigeria," 2.

19. CRL M/E/L/1/1, "Address by Dr. E Downes," 7.

20. CRL CMS, *The Mission Hospital: A Record of Medical Missions of the C.M.S.* XXXII (1928): 171; CRL CMS, *The Mission Hospital* XXXII (1929): 18.

21. "The Education of the African Woman (Final Article)," *Nigerian Daily Times*, November 2, 1928, 6.

22. See Helen Callaway, *Gender, Culture and Empire: European Women in Colonial Nigeria* (London: Oxford and Macmillan, 1987); Margaret Strobel, *European Women and the Second British Empire* (Bloomington: Indiana University Press, 1991).

23. CRL CMS, *The Mission Hospital: A Record of Medical Missions of the CMS* XXXI (1927): 172–173; CRL CMS, *The Mission Hospital: A Record of Medical Missions of the CMS* XXXIV (1930): 32–33.

24. CRL CMS M/C 2/1/7 (1898–1905), 1905. See also M. Roseveare, *High Spring: The Story of Iyi Enu Hospital* (London: Church Missionary Society, 1946).

25. CRL CMS M/C 2/1/7 (1898–1905), 1898–1900; CRL CMS M/C 2/1/7 (1898–1905), April 8, 1902; CRL CMS M/C 2/1/7 (1898–1905), November 7, 1902, 132–133.

26. CRL CMS M/C 2/1/7 (1898–1905), June 23, 1900.

27. CRL CMS M/Y/A3/1, 1916–1933, "Iyi-Enu Medical Mission Report, 1919," 2.

28. CRL CMS M/Y/A3/1, 1916–1933, "In Nigeria. Dated Achimota, 28 May, 1927," 3.

29. CRL M/Y/A3/1, 1916–1933, "Extract from the Letter from Archdeacon Basden to Rev. H.D. Hooper, Dated, Onitsha, July 29, 1932 (Despatch [sis], Niger No. 24 of 1932)."

30. CRL M/Y/A3/1, 1916–1933, "Notes of Interview between Dr. Sybil K. Batley and Medical Committee, March 22, 1932."

31. CRL M/Y/A3/2, 1934–1937, "Iyi Enu C.M.S. Hospital Onitsha 2.3.37."

32. CRL M/Y/A3/2, 1934–1937, "Extract from the Letter from Archdeacon Basden to Rev. H.D. Hooper."

33. CRL CMS, *The Mission Hospital: A Record of Medical Missions of the CMS* XXXIV (1930): 112.

34. CRL M/Y/A2/1, 1918–1945, "Memorandum Re Medical Work in the Niger Mission," 3.

35. CRL M/Y/A2/1, 1918–1945, "Memorandum Re Medical Work in the Niger Mission."

36. CRL, *The Mission Hospital* XXIX (1925): 299; CRL M/Y/A3/1, 1916–1933, *Notes of Interview between Dr. Sybil K. Batley and Medical Committee*, March 22, 1932, 2; CRL M/Y/A2/1, 1918–1945, "Diocese on the Niger Annual Conference," 2–3. For more information on missionary actions against twin killing, see CRL CMS, *Mercy and Truth*, vol. 9, 6–7.

37. CRL M/Y/A3/1, 1916–1933, *Notes of Interview Between Dr. Sybil K. Batley and Medical Committee*, March 22, 1932, 2–3; CRL M/Y/A2/1 1918–1945, "Diocese on the Niger Annual Conference," 2–3.

38. Similar tactics played out in northern Nigeria through formerly enslaved women. See Shankar, *Who Shall Enter Paradise*, xvii–ix; G. O. Olusanya, "The Freed Slaves' Homes—An Unknown Aspect of Northern Nigerian Social History," *Journal of the Historical Society of Nigeria* 3, no. 3 (1966): 523–538. For more on the northern slave trade, see Paul Lovejoy and Jan Hogendorn, *Slow Death of Slavery: The Course of Abolition in Northern Nigeria, 1897–1936* (Cambridge, UK: Cambridge University Press, 1993); C. N. Ubah, "The Colonial Administration in Northern Nigeria and the Problem of Freed Slave Children," *Slavery and Abolition* 14, no. 3 (1993): 208–233; Paul Lovejoy, "Concubinage and the Status of Women Slaves in Early Colonial Northern Nigeria," *The Journal of African History* 29, no. 2 (1988): 245–266; Humphrey J. Fisher, "Slavery and Seclusion in Northern Nigeria: A Further Note," *The Journal of African History* 32, no. 1 (1991): 123–135.

39. CRL CMS, *The Mission Hospital* XXXII (1928): 171.

40. CRL CMS, *The Mission Hospital* XXXII (1928).

41. MH (FED) 1/1/4075, *Infant Welfare Center Ondo Province*, "Training of Midwives Grade II," 1.

42. For more on Baby Week in Britain, see Davin Anna, "Imperialism and Motherhood," *History Workshop* 5 (Spring 1978): 9–65; Dwork Deborah, *War Is Good for Babies and Other Young Children: A History of the Infant and Child Welfare Movement in England 1898–1918* (London: Tavistock, 1987); Ross Ellen, *Love and Toil: Motherhood in Outcast London 1870–1918* (New York: Oxford University Press, 1993); Susan R. Grayzel, *Women and the First World War* (Harlow: Longman, 2002).

43. "Editorial," *British Journal of Nursing*, June 30, 1917, n.p.

44. CRL CMS, *The Mission Hospital* XXXII (1927): 172.

45. G. T. Basden, *Among the Igbo of Nigeria*, 2nd ed. (Gloucestershire: Nonsuch Publishing Limited, 2006), 53.

46. CRL CMS, *The Mission Hospital* xxxi (1927): 172, 272; CRL CMS, *The Mission Hospital* xxxiv (1930): 172–173.

47. CRL CMS, *The Mission Hospital* xxxiv (1930): 173.

48. "Baby Show at Abeokuta," *Daily Times*, January 14, 1938, 1.

49. CRL CMS, *The Mission Hospital* xxxi (1927), 171

50. CRL CMS, *The Mission Hospital* XXX (1926): 173.

51. See Roseveare, *High Spring*, 22.

52. See CRL CMS, *The Mission Hospital*, 1927, 272.

53. CRL M/Y/A3/1, 1916–1933, 2; CRL M/Y/A2/1, 1918–1945, "Memorandum Re," 2–3.

54. CRL G/Y/A/9/2, *Northern Nigeria Missions*, ". . . in Nigeria, dated Achimota, 28th May 1927," 2.

55. CRL CMS G/Y/A9/2, "20 Years of an African Diocese 1919–1939. 'Out of Darkness,'" 3.

56. CRL CMS G/Y/A9/2, "20 Years of an African Diocese."

57. CRL CMS G/Y/A9/2, , "Iyi Enu Hospital 8.12.36," 1–3; CRL CMS, *The Mission Hospital* XXX (1926): 58–59.

58. See NAE ONPROF 7/11/46, *The Marriage Ordinance*, 1929, 1–6. See also NAE ONDIST 12/1/854, "Conflict between Christian Rites and Pagan Customs," 1930s and 1940s.

59. CRL M/Y/A2/1 1918–1945, "Diocese on the Niger," 4.

60. Roseveare, *High Spring*, 41.

61. Interview with Philip Nnatu, June 7, 2014. Philip's account is collaborated by the missionary, Roseveare, in *High Spring*, 44.

62. W. H. S. Curryer, "Mothercraft in Southern Nigeria," *Nigerian Daily Times*, March 4, 1927, 2.

63. Roseveare, *High Spring*, 31–32.

64. CRL CMS, *The Mission Hospital* XXXII (1928): 172.

65. CRL CMS, *The Mission Hospital* xxxiv (1930): 172.

66. Roseveare, *High Spring*, 46.

67. Roseveare, *High Spring*.

68. CRL CMS, *The Mission Hospital* xxxiii (1929): 172.

69. CRL CMS, *The Mission Hospital* xxxiv (1930): 171.

70. CRL CMS, *The Mission Hospital* xxxiv (1930): 172.

71. CRL M/Y/A2/1, 1918–1945, "Memorandum Re Medical Work in the Niger Mission," 61.

72. CRL M/Y/A2/1, 1918–1945, Dr. Anderson, "Extract from Letter from Miss D. Jewitt, Dated 4/11/42."

73. CRL CMS, *The Mission Hospital* xxxiv (1930): 172.

74. BNA, CO 917/2, *Pan African Health Conference*, 1935 file; "Misunderstanding Cleared on Colonial Question," *Daily Times*, December 19, 1949, 3; "Developing Britain's Colonies," *Daily Times*, December 28, 1949, 3.

75. CRL M/Y/A3/1, 1916–1933, "CMS Onitsha, March 28, 1933," 2.

76. CRL M/Y/A3/1, 1916–1933, "From the Secretary, Niger Mission, November 7, 1933," 1–2; "July 31 1933," 1.

77. CRL M/Y/A3/1, 1916–1933, "From the Secretary," 2.

78. CRL M/Y/A3/1, 1916–1933, "CMS Onitsha, May 30, 1933," 1.

79. CRL M/Y/A3/1, 1916–1933, "From the Secretary, Niger Mission," November 7, 1933, 1–2.

80. CRL M/Y/A3/1, 1916–1933, "Travelling Lady Doctor for Ibo Country," July 31, 1933, 1.

81. CRL M/Y/A3/1, 1916–1933, "CMS Onitsha, March 28, 1933," 2.

82. CRL G/Y/A/9/2, *Northern Nigeria Missions*, ". . . in Nigeria, dated Achimota, 28th May 1927," 2.

83. NAI OYO PROF 1/1129, *Domestic Training for Girls-Suggestions as to*, 3.

84. NAI OYO PROF 1/1129, *Domestic Training for Girls-Suggestions as to*.

85. NAI OYO PROF 1/1129, *Domestic Training for Girls-Suggestions as to*, 3; "Training Women Teachers in Western Division," 1–2.

86. CRL CMS, *Mercy and Truth: A Record of C.M.S Medical Missions* III (1899): 216–217.

87. CRL CMS ACC 780/F1, Dorothy Ross, *The Pattern of a Life*, 19.

88. BNA CO 583/248/6, *Training of Subordinate Staff in the Medical Department*, "Mission Activities African Missions," 2.

89. CRL CMS, *The Mission Hospital: A Record of C.M.S Medical Missions* xxxiii (1929): 18.

90. BNA CO 583/266/4, *Higher College of Yaba. Medical Training for Girls*, "Colonial Social Welfare Advisory Committee," 1945, 2.

91. BNA, CO 917/2, *Pan African Health Conference*, 1935 file; "Misunderstanding Cleared on Colonial Question," *Daily Times*, December 19, 1949, 3.

92. "Developing Britain's Colonies," *Daily Times*, December 28, 1949, 3.

93. NAI J/1/a, "Medical Policy in the Colonial Empire," 1942.

94. CRL M/Y/A2/1, 1918–1945, "Diocese on the Niger. C.M.S. Annual Conference Standing Committee. September 1939," 1–2.

95. NAI J/1/a, *Medical Policy in the Colonial Empire*, 1.

96. M/Y/A3/1, 1916–1933, "Interview between Dr. H. Lankester and Miss M.E. Elms," 1–2.

97. M/Y/A2/1, 1918–1945, "Diocese on the Niger," 1–3.

98. See Davin, *Imperialism and Motherhood*, 24–29, 36–38, 47.

99. NAI J/1/a, *Medical Policy in the Colonial Empire*, 2.

100. NAI J/1/a, *Medical Policy in the Colonial Empire*.

101. NAI OYO PROF 1/1129, "Training of Women," 41.

102. NAI J/1/a, *Medical Policy in the Colonial Empire*, 1943, 3.

103. NAE MINHEALTH 30/1/253, "Co-operation with Voluntary Bodies"; NAE MINHEALTH 30/1/253, "The Relationship between Government and the Missionary and Other Voluntary Societies Regarding the Development of Medical and Health Services"; NAE MINHEALTH 30/1/253, "To the Secretary of States for the Colonies," London, January 22, 1948.

104. NAE MINHEALTH 30/1/253, "Medical Development Nigeria," June 24, 1947, 169.

105. NAE MINHEALTH 30/1/253, "Medical Development Nigeria," June 24, 1947, 169.

106. *Practicing Midwifery in Nigeria (Ordinances and Laws) 1930–1992*, compiled by P. N. Ndatsu (Abuja: Nursing and Midwifery Council of Nigeria, 1999), 4–10. For more on the Midwifery Ordinance, see CRL M/Y/A/3, 1916 to 1933, *Despatch Niger No. 16 of 1933*, 1; WL, *Annual Medical and Sanitary Report*, 1930, 30.

107. *Practicing Midwifery in Nigeria*, 4–5.

108. NAI MH (FED)1/1/4075, *Infant Welfare Center, Ondo Province*, 1.

109. NAI MH (FED)1/1/4075, *Infant Welfare Center, Ondo Province*.

110. NAE MINHEALTH 30/1/253, "Medical Development Owerri Province," 8; Bright, *Daily Times*, April 10, 1950, 5.

111. NAI MH (FED)/1/1/4075, *Infant Welfare Center Ondo Province*, "The Training of Midwives in Nigeria, 1.6.42," 9.

112. NAI MH (FED)/1/1/4075, "The Training of Midwives in Nigeria," June 16, 1942, 2.

113. CRL G/Y/A/9/2, *Northern Nigeria Mission*, "Notes Made by E.M.F. after a Talk with Dr. Mess, Northern Nigeria, 22.3.49," 2–3.

114. NAI J/1/a, "Minutes by His Honour, the Acting Chief Commissioner, Northern Provinces (MR. J.R. Patterson D.M.G.)," 16–17.

115. London Correspondent, "Training of Women Reviewed," *Daily Times*, August 15, 1949, 15.

116. NAI MH (FED)/1/1/4075, "The Training of Midwives in Nigeria, 1.6.42," 9–10.

117. NAI MH (FED)/1/1/4075, "The Training of Midwives in Nigeria, 1.6.42," 12.

118. CRL G/Y/A/9/2, *Northern Nigeria Mission*, "Notes Made by E.M.F. after a Talk with Dr. Mess, Northern Nigeria, 22.3.49," 3; NAE MINHEALTH 30/1/253, "Ref. No. E.1.84," 84.

119. NAI J/1/a, *Medical Policy in the Colonial Empire*, "No. 19996/7," 12.

120. For further information, see CRL CMS ACC/165/F27, *The Private Owned Maternity Home in Nigeria*, 1–2.

121. NAI CSO 26/3, *Infant and Maternity Work in Nigeria II*, 133. See also *Daily Times* Photo Interview, "Boys and Girls Must Be Given Equal Education," *Daily Times*, December 21, 1949, 6; "Misunderstanding Cleared on Colonial Question," *Daily Times*, December 19, 1949, 3; Mrs. Ibiyemi Bright, "Should Married Women Work," *Daily Times*, April 10, 1950, 5; D. O. Dinyo, "Women Should Pay No Income Tax," *Daily Times*, April 17, 1950, 4.

122. NAI MH (FED)/1/1/4075, *Infant Welfare Center Ondo Province*, "Training of Midwives Grade II," 2–3.

123. NAI MH (FED)/1/1/4075, *Infant Welfare Center Ondo Province*.

124. NAI MH (FED)/1/1/4075, *Infant Welfare Center Ondo Province*, 3.

125. NAE MINHEALTH 30/1/253, "A Bulletin for Community Nurses in Eastern Nigeria," 37; NAI J/1/a, 3–4.

126. BNA CO 859/62/17, *Birth Control West Africa*, "Ministry of Health Annual Report, 1957."

127. BNA, *Ministry of Health Annual Report 1957–1958*, vol. 1, 1.

128. BNA, *Ministry of Health Annual Report 1957–1958*, vol. 2, 6.

129. BNA, *Ministry of Health Annual Report 1957–1958*, vol. 2.

130. WL HIB948, *Annual Report of the Federal Medical Services 1958*, 3.

131. L. J. Bruce-Chwatt, "Obituary: Sir Samuel L.A. Manuwa," *Transactions of the Royal Society of Tropical Medicine and Hygiene* 70, no. 2 (1976): 173.

132. See NAI J/1/a, *Medical Policy in the Colonial Empire*, 6.

133. BNA, *Ministry of Health Annual Report 1957–1958*, vol. 2, 6.

134. BNA, *Ministry of Health Annual Report 1957–1958*, vol. 2, 6, 51.

135. NAI J/1/a, *Medical Policy in the Colonial Empire*, 2.

136. "The Education of the African Woman," *Nigerian Daily Times*, November 1, 1928, 6.

137. "The Education of the African Woman."

138. CRL M/Y/A2/1, 1918–1945, "Annual Conference Held at Onitsha," 7; M/FL1 N1/1, "Onitsha May 1919."

Chapter 3. "Attendants Mostly Women"

1. See National Archives Ibadan (NAI), OYOPROF 662, *The Faith Healer—Babalola and Faith Tabernacle, Otherwise Known as the Aladura Religious Movement, Operation of in Oyo Province*, 3.

2. NAI, OYOPROF 662, *The Faith Healer—Babalola*.

3. NAI, OYOPROF 662, *The Faith Healer—Babalola*.

4. NAI, OYOPROF 662, *The Faith Healer—Babalola*, 3–5. See also J. D. Y. Peel, *Aladura: A Religious Movement among the Yoruba* (Oxford: Oxford University Press, 1968), 95.

5. NAI, OYOPROF 662, *The Faith Healer—Babalola*, 2.

6. Wellcome Library (WL), MEDK22987, Robert Rene Kuczynski, *Demographic Survey of the British Colonial Empire, Vol. 1 (West Africa)* (Oxford: Oxford University Press, 1948), 660; Government of Nigeria, *Census of Nigeria 1931*, vol. I (London: Government of Nigeria, 1932), 126.

7. Government of Nigeria, *Census of Nigeria 1931*, 126.

8. R. Galletti, K. D. S. Baldwin, and I. O. Dina, *The Nigerian Cocoa Farmer* (Oxford: Oxford University Press, 1956), 203; C. R. Barber et al., "Vital Statistics at Igbo-Ora," *First African Population Conference* (Ibadan: University of Ibadan), 1966.

9. WL MEDK22987, Kuczynski, *Demographic Survey*, 689.

10. Government of Nigeria, *Census of Nigeria 1931*, 8–9.

11. Government of Nigeria, *Census of Nigeria 1931*, 126.

12. WL MEDK22987, Kuczynski, *Demographic Survey*, 689.

13. Joseph Babalola, *Joseph Ayo Babalola, Thoughts of an Apostle: His Collected Works and Teachings*, compiled and translated by Moses Idowu (Lagos: Artillery Christian Ministries, 2000), 76.

14. Joshua Alokan, *Christ Apostolic Church @ 90, 1918–2008* (Ile-Ife: Timade Ventures, 2010), 37.

15. Cadbury Research Library (CRL) ACC 716/F8, *Church Missionary Outlook* LIX (January 1932): 3.

16. NAI, OYOPROF 662, *The Faith Healer—Babalola*, 4.

17. Babalola, *Joseph Ayo Babalola*, 75–76.

18. A note on usage: I use *faith delivery homes* and *faith homes* interchangeably to describe the form of midwifery that the CAC created. In some CAC congregations, especially in Ibadan, the maternity facilities were commonly referred to as faith delivery homes while those in Lagos were frequently called faith homes. Both names are acceptable in all CAC branches. The CAC midwives specifically used these names to distinguish themselves from the biomedical maternity centers and promptly corrected my description of their facilities during the early stage of this research as a maternity center.

19. J. D. Y. Peel discusses these secessions, the earliest of which occurred in the 1880s, in detail in *Aladura: A Religious Movement among the Yoruba* (Oxford: Oxford University Press, 1968), 55–62. For more information, see J. B. Webster, *The African Churches among the Yoruba* (Oxford: Clarendon Press, 1964); J. F. Ade Ajayi, *Christian Missions in Nigeria, 1841–1891: The Making of a New Élite* (Evanston, IL: Northwestern University Press, 1965); E. A. Ayandele, *The Missionary Impact on Modern Nigeria 1842–1914: A Political and Social Analysis* (London: Longman Group LTD, 1966), 3–5; Jude Aguwa, "Mission, Colonialism, and the Supplanting of African Practices," in *Missions, States, and European Expansion in Africa,*

edited by Chima J. Korieh and Raphael Chijioke Njoku (New York: Routledge, 2007), 128; Clement Chesterman, *In the Service of the Suffering: Phases of Medical Missionary Enterprise* (London: Edinburgh House Press, 1940); Andrew Walls, "The Legacy of Samuel Ajayi Crowther," *International Bulletin of Missionary Research* 16, no. 1 (1992): 19–20; Andrew F. Walls, "Crowther, Samuel Adjai (or Ajayi)," in *Biographical Dictionary of Christian Missions*, edited by Gerald H. Anderson (New York: Macmillan Reference USA, 1998), 160–161.

20. A similar short-lived movement emerged for the same reasons in Nigeria's Niger Delta region in 1915 under the leadership of Garrick Braid. There were smaller equivalents of the Aladura movement in areas across Africa with similar early exposure to pronounced missionary activities, such as former Nyasaland (Malawi) under John Chilembwe between 1900 and 1915 (see Jane Linden and Ian Linden, "John Chilembwe and the New Jerusalem," *Journal of African History* 12, no. 4 (1971): 629–651) and the 1921 religious movement of Joseph Kimbangu in Belgian Congo (Congo DRC). For *Kimbanguism*, see Aurelien Mokoko Gampiot, "Kimbanguism: An African Initiated Church," *Scriptura: International Journal of Bible, Religion and Theology in Southern Africa* 113 (2014): 1–11. See also Philip Jenkins, *The Next Christendom: The Coming of Global Christianity* (Oxford: Oxford University Press, 2002), 48–50, for the movement of William Wade Harris in Ivory Coast. These religious movements varied in their political nature and adherence to faith-healing. None were as large-scale and sustained as that of Nigeria's Aladura.

21. University of Illinois (UI), *Colonial Annual Reports, No. 1030, Nigeria*, "Reports for 1918," 18; WL, *Nigeria. Southern Provinces. Annual Medical and Sanitary Report for the Year Ended 31st December 1918*, 29.

22. UI *Colonial Annual Reports, No. 1030*, 18; WL, *Nigeria. Southern Provinces. Annual Medical and Sanitary Report 1918*, 29.

23. WL, *Nigeria. Southern Provinces. Annual Medical and Sanitary Report 1918*, 28. The colonial annual report put the number of casualties in Lagos at 2%. See UI, *Colonial Annual Reports, No. 1030, Nigeria*, "Reports for 1918," 18.

24. WL, *Nigeria. Southern Provinces. Annual Medical and Sanitary Report 1918*, 18. See also WL ANN REP WA28 NH5 N68 1922–1925, *Annual Medical and Sanitary Report for the Year 1922*, 18–20.

25. WL, *Nigeria. Southern Provinces. Annual Medical and Sanitary Report for the Year Ended 31st December 1915*, 38; WL, *Nigeria. Southern Provinces. Annual Medical and Sanitary Report for the Year Ended 31st December 1916*, 6.

26. WL, *Nigeria. Southern Provinces. Annual Medical and Sanitary Report for the Year Ended 31st December 1918*, 27.

27. UI, *Colonial Annual Reports, No. 1315, Nigeria*, "Reports for 1925," 12; WA28 HN5 N68, *Nigeria. Annual Medical and Sanitary Report*, 1925, 8; WA28 HN5 N68, *Nigeria. Annual Medical and Sanitary Report*, 1924, 9.

28. WA28 HN5 N68, *Nigeria. Annual Medical and Sanitary Report*, 1924, 9.

29. WA28 HN5 N68, *Nigeria. Annual Medical and Sanitary Report*, 1925, 8.

30. CRL, H7/B/7/2, *West Africa*, 3.

31. H. W. Turner, *History of an African Independent Church* (Oxford: Clarendon Press, 1967), 9; Peel, *Aladura*, 62–63.

32. See H. W. Turner, *History of an African Independent Church* (Oxford: Clarendon Press, 1967), 9; Peel, *Aladura*, 62–63; Alokan, *Christ Apostolic Church*, 18–19.

33. See OYO PROF 662, "Cherubim and Seraphim Society," 1–3, 11.

34. OYO PROF 662, "Aladura Movement," 45; CRL ACC 716 F8, "The Prophet Movement in Ekiti and Beyond by Archdeacon Dallimore, Lagos Diocese," *Church Missionary Outlook* LIX (January 1932): 1; Alokan, *Christ Apostolic Church*, 36–38; Babalola, *Joseph Ayo Babalola*, 74–77.

35. Babalola, *Joseph Ayo Babalola*, 75.

36. NAI OYOPROF 662, *The Faith Healer-Babalola*, 9.

37. CRL ACC 716 F8, "The Prophet Movement in Ekiti and Beyond," January 1932, 1; CRL ACC 716 F8, "The Aladura Movement in Ekiti," *Church Missionary Outlook*, May 1931, 94; Babalola, *Joseph Ayo Babalola*, 75–77.

38. CRL ACC 716 F8, "The Prophet Movement in Ekiti and Beyond," 1; CRL ACC 716 F8, "The Aladura Movement in Ekiti," 94; Babalola, *Joseph Ayo Babalola*, 75–77.

39. CRL ACC 716 F8, "The Aladura Movement in Ekiti," 94; CRL ACC 716 F8, "The Prophet Movement in Ekiti and Beyond," 2.

40. CRL ACC 716 F8, "The Prophet Movement in Ekiti and Beyond," 2.

41. CRL ACC 716 F8, "The Aladura Movement in Ekiti," 94.

42. CRL ACC 716 F8, "The Aladura Movement in Ekiti."

43. Other converts joined new and existing African Independent Churches that either emerged during Babalola's prophetic movement or gained widespread attention during that period.

44. NAI OYOPROF 1/28, *Aladura Movement (Apostolic Church)*, "The Apostolic Church in Ilesha. Your Confidential Memo," 3–4.

45. CRL CMS ACC 716 F8, *The Church Missionary Outlook*, 182–183; "The Aladura Movement in Ekiti," 96–97.

46. NAI OYO PROF 662, "Faith Tabernacle, Ilesha," 9.

47. CRL CMS ACC 716 F8, "The Prophet Movement in Ekiti and Beyond," September 1932, 182.

48. CRL CMS ACC 716 F8, "The Prophet Movement in Ekiti and Beyond," 182–183; CRL CMS ACC 716 F8, "The Aladura Movement in Ekiti," 96–97.

49. CRL CMS G/Y/A/2/2, "Extract from Minutes of the Missionary Conference of the CMS Yoruba Mission Held in Lagos, January 7 to 16, 1932. (Despatch, Yoruba No. 15 of 1932.)"; CRL CMS ACC 716 F8, "The Prophet Movement in Ekiti and Beyond," September 1932, 183.

50. CRL H7/B/51/3/21 *Nigeria*, "The Social Impacts of New Religious Movements on Yoruba Life," 41.

51. NAI OYOPROF 662, *The Faith Healer—Babalola*, 9–16.

52. NAI OYOPROF 662, *The Faith Healer—Babalola*; "*Aladura* Religious Movement," 30.

53. NAI OYO PROF 662, "Extract from Memorandum NO. 404/30/1930 of 20th April, 1931, from A.D.O. Ilesha to District Officer, Ife," 13.

54. NAI OYO PROF 662, *The Faith Healer—Babalola*, 22–23, 31–38, 46.

55. NAI OYO PROF 662, "Extract from Memorandum NO. 404/30/1930 of 20th April, 1931, from A.D.O. Ilesha to District Officer, Ife," 13.

56. NAI OYO PROF 662, *The Faith Healer—Babalola*, 22–23, 31–38, 46.

57. NAI OYO PROF 662, *The Faith Healer—Babalola*, 30.

58. NAI OYO PROF 662, *The Faith Healer—Babalola*, 32–33.

59. Earlier African church movements like the Garrick Braide movement of 1915 in the Niger Delta and other movements that the colonial government classified as "Spirit Movement" existed but neither spread nor endured like the Aladura movement.

60. OYO PROF 1 662, *The Faith Healer—Babalola*, 3–6.

61. OYO PROF 1 662, *The Faith Healer—Babalola*, 3.

62. CRL CMS ACC 716 F8, "The Aladura Movement in Ekiti," 96.

63. NAI OYOPROF 662, "Aladura Religious Movement," 30; NAI OYOPROF 662, "Aladura Movement," 32.

64. CRL CMS ACC 716 F8, "The Prophet Movement in Ekiti and Beyond," January 1932, 2–3; CMS ACC 716 F8, "The Prophetic Movement in Ekiti and Beyond," September 1932, 184; OYOPROF 662, *The Faith Healer—Babalola* 3–5.

65. Government of Nigeria, *Census of Nigeria, 1931*, 22–23.

66. Government of Nigeria, *Census of Nigeria, 1931*, vol. vi, 31.

67. Nekpen Ebohon and Pat Ibude, "Childless Marriage: Is the Woman to Blame," *Sunday Times*, October 18, 1992, 13; Tola Olu Pierce, "She Will Not Be Listened to in Public: Perceptions among the Yoruba of Infertility and Childlessness in Women," *Reproductive Health Matters* 7, no. 13 (1999): 69.

68. Ebohon and Ibude, "Childless Marriage," 13.

69. Interview with Victoria Ayobola, Oke-Ola, January 23, 2021.

70. WL ANN REP WA28 NH5 N68 1922–1925, *Annual Medical and Sanitary Report for the Year 1922*, 19; WL ANN REP WA28 NH5 N68 1926–1928, *Annual Medical and Sanitary Report for the Year 1926*, 37.

71. WL ANN REP WA28 NH5 N68 1922–1925, *Annual Medical and Sanitary Report for the Year 1922*, 19.

72. WL Nigeria, *Southern Provinces. Annual Medical and Sanitary Report for the Year Ended 31st December 1918*, 37.

73. CRL CMS ACC 716 F8, "The Prophet Movement in Ekiti and Beyond," January 1932, 3.

74. For some missionary references to Babalola's maternity services, see CRL CMS ACC 716 F8, "The Prophetic Movement in Ekiti and Beyond," January 1932, 3; CMS ACC 716 F8, "The Prophetic Movement in Ekiti and Beyond," September 1932, 184, OYOPROF 662, 3–5.

75. CRL CMS ACC 716 F8, "The Prophetic Movement in Ekiti and Beyond," January 1932, 3.

76. WL, *Nigeria. Southern Provinces. Annual Medical and Sanitary Report for the Year Ended 31st December 1915*, 38; WL, *Nigeria. Southern Provinces. Annual Medical and Sanitary Report for the Year Ended 31st December 1916*, 6; WL, *Nigeria. Southern Provinces. Annual Medical and Sanitary Report for the Year Ended 31st December 1929*, 11.

77. NAI OYO PROF 662, "Faith Tabernacle, Ilesha," 9; CRL CMS ACC 716 F8, "The Prophetic Movement in Ekiti and Beyond," September 1932, 182.

78. CRL CMS ACC 716 F8, "The Prophetic Movement in Ekiti and Beyond," September 1932, 182.

79. See WL, *Nigeria. Southern Provinces. Annual Medical and Sanitary Report for the Year Ended 31st December 1929*, 34–36.

80. WL, *Nigeria. Southern Provinces. Annual Medical and Sanitary Report for the Year Ended 31st December 1930*, 31–32.

81. BNA MH 55/269, *Maternal Mortality Departmental Committee Memorandum on Antenatal Clinics*, "Maternal Mortality in Childbirth," 3.

82. "Exodus," chapter 1, verse 19, *Holy Bible*, New International Version.

83. See CRL H7/B/42/101 CAC, "The Christ Apostolic Church, Its History, Beliefs and Organization," *Ecumenical Review* 28, no. 4 (1976): 418–424; E. O. A. Adejobi, *An Address Entitled "Facts about Faith, Psychic or Spiritual Healing" Delivered to the Teachers in Theological Colleges at the Emmanuel College, Ibadan*, May 1974, 4–5; CRL H7/B/42/101, Africa, Nigeria, John Ferguson, "Christianity in Interaction with Yoruba Culture," 6.

84. Babalola, *Joseph Ayo Babalola*, 6–7, 75–76; CRL H7/B/42/101 CAC, "The Christ Apostolic Church," 419.

85. Interview with M. A. Adeleye, Lagos, July 2, 2018; interview with E. O. T. Olorunwa, Lagos, March 23, 2016; interview with Moses Olowe, Oke-Ife, November 18, 2015; Babalola, *Joseph Ayo Babalola*, 6.

86. See Babalola, *Joseph Ayo Babalola*, 6.

87. Babalola, *Joseph Ayo Babalola*, 10.

88. CRL CMS ACC 716 F8, "The Prophetic Movement in Ekiti and Beyond," January 1932, 1.

89. Interview with Olowe; interview with Adeleye; interview with Olorunwa.

90. See CMS's CRL ACC 716 F8, "The Aladura Movement in Ekiti," 94; Babalola, *Joseph Ayo Babalola*, 48–55.

91. Interview with Olowe.

92. NAE, MISF 257, Box 161, F. A. M. Adewale-Abayomi, "African Traditional Healing through Ohun Ife," *Orunmila* 2 (1986): 25–26.

93. Adewale-Abayomi, "African Traditional Healing through Ohun Ife," 25. See also Sanya Onabamiro, *Why Our Children Die: The Causes and Suggestions for Prevention of Infant Mortality in West Africa* (London: Methuen, 1949), 17–20, for further description of this process among the Yoruba.

94. Adewale-Abayomi, "African Traditional Healing through Ohun Ife," 25; Onabamiro, *Why Our Children Die*, 17–20.

95. See NAE, MISF 257, Box 161, Adeboye Oyesanya, "Ifa: The Do It Yourself for the Beginners," 8–9.

96. CRL ACC 716 F8, "The Prophet Movement in Ekiti," 94.

97. CRL ACC 716 F8, "The Prophet Movement in Ekiti"; interview with Olorunwa; interview with Lydia Ajayi, Ofatedo, October 18, 2020.

98. CRL H7/B/42/101 CAC, "Christ Apostolic Church," 419–420.

99. Babalola, *Joseph Ayo Babalola*, 13.

100. Babalola, *Joseph Ayo Babalola*, 7.

101. Babalola, *Joseph Ayo Babalola*, 2–7, 10, 13–14.

102. Babalola, *Joseph Ayo Babalola*, 14.

103. Babalola, *Joseph Ayo Babalola*, 9.

104. Babalola, *Joseph Ayo Babalola*.

105. Babalola, *Joseph Ayo Babalola*, 11.

106. Babalola, *Joseph Ayo Babalola*, 10.

107. Babalola, *Joseph Ayo Babalola*, 8, 13–14.

108. This letter is reproduced in full on the website of The Apostolic Church Nigeria (TACN). Available: https://tacnlawna.org/the-great-schism-and-emergence-of-cac/#_ftn11. Accessed February 26, 2021.

109. Christ Apostolic Church, *The Constitution and the Order of Service* (Nigeria, n.d.), 42. The CAC's publication in *Ecumenical Review* places the date of their first constitution at 1946.

110. The expansion of female education and maternity services is discussed extensively in the previous chapter.

111. *Daily Times* Photo Interview, "Boys and Girls Must Be Given Equal Education," *Daily Times*, December 21, 1949, 6; "Misunderstanding Cleared on Colonial Question," *Daily Times*, December 19, 1949, 3; Mrs. Ibiyemi Bright, "Should Married Women Work," *Daily Times*, April 10, 1950, 5; London Correspondent, "Training of Women Reviewed," *Daily Times*, August 15, 1949, 15.

112. Interview with Adeleye; interview with Comfort Aluko, Ibadan, November 20, 2015.

113. Grade II midwifery originally allowed people with very limited Western education to qualify as midwives. For more on Grade I and Grade II midwifery, see chapter 3.

114. WL, HIB/948, *Annual Report of the Federal Medical Services 1958*, 4.

115. WL, HIB/948, *Annual Report of the Federal Medical Services 1958*.

116. Crab Ewulu, "Nursing and Midwifery," *West African Pilot*, December 20, 1963.

117. CRL H7/B/42/101, CAC, "Christ Apostolic Church," 420.

118. Interview with Victoria Alabi, Ede, October 17, 2020.

119. "Lagos Clinic Critics Are Replied," *Daily Times*, April 28, 1950, 11. See also similar accounts in Sunday Abukuru, "Hospitals without Doctors," *Daily Times*, April 14, 1978, 21; Festus Ijilade, "Stories of Woe in State Hospitals," *Daily Times*, April 1978, 3.

120. Alokan, *Christ Apostolic Church*, 353–354. See also 221, 234.

121. See H7/B/42/124, *Africa Nigeria, Recent Developments in the Healing Concepts and Activities of Aladura Churches*, 9.

122. Interview with Funmilola Awoyungbo, Ede, October 27, 2020.

123. Interview with Funmilola Awoyungbo.

124. Interview with Alabi.

125. This training center at Ede is popularly called the CAC Faith Home, Faith Home Training Center, and Faith Home School of Midwifery. Its official title is Faith Home, Childbirth, and Missionary Health Workers Training Center. I refer to the training center interchangeably as the faith home training center and faith home school of midwifery.

126. Interview with Olorunwa; interview with Deaconess Oyewo, Idi-Oro, July 2, 2018.

127. Interview with Adeleye.

128. For more on gender in Aladura churches, see Brigid Sackey, *New Directions in Gender and Religion: The Changing Status of Women in African Independent Churches* (Lanham, MD: Lexington Books, 2006); Isabel Mukonyora, *Wandering a Gendered Wilderness: Suffering and Healing in an African Initiated Church* (New York: Peter Lang, 2007); Deidre Helen Crumbley, *Spirit, Structure, and Flesh: Gendered Experiences in African Instituted Churches among the Yoruba of Nigeria* (Madison: University of Wisconsin Press, 2008); Adam Mohr, "Faith Tabernacle Congregation and the Emergence of Pentecostalism in Colonial Nigeria, 1910s–1941," *Journal of Religion in Africa* 43 (2013): 196–221.

129. For more information on Mama Ogunranti (Joanah Ogunranti), see her profile on her congregation's webpage: https://mountbethelministry.tripod.com/joanah1.htm. Accessed November 20, 2020. She founded several CAC Bethel congregations in Nigeria and abroad. See also Crumbley, *Spirit, Structure, and Flesh*, 105–106.

130. Interview with Dorcas Olaniyi, Ibadan, November 23, 2015; Gabriel Adeyemi and Freeman Okosun, *The Great Woman of God Archbishop (Dr.) Dorcas Siyanbola. Olaniyi at 70* (Ibadan: Freeman Productions, 2004).

131. Interview with Midwife Oluwaleye Ara, Odi Olowo, March 22, 2016; interview with Adeleye.

132. Interview with Awoyungbo.

133. Interview with Midwife Alu, 60+, Ibadan, November 20, 2015.

134. Interview with Comfort Aluko.

135. Interview with Alabi.

136. Interview with Victoria Ayobola, Ejigbo, January 23, 2021.

137. Interview with Alabi.

138. Interview with Adeleye; interview with Awoyungbo.

139. Interview with Aluko.

140. Interview with Aluko.

141. Interview with Aluko.

142. Interview with Aluko.

143. Interview with Adeleye.

144. Interview with Adeleye.

145. Interview with Esther Oluwafemi, Okeife, November 18, 2016.

146. Interview with Ara; interview with Olowe; interview with Aluko.

147. "Exodus," chapter 1, verse 19.

148. CRL ACC 716/F8, "The Prophetic Movement in Ekiti and Beyond," January 1932, 3.

149. See H7/B/42/124, *Africa Nigeria, Recent Developments*, 9.

150. Interview with Aluko.

Chapter 4. "Birth Control Under Whatever Name"

1. British National Archives (BNA), CO 859/52/17, *Birth Control West Africa*, "Extract from Letter from Dr. Julian Huxley to the Colonial Secretary of State dated 17th July, 1943," 1.

2. See Matthew Connelly, *Fatal Misconception: The Struggle to Control World Population* (Cambridge, MA: Harvard University Press, 2008), 18–45; Nicole Bourbonnais, *Birth Control in the Decolonizing Caribbean: Reproductive Politics and Practice on Four Islands, 1930–1970* (Cambridge, UK: Cambridge University Press, 2016), 10–11; Dudley Kirk, "Population Changes and the Postwar World," *American Sociological Review* 9, no. 1 (1944): 148–157.

3. For more on eugenics, see Edwin Black, *War against the Weak: Eugenics and America's Campaign to Create a Master Race-Expanded* (Washington, DC: Dialog Press, 2008); Harry Bruinius, *Better for All the World: The Secret History of Forced Sterilization and America's Quest for Racial Purity* (New York: Vintage Press, 2007); Wendy Kline, *Building a Better Race: Gender, Sexuality, and Eugenics from the Turn of the Century to the Baby Boom* (Berkeley: University of California Press, 2005).

4. BNA CO 859/52/17, *Birth Control West Africa*, "Extract from Letter," 1.

5. BNA CO 859/52/17, *Birth Control West Africa*, "Extract from Letter," 1–2.

6. BNA CO 859/52/17, *Birth Control West Africa*, "Extract from Letter."

7. BNA CO 859/52/17, *Birth Control West Africa*, "Response to Letter from Julian Huxley," 1.

8. See BNA CO 859/62/16, *Birth Control: West Indies, 1941–1942*. See also Bourbonnais, *Birth Control*, 21–26; Juanita de Barros, *Reproducing the British Caribbean: Sex, Gender, and Population Politics after Slavery* (Chapel Hill: University of North Carolina Press, 2014); Nicholas Bourbonnais, "Reproductive Rights and Race Struggle in the Decolonizing Caribbean, Black Perspectives," April 1, 2017, https://www.aaihs.org/reproductive-rights-and -race-struggle-in-the-decolonizing-caribbean/; BNA CO 859/52/17, *Birth Control West Africa*, "Response to Letter from Julian Huxley," 1; Dorothy Roberts, *Killing the Black Body: Race, Reproduction, and the Meaning of Liberty* (New York: Pantheon Books, 1997); Chloe Campbell, *Race and Empire: Eugenics in Colonial Kenya* (Manchester: Manchester University Press, 2007); Betsy Hartmann, *Reproductive Rights and Wrongs: The Global Politics of Population Control* (Boston: South End Press, 1995); Harriet Washington, *Medical Apartheid: The Dark History of Medical Experimentation on Black Americans from the Colonial Times to the Present* (New York: Harlem Moon, 2008).

9. Roberts, *Killing the Black Body*; Campbell, *Race and Empire*; Hartmann, *Reproductive Rights and Wrongs*; Washington, *Medical Apartheid*.

10. Connelley, *Fatal Misconception*, 122.

11. Wellcome Library (WL), MEDK22987; Robert Rene Kuczynski, *Demographic Survey of the British Colonial Empire: Vol. 1. West Africa* (Oxford: Oxford University Press, 1948).

12. BNA CO 859/52/17, *Birth Control West Africa*, "Response to," 1.

13. BNA CO 859/52/17, *Birth Control West Africa*, "Response to."

14. RAC JDR III 80/667/670, *Population Interests General*, "Summary Report, Conference on Population Problems, 1952," 1952–1961, 6–10; RAC JDR III 85/718-719/FA108, 104.54.1, *Population Council Williamsburg Conference*, 1952, 1–10. See Connelley, *Fatal Misconception*, 155–156, for more details of how this conference materialized.

15. RAC JDR III 80/667/670, *Population Interests General*, "Summary Report," 6.

16. RAC JDR III 80/667/670, *Population Interests General 1952–1961*, "The Population Problem. A Tentative Analysis," 1952, 2.

17. RAC JDR III 80/667/670, *Population Interests General 1952–1961*, "The Population Problem. A Tentative Analysis."

18. RAC JDR III 80/667/670, *Population Interests General*, "Summary Report," 8.

19. BNA CO 859/52/17, *Birth Control West Africa*, "Response to Letter from Julian Huxley," 2.

20. BNA CO 859/52/17, *Birth Control West Africa*, "Response to Letter from Julian Huxley," 1.

21. BNA, CO 917/2, *Pan African Health Conference*, 1935 file; "Developing Britain's Colonies," *Daily Times*, December 28, 1949, 3.

22. BNA CO 323/1463/5, *Medical Miscellaneous: Abortion in the Colonies*, 2.

23. WL MEDK22987, Kuczynski, *Demographic Survey*, vi.

24. See WL MEDK22987, Kuczynski, *Demographic Survey*, 542–555.

25. Government of Nigeria, *Census of Nigeria, 1931*, vol. iii (London: Government of Nigeria, 1932), 1.

26. Kuczinsky arrives at a similar conclusion in WL MEDK22987, HH 3/West Africa, "Population of," Kuczynski, *Demographic Survey*, 655.

27. University of Illinois (UI) 3064634, *Annual Report of the Social and Economic Progress of the People of Nigeria, 1931*, "Population."

28. BNA MH 55/269, *Maternal Mortality Departmental Committee Memorandum on Antenatal Clinics*, "Maternal Mortality in Childbirth," 2–5.

29. "The Education of the African Woman (Final Article)," *Nigerian Daily Times*, November 1, 1928, 6.

30. "Childlife in Nigeria," *Nigerian Daily Times*, August 20, 1928, 4.

31. WL MEDK22987, HH 3/West Africa, "Population of," Kuczynski, *Demographic Survey*, 677–678.

32. WL 954574379, *Lagos Health and Baby Week*, April 22–29, 6.

33. BNA CO 583/296/4, *Resettlement of Africans in Overpopulated Areas*, "Mass Transfer of Populations," 5. See also UI 3064634, *Annual Report*, "Population," 6.

34. BNA CO 583/296/4, *Resettlement of Africans*, 5.

35. BNA CO 583/296/4, *Resettlement of Africans in Overpopulated Areas*, "Nigeria. Order in Council," 1432.

36. Interview with Mrs. Omolayo Adeyemi, Lagos, December 5, 2021.

37. Locals sought labor for their own benefits and sustenance while the government's objective was geared toward imperial extraction, by force or by mutual agreement, for the benefit of the British colony and its allies.

38. Interview with Ichie Nwezefunamba, Onitsha, July 7, 2019.

39. Interview with Mrs. Adedeji, November 3, 2021.

40. Interview with Mrs. Adedeji, November 3, 2021.

41. Interview with Mrs. Omotosho, Ibadan, November 25, 2021. For more on breastfeeding as a traditional birth control method, see also NACP R286/P792/4-7, *Nigeria-Reports, Correspondence*, "Family Planning at the University College Hospital, Ibadan 1965–1982, Planners Forum Magazine," 3; NACP R286/P811/3, *Nigeria 08 Birth Spacing Project*, "USAID/Nigeria Population Officer," 13.

42. Interview with Mrs. Balogun, Ibadan, November 26, 2021.

43. Interview with Mrs. Adedeji.

44. Interview with Dr. Alalaye, Ibadan, February 2, 2022.

45. Interview with Dr. Alalaye, Ibadan, February 2, 2022.

46. Interview with Mrs. Balogun.

47. Interview with Mrs. Balogun.

48. Interview with Mrs. Isiak.

49. Interview with Mrs. Isiak; interview with Alalaye.

50. Interview with Mrs. Adeyemi; interview with Mrs. Omotosho, Oke Ife, November 25, 2021; interview with Mrs. Adedeji; interview with Mrs. Balogun.

51. Interview with Mrs. Adeyemi.

52. Interview with Mrs. Adeyemi.

53. References on the global powershift in the Cold War era as well as the increased oversight that Britain began to have from international organizations in Nigeria.

54. RAC JDR III 80/667/670, *Population Interests General 1952–1961*, "The Population Problem. A Tentative Analysis," 1–12.

55. RAC JDR III 80/667/670, *Population Interests General 1952–1961*, "The Population Problem. A Tentative Analysis," 4–5.

56. RAC JDR III 80/667/670, *Population Interests General 1952–1961*, "Conference on Population Problems," 6.

57. RAC JDR III 80/667/670, *Population Interests General 1952–1961*, "Conference on Population Problems," 7.

58. RAC JDR III 80/667/670, *Population Interests General 1952–1961*, "Conference on Population Problems," 8.

59. RAC JDR III 80/667/670, "The Population Problem. A Tentative Analysis," 2. See also RAC JDR III 80/667/670, *Population Interests General 1952–1961*, "Conference on Population Problems," 9, for a definite statement on the Population Council's mandate. Connelly writes that the Williamsburg conference gave Rockefeller III a license to do what he liked, resulting in his funding of PC. See *Fatal Misconception*, 159. See also Donald Critchlow, *Intended Consequences: Birth Control, Abortion and the Federal Government in Modern America* (Oxford: Oxford University Press, 1999), 14–30, for more information of JDR III and the Population Council.

60. NACP R286/P822/4, *Economic Assistance Task Force FY 61*, "Nigeria. Program Development Task Force," 1.

61. See RAC JDR III 80/667/670, *Population Interests General 1952–1961*, "Conference on Population Problems," 1–10; NACP R286/P822/4, *Economic Assistance Task Force FY 61*, "Nigeria. Program Development Task Force," 1.

62. See Ibid.; NACP R286/P792/4-7, "Nigeria-Reports."

63. NACP R286 P606, *AHEA Consultations, Field Visits, Workshops (Nigeria-Panama)*, "The Possibility of a POPLAB in Nigeria," 1972, 1.

64. NACP R286 P606, *AHEA Consultations*, 1972, 1; NACP R286/P792/4-7, "Nigeria-Reports"; International Planned Parenthood Federation Archives (IPPFA), *IPPF Governing Body, 14th Meeting (Special Meeting) 5th–7th November*, "Discussion on Additional Grant Support," 19.

65. International Planned Parenthood Federation Archives (IPPFA), *IPPF Governing Body, 14th Meeting (Special Meeting) 5th–7th November*, "Discussion on Additional Grant Support."

66. Robert Morgan, "Family Planning Acceptors in Lagos, Nigeria," *Studies in Family Planning* 3, no. 9 (1972): 221–222.

67. See Morgan, "Family Planning Acceptors in Lagos, Nigeria," 221–223.

68. NACP R286/P792/4-7, *Nigeria-Reports, Correspondence*, "Family Planning at the University College Hospital, Ibadan 1965–1982, Planners Forum Magazine," 3.

69. NACP R286/P792/4-7, *Nigeria-Reports, Correspondence*, "Family Planning at the University College Hospital, Ibadan 1965–1982, Planners Forum Magazine," 3.

70. Layi Olajide, "Family Planning Is Very Necessary," *Daily Times*, January 20, 1973, 13; Air Iyare, "Birth Control through Family Planning," *Nigerian Observer*, September 7, 1973, 10.

71. G. B. Ajayi, "Birth Control Controversy. Extended Family: Core of African Society," *Daily Times*, January 8, 1973, 7.

72. NACP R286/P822/4, *Economic Assistance Task Force*, "Nigeria. Program Development Taskforce," 1961–1972, 2.

73. Layi Olajide, "Family Planning Is Very Necessary," *Daily Times*, January 20, 1973, 13.

74. S. C. Onoguwe, "Family Planning and Our Social Problems," *Nigerian Observer*, October 8, 1973, 9.

75. O. A. Ojo (Jr.), "Population Growth and Its Problems," August 20, 1972, *Sunday Sketch*, 2.

76. Kenule Sarowiwa, "We Need More Babies Here," *Daily Times*, November 12, 1971.

77. Alexander Akinyele, "Pill Pedlars Are Welcome," *Daily Times*, December 11, 1971, 7.

78. For instance, the series of responses to Tsaro-Wiwa's article on birth control were featured in *Daily Times*' Birth Control Row. See Felix Adenaike, "We Want More Babies Here But . . . ," *Daily Times*, December 11, 1971, 7; I. B. Abodunrin, "Where Tsaro-Wiwa Is Wrong," *Daily Times*, December 11, 1971, 7; Akinyele, "Pill Pedlars Are Welcome," 7.

79. "Dr. Adetoro on Family Planning," *The Truth Weekly*, November 8–14, 1968, 1.

80. "Chief Awolowo on Family Planning," *The Truth Weekly*, October 25–31, 1968, 8.

81. "Birth Control," *The Truth Weekly*, November 8–14, 1968, 7.

82. "Birth Control," *The Truth Weekly*, November 8–14, 1968.

83. Federal Republic of Nigeria, *Second National Development Plan 1970–74* (Lagos: Federal Ministry of Information, 1970), 77–78.

84. "The Role of Family Planning in Nigeria," *Lagos Weekend*, September 30, 1977, 16.

85. RAC Ford Foundation (RAC FF) FA571/3/7, *Family Planning Communications in Nigeria*, 7.

86. See NACP R 286 P811 5, *Education THRU Programs*, 2.

87. RAC Population Council (PC) S 107/FA432, *Nigeria, Post-partum Program D&I-S*, "Lagos Island Maternity Hospital Proposal," 1967, 1.

88. RAC Population Council (PC) S 107/FA432, *Nigeria, Post-partum Program D&I-S*, "Lagos Island Maternity Hospital Proposal," 1967.

89. RAC (PC), S 107/FA432, *Nigeria, Postpartum Program*, "Site Visit to Lagos Island Maternity Hospital," 6.

90. RAC (PC), S 107/FA432, *Nigeria, Postpartum Program*, "Site Visit to Lagos Island Maternity Hospital," 2.

91. Iyare, "Birth Control through Family Planning," 10.

92. RAC Ford Foundation (FF) FA571/4/4, *A Report on a Visit to Nigeria to Consult on Communications Activities of the Family Planning Council of Nigeria*, "Proposed FPCH Education/Motivation Campaign for Men," 1973, 4. This is also reported in Iyare, "Birth Control through Family Planning," 10.

93. Ebele Ene, "Family Planning, Fertility Control and the Law in Nigeria—The Choices for a New Century," *African Journal of Reproductive Health* 2, no. 2 (1998): 90. See also Arthur Erken, ed., *My Body Is My Own: Claiming the Right to Autonomy and Self-Determination* (New York: UNFPA, 2021).

94. Interview with Mrs. Adedeji.

95. Promiscuity as the basis of opposition to family planning recurs multiple times in Nigerian newspapers. Examples include Iyare, "Birth Control through Family Planning," 10; Onoguwe, "Family Planning," 9; Bose Orishawo, "Times Woman," *Daily Times*, September 30, 1991, 32; Pat Odedina, "Should Teenagers Use Contraceptives?" *Daily Times*, September 29, 1991, 13.

96. Bose Orishawo, "Times Woman," *Daily Times*, September 30, 1991, 32.

97. RAC Ford Foundation (FF) FA571/4/4, *A Report on a Visit to Nigeria to Consult on Communications Activities of the Family Planning Council of Nigeria*, "Proposed FPCH Education/Motivation Campaign for Men," 1.

98. Clarkson de Majomi, "Africa Accepts Birth Control," *Daily Times*, January 8, 1973, 7.

99. Odedina, "Should Teenagers Use Contraceptives?" 13.

100. RAC PC, S 107/FA432, *Postpartum Program*, "Recommendations," 2.

101. RAC PC, S 107/FA432, *Postpartum Program*, "Recommendations."

102. RAC PC, S 107/FA432, *Postpartum Program*, "Recommendations."

103. RAC PC, S 107/FA432, *Postpartum Program*, "Recommendations."

104. RAC PC, S 107/FA432, *Postpartum Program*, "Recommendations," 2; RAC Ford Foundation (FF) FA571/4/4, *A Report on a Visit*, 5.

105. RAC Ford Foundation (FF) FA571/4/4, *A Report on a Visit*.

106. RAC Ford Foundation (FF) FA571/4/4, *A Report on a Visit*, 4.

107. RAC Ford Foundation (FF) FA571/4/4, *A Report on a Visit*.

108. WL 7720600, *Choices. Lyrics*.

109. RAC FF FA571/3/7, *Family Planning Communications in Nigeria*, 5.

110. "Training in Family Planning," *Daily Times*, December 2, 1972.

111. NACP R286 P606, *AHEA Consultations, Field Visits, Workshops (Nigeria-Panama)*, "The Possibility of a POPLAB in Nigeria," 1972, 1.

112. NACP R286 P606, *AHEA Consultations, Field Visits, Workshops (Nigeria-Panama)*, "February 21, 1973. For the Attention of: The Chief Inspector of Education, 1"; "December 6, 1972," 2.

113. NACP R286 P606, *AHEA Consultations*, "AHEA NEWS," 1–2.

114. See NAI OYO PROF 1/1129, *Domestic Training for Girls-Suggestions as to*, 1933, 3; CRL G/Y/A/9/2, *Northern Nigeria Missions*, ". . . in Nigeria, dated Achimota, 28th May 1927," 2.

115. NACP R286 P606, *AHEA International Family Planning Conference*, "AID Project-The Role of Home Economics in Family Planning," 6.

116. NACP R286/P646/11, *AHEA IPF Workshop London*, "Home Economics and Family Planning: Pathways for Change," 1975, 2.

117. Henry Kamm, "Pope to Nigerians: Defend the Family," *New York Times*, February 14, 1982, 4.

118. NACP R286/P811/3, *Nigeria 08 Birth Spacing Project*, 1981, 3.

119. See NACP R286/P811/3, *Nigeria 08 Birth Spacing Project*.

120. NACP R286/P811/3, *Nigeria 08 Birth Spacing Project*, "USAID/Nigeria Population Officer," 1.

121. See Frederick John Dealtry Lugard, *The Dual Mandate in British Tropical Africa* (London: William Blackwood and Sons, 1922), 594; CMS G/3/A/9/0 *Map of Northern Nigeria*, 9; Andrew Barnes, *Making Headway: The Introduction of Western Civilization in Colonial Northern Nigeria* (Rochester, NY: University of Rochester Press, 2009), 133; Shobana Shankar, *Who Shall Enter Paradise: Christian Origins in Modern Northern Nigeria, ca. 1890–1975* (Athens: Ohio University Press, 2014), 72, 78–79; G/Y/A/9/2, "Memorandum on Missionary Work in Northern Nigeria," 6.

122. NACP R286/P811/3, *Nigeria 08 Birth Spacing Project*, "USAID/Nigeria Population Officer," 13.

123. Interview with Mrs. Omotosho, Oke Ife, November 25, 2021.

124. Interview with Mrs. Adedeji.

125. Interview with Mrs. Adedeji.

126. Interview with Mrs. Olaoba, Odo-Ona, December 14, 2021.

127. Interview with Mrs. Olaoba.

128. Interview with Mrs. Adedeji.

129. Interview with Mrs. Omotosho, Ibadan, November 25, 2021.

130. Interview with Mrs. Omotosho; interview with Dr. Alalaye; interview with Mrs Olaoba.

131. Interview with Mrs Olaoba.

132. "Beware of the Pill," *Nigerian Tide*, September 2, 1981, 8.

133. "Beware of the Pill," *Nigerian Tide*, September 2, 1981.

134. Awusinba Iyalla, "Contraception and What It Does to Your Health," *Sunday Tide*, August 30, 1981, 13.

135. Interview with Mrs. Isiaka; interview with Mrs. Adeyemi; interview with Mrs. Balogun; interview with Mrs. Ajibade.

136. Interview with Mrs. Balogun.

137. Interview with Mrs. Adeyemi.

138. Interview with Mrs. Ajibade.

139. Francis Agbo, "Family Planning Has Its Advantage," *Nigerian Standard*, June 20, 1977.

140. "Family Planning Helps Families," *Lagos Weekend*, August 8, 1980, 10.

141. K. Mazzocco, "Nigeria's New Population Policy," *International Health News*, March 9, 1988, 1–12; "Nigeria Chief Urges 4-Child Limit," *Deseret News*, April 16, 1989.

142. WL SA/ICM/7/1/1, *JSG 1970–1980*, "International Federation of Gynecology and Obstetrics. International Confederation of Midwives," 3.

143. WL SA/ICM/7/1/1, *JSG 1970–1980*, "International Federation of Gynecology and Obstetrics. International Confederation of Midwives."

144. WL SA/ICM/7/1/1, *JSG 1970–1980*, "International Federation of Gynecology and Obstetrics. International Confederation of Midwives," 2.

145. See "Family Planning Helps Families," *Lagos Weekend*, August 8, 1980, 10; "The Role of Family Planning in Nigeria," *Lagos Weekend*, September 30, 1977, 15.

146. Karen Otsea and Family Care International, *Progress and Prospects: The Safe Motherhood Initiative, 1987–1992* (Washington, DC: The World Bank, 1992), 3, 6.

Chapter 5. Reinventing Themselves

1. Interview with Ademola Saheed on behalf of Durodola Abimbola, Ibadan, November 15, 2015.

2. J. O. Mume, *Tradomedicalism: What Is It?* (Warri: Jom Nature Cure Center, 1980), 60.

3. See E. A. Ayandele, *The Missionary Impact on Modern Nigeria 1842–1914: A Political and Social Analysis* (London: Longman Group LTD, 1966).

4. Interview with Abimbola Durodola, January 23, 2022.

5. British National Archives (BNA) CO 583/248/6, *Training of Subordinate Staff in the Medical Department*, "Mission Activities African Missions," 1930, 13.

6. Stacey Langwick, *Bodies, Politics, and African Healing: The Matter of Maladies in Tanzania* (Bloomington: Indiana University Press, 2011), 121–150.

7. See Karen Otsea and Family Care International, *Progress and Prospects: The Safe Motherhood Initiative, 1987–1992* (Washington, DC: The World Bank, 1992).

8. See Cadbury Research Library (CRL) CMS, *The Mission Hospital* xxxiv (1930): 172; CRL M/Y/A2/1, 1918–1945, "Extract from Letter from Miss D. Jewitt, dated 4/11/42," 1942; National Archives Enugu (NAE) MINHEALTH 30/1/253, *Medical Development in Nigeria*, 1946, 127, 235; NSUDIV 12/1/38, *Midwives General*, 1955–1960.

9. NAE MINHEALTH 30/1/253, *Medical Development in Nigeria*, "Co-operation with Voluntary Bodies," 28.

10. NAE MINHEALTH 30/1/253, *Medical Development in Nigeria*, "Proceedings of a Meeting of District Officers and Local Heads of Regionalized Departments of the Rivers Province Held at Resident's Office, Port Harcourt on 19th June, 1947," 178.

11. NAE MINHEALTH 30/1/253, *Medical Development in Nigeria*, 127.

12. NAE MINHEALTH 30/1/253, *Medical Development in Nigeria*, 235.

13. NSUDIV 12/1/38, *Midwives General*, "Community Nurse Training Center at School of Hygiene, Aba," 1954–1960, 1.

14. NSUDIV 12/1/38, *Midwives General*, "Community Nurse Training Center at School of Hygiene, Aba," 1954–1960.

15. NSUDIV 12/1/38, *Midwives General*, "Community Nurse Training Center at School of Hygiene, Aba," 1954–1960.

16. NSUDIV 12/1/38, *Midwives General*, "The Future of the Community Nurse in an Independent Nigeria by Dr. E.M. Poulton," 9.

17. NSUDIV 12/1/38, *Midwives General*, "Community Nursing Report by Patricia Eze," 5.

18. NSUDIV 12/1/38, *Midwives General*, "Community Nurse Training Center at School of Hygiene, Aba," 85; see also NSUDIV 12/1/38, *Midwives General*, "Community Nurse Training Course Aba: Bond of Agreement with Miss Eunice Aririguzo Completion of," 2–3.

19. BNA DV 12/68, *Nigeria: Lagos Island Maternity Hospital*, 1959, 3.

20. BNA DV 12/68, *Nigeria: Lagos Island Maternity Hospital*, 1959.

21. NSUDIV 12/1/38, *Midwives General*, "The Future of the Community Nurse," 9.

22. NSUDIV 12/1/38, *Midwives General*, "The Future of the Community Nurse."

23. NSUDIV 12/1/38, "Community Nurses Report by Patricia Eze," 212.

24. NSUDIV 12/1/38, "Community Nurses Report by Patricia Eze."

25. Wellcome Library (WL) H1B 948, *Annual Report of the Federal Medical Service, Nigeria*, 1958, 33–34.

26. Wellcome Library (WL) H1B 948, *Annual Report of the Federal Medical Service, Nigeria*, 1958.

27. Wellcome Library (WL) H1B 948, *Annual Report of the Federal Medical Service, Nigeria*, 1958.

28. Interview with Roseline Ezekwem, March 28, 2016.

29. Testimony at Fire Falls Assembly, Onitsha, June 2009. I write about this story in Ogechukwu Williams, "A Blur between the Spiritual and the Physical: Birthing Practices among the Igbo of Nigeria in the Twentieth Century," in *Sacred Inception: Reclaiming the Spirituality of Birth in the Modern World*, edited by Marianne Delaporte and Morag Martins (Lanham, MD: Lexington Books, 2018), 97–112.

30. Interview with Saheed Durodola, Ibadan, January 23, 2022.

31. Interview with Banire Alalaye, Ibadan, February 2, 2022.

32. Interview with Mary Ugwuanyi, Nsukka, June 26, 2013.

33. Interview with Chizoba, Nsukka, April 9, 2016.

34. NAE MINHEALTH 30/1/253, "Proceedings of a Meeting of District Officers and Local Heads," 157.

35. NAE MINHEALTH 30/1/253, "Proceedings of a Meeting of District Officers and Local Heads," 157.

36. CRL CMS ACC 165 F27, *The Private Owned Maternity*, 1959, 1–3.

37. CRL, *Medical Missions Quarterly, Nos IX to XVI January 1895 to October 1896* (London: Church Missionary Society, Salisbury Square, E.C., 1897), 88.

38. Osseo-Asare argues that access to Western pharmaceuticals and the attending technology became a tool for unmaking TBAs. See Abena Osseo-Asare, "'Don't Use Herbs in Labor!': Plants, Pharmaceuticals, and the Unmaking of Traditional Birth Attendants in Ghana, 1970–2000," *Social Science and Medicine* 329 (2023), https://doi.org/10.1016/j.socscimed.2023.

39. Interview with Dr. Alalaye.

40. Interview with Ngozi Ikwueze, Orloto, April 2, 2016.

41. Interview with Felicia Eze, Enugu, April 2, 2013.

42. Interview with Mary Ugwuanyi.

43. National Archives Ibadan (NAI) OYOPROF 105/1921, *Native Herbal Medicine Dealers: Practice and Sale of Herbal Preparations*, 31.

44. "Give Traditional Medicine a Chance, NMA," *Daily Times*, April 2, 1981, 15.

45. "Give Traditional Medicine a Chance, NMA," *Daily Times*, April 2, 1981.

46. "Give Traditional Medicine a Chance, NMA," *Daily Times*, April 2, 1981.

47. Inatimi Spiff, "The Trials of Traditional Medicine," *Daily Times*, December 31, 1991, 36.

48. Mume, *Tradomedicalism*, 5.

49. For these stereotypes, see Ogechukwu E. Williams, "The Politics of Labels: Imperial Categorizations and the Marginalisation of Ethnomedicine in Nigeria during the 20th Century," *Social History of Medicine* 34, no. 1 (2021): 1297–1316.

50. Inatimi Spiff, "The Trials of Traditional Medicine," *Daily Times*, December 31, 1991, 36.

51. Spiff, "The Trials of Traditional Medicine."

52. See Mume, *Tradomedicalism*, 15–16.

53. See Mume, *Tradomedicalism*, 7–10.

54. Mume, *Tradomedicalism*, 15.

55. Interview with Saheed.

56. Interview with Saheed.

57. NAE MINHEALTH 30/1/243, "Native Medicine," 14.

58. NAI OYOPROF 105/1921, *Native Herbal Medicine Dealers*, 31.

59. NAE MINHEALTH 30/1/243, "Native Medicine," 14.

60. Interview with Dr. Alalaye; interview with Saheed Durodola.

61. Interview with Dr. Alalaye.

62. Otsea, Family Care International, *Progress and Prospects*, 1–2.

63. Otsea, Family Care International, *Progress and Prospects*, 17.

64. Magdalene Ohaja, Jo Murphy-Lawless, and Margaret Dunlea, "Midwives Views of Traditional Birth Attendants within Formal Healthcare in Nigeria," *Women and Birth* 32, no. 2 (2020): 111.

65. Interview with Anonymous staff at the Ministry of Health, Enugu State, June 24, 2013.

66. Interview with M. A. Adeleye, Lagos, July 2, 2018; Interview with Lydia Ajayi, Ofatedo, October 18, 2020; Interview with Comfort Aluko, Ibadan, November 20, 2015; Interview with Folashade Akande, Ede, October 16, 2020.

67. Interview with Grace Abiala, Ede, January 17, 2021.

68. Interview with Isaac Yemi, Ibadan, November 18, 2015.

69. Cofie Annan and Kehinde Opadeji, "75,000 Nigerian Women Die Yearly from Pregnancy Problem," *Daily Times*, September 24, 1991, 2. See also WHO, *World Health Day, Safe Motherhood 7 April 1998* (Geneva: Division of Reproductive Health, 1998), 2. See also F. T. Sai, "The Safe Motherhood Initiative: A Call for Action," *IPPF Medical Bulletin* 21, no. 3, (1987): 1–2.

70. Our Reporter, "Treatment of the Sick in Churches: Aladuras Warned," *Sunday Observer*, July 1, 1973, 1.

71. Interview with M. A. Adeleye.

72. Interview with Dr. Ajuwon, Ede, October 20, 2020. Dr. Thomas Odejide, who presently serves the faith home as its internal consultant (doctor-in-charge), affirms that this view is the only bias that hospitals have against the faith homes. Interview with Dr. Thomas Odejide, Faith Home Doctor-in-Charge, February 6, 2021.

73. Interview with Lydia Ajayi.

74. Interview with Lydia Ajayi; interview with M. A. Adeleye; interview with Oluwaleye Ara, Odi Olowo, March 22, 2016.

75. Interview with Esther Oluwafemi, Okeife, November 18, 2016; interview with Oluwaleye Ara; interview with Comfort Aluko.

76. Interview with M. A. Adeleye.

77. Interview with Victoria Alabi.

78. See Bolaji Olaribigbe, "Surrogate Mom and the African Tradition," *Daily Times*, February 20, 1991, 16, for some discussion of the social tensions around assisted reproduction.

79. Interview with E. O. T. Olorunwa, Lagos, March 23, 2016; Joshua Alokan, *Christ Apostolic Church @ 90, 1918–2008* (Ile-Ife: Timade Ventures, 2010), 71–72.

80. Interview with Moses Olowe, Oke-Ife, November 18, 2015.

81. Interview with M. A. Adeleye.

82. Interview with Victoria Alabi.

83. Interview with Victoria Alabi.

84. See Babalola, *Joseph Ayo Babalola*, 8, 13–14. See also the letter by CAC leaders in the late 1930s explaining their stance on the use of biomedicine. https://tacnlawna.org/the-great-schism-and-emergence-of-cac/#_ftn11. Accessed February 26, 2021.

85. Interview with Victoria Alabi.

86. Before this formal ratification, some doctors who were CAC members assisted in the faith home when necessary.

87. Interview with Victoria Alabi.

88. Interview with Funmilola Awoyungbo, Ede, October 27, 2020; interview with Dr. Thomas Odejide.

89. Interview with Funmilola Awoyungbo. It is not clear when this registration first occurred, but Osun State made provisions for registration under the State of Osun Registration of Private Hospitals and Other Health Institutions Law of 2002. Before this provision, faith homes in Ede and elsewhere could register with Nigeria's Federal Ministry of Health.

90. Interview with Funmilola Awoyungbo.

91. Soji Akinrinade, "The Snarl of Fortune: Structural Adjustment Program Brings Mixed Blessings to Industries, Others," *Newswatch*, August 29, 1988, 17–19; Bala Dan Abu, "A Bog on the Path: Babangida's Well-Laid Social Programs Are Frustrated by Poor Execution," *Newswatch*, August 29, 1988, 20–22.

92. Akinrinade, "The Snarl of Fortune," 19.

93. Abu, "A Bog on the Path," 22.

94. Abu, "A Bog on the Path."

95. "Patients Ejected as Nurses Join Strike," *Daily Times*, December 28, 1991, 1; "Doctors in Edo Continue Strike," *Daily Times*, December 27, 1991, 3; "The Nurses' Strike," *Daily Times*, February 22, 1991, 14.

96. "Patients Now Wait for 3 Months before Getting Treatment . . . As Hospital Lacks Facilities," *Daily Times*, March 5, 1990, 4; "New Deal for Doctor," *Daily Times*, October 31, 1990, 14; Dr. Friday Njoku, "Overseas Medical Checkup Should Be Discouraged," *Daily Times*, April 4, 1981, 15; Daily Times Opinion, "The Quality of Private Medicine," *Daily Times*, April 4, 1981, 16.

97. Annan and Opadeji, "75,000 Nigerian Women Die Yearly," 2.

98. Annan and Opadeji, "75,000 Nigerian Women Die Yearly."

99. Lydia Ajala, Focus Group Session with seven past and current faith home users.

100. Lydia Ajala, Focus Group Session with seven past and current faith home users.

Coda

1. Interview with Moses Olowe, Oke-Ife, November 18, 2015.

2. Interview with Omolayo, Lagos, December 5, 2021.

3. The focus group session was conducted in Lagos on March 23, 2016, and included thirty-five pregnant women.

4. Interview with Isaac Yemi, Ibadan, November 18, 2015.

5. Focus Group Interview, ESUT School of Post-Basic Midwifery, Enugu, April 6, 2016.

6. Olusegun, Mimiko, "Experiences with Universal Health Coverage of Maternal Health Care in Ondo State, Nigeria, 2009–2017," *African Journal of Reproductive Health* 21, no. 3 (2017): 9–26.

7. Jennifer Cooke and Farha Tahir, *Maternal Health in Nigeria: A Report of the CSIS Global Health Policy Center* (Washington, DC: Center for Strategic & International Studies, 2013), 11–12.

8. Cooke and Tahir, *Maternal Health in Nigeria*; "World Band Lauds Ondo Governor over Safe Motherhood Project," http://www.ondostate.gov.ng/press_release/WORLD%20BANK.pdf, accessed March 20, 2017.

9. Adeyanju, "How Ondo Govt's Agbebiye Project Improves Maternal Healthcare," *Vanguard*, May 25, 2015.

10. Cooke and Tahir, *Maternal Health in Nigeria*, 11–14.

11. National Population Commission, *Nigeria Demographic and Health Survey 2008* (Abuja: National Population Commission, Federal Republic of Nigeria and MEASURE DHS+ ORC Macro, 2009).

Bibliography

Interviews

Interview with Dr. Alalaye, Ibadan, February 2, 2022.

Interview with Abimbola Durodola, January 23, 2022.

Interview with Saheed Durodola, Ibadan, January 23, 2022.

Interview with Banire Alalaye, Ibadan, February 2, 2022.

Interview with Mrs. Omolayo Adeyemi, Lagos, December 5, 2021.

Interview with Victoria Ayobola, Ejigbo, January 23, 2021.

Interview with Mrs. Adedeji, November 3, 2021.

Interview with Mrs. Omotosho, Ibadan, November 25, 2021.

Interview with Mrs. Balogun, Ibadan, November 26, 2021.

Interview with Mrs. Olaoba, Odo-Ona, December 14, 2021.

Interview with Grace Abiala, Ede, January 17, 2021.

Interview with Dr. Thomas Odejide, Faith Home Doctor-in-Charge, February 6, 2021.

Interview with Omolayo, Lagos, December 5, 2021.

Interview with Victoria Alabi, Ede, October 17, 2020.

Interview with Funmilola Awoyungbo, Ede, October 27, 2020.

Interview with Lydia Ajayi, Ofatedo, October 18, 2020.

Interview with Folashade Akande, Ede, October 16, 2020.

Interview with Dr. Ajuwon, Ede, October 20, 2020.

Interview with Ichie Nwezefunamba, Onitsha, July 7, 2019.

Interview with M. A. Adeleye, Lagos, July 2, 2018.

Interview with Deaconess Oyewo, Idi-Oro, July 2, 2018.

Interview with Onyeugwu nwa Ogwo, Nsukka, April 6, 2016.

Interview with Roseline Ezekwem, March 28, 2016.

Interview with Chizoba, Nsukka, April 9, 2016.

Interview with Ezechikwelu, Adazi-Enu, May 4, 2016.

Interview with Philip Nnatu, Enugwu-Ukwu, April 9, 2016.

Interview with Ogidija Ugwuole, Lejja, April 5, 2016.

Interview with Gloria, Nsukka, April 5, 2016.

Interview with Amalugo, Umuabu, May 4, 2016.

Interview with Ngozi Ikwueze, Orloto, April 2, 2016.

Interview with E. O. T. Olorunwa, Lagos, March 23, 2016.

Interview with Midwife Oluwaleye Ara, Odi Olowo, March 22, 2016.

Interview with Esther Oluwafemi, Okeife, November 18, 2016.

Interview with Chizoba, Nsukka, April 9, 2016.

Interview with Ngozi Ikwueze, Orloto, April 2, 2016.

Interview with Oluwaleye Ara, Odi Olowo, March 22, 2016.

Interview with Esther Oluwafemi, Okeife, November 18, 2016.

Focus group session, CAC Idi Oro, Lagos, March 23, 2016.

Focus Group Interview, ESUT School of Post-Basic Midwifery, Enugu, April 6, 2016.

Interview with Comfort Aluko, Ibadan, November 20, 2015.

Interview with Moses Olowe, Oke-Ife, November 18, 2015.

Interview with Dorcas Olaniyi, Ibadan, November 23, 2015.

Interview with Ademola Saheed on behalf of Durodola Abimbola, Ibadan, November 15, 2015.

Interview with Isaac Yemi, Ibadan, November 18, 2015.

Interview with Comfort Aluko, Ibadan, November 20, 2015.

Interview with Midwife Alu, 60+, Ibadan, November 20, 2015.

Interview with Moses Olowe, Oke-Ife, November 18, 2015.

Interview with Philip Nnatu, June 7, 2014.

Interview with Mary Ugwuanyi, Nsukka, June 26, 2013.

Interview with Felicia Eze, Enugu, April 2, 2013.

Interview with Anonymous staff at the Ministry of Health, Enugu State, June 24, 2013.

Interview with Nnanna Okorom, Imo State, March 2, 2011.

Interview with Felicia Agu, Imo State, March 5, 2011.

Interview with Rita Ewereji, Imo State, March 5, 2011.

Interview with Mrs. Obijelu Okpalaeze, Adazi-Enu, January 29, 2009.

Interview with Roseline Ezekwem, Adazi-Enu, January 27, 2009.

Interview with Mrs. Patty Iloghalu, Umuabu, January 28, 2009.

Interview with Ichie Ezedum, Ogweni Ocha, January 29, 2009.

Congregant Testimony at Fire Falls Assembly, Onitsha, June 2009.

Interview with Florence Odo, Enugu, April 4, 2008.

Archives

National Archives, Enugu

ON DIST 12/1/1244, *Human Sacrifices and Destruction of Twin Children*, 1955.

ONDIST 12/1/854, "Conflict between Christian Rites and Pagan Customs," 1930s and 1940s.

ON DIST 12/1/1247, *Triplets: Queens Bounty for the Birth of Triplets.*

ON PROF 7/13/97, *Trial Exposure of Twins*, 1926.

ONPROF 7/11/46, *The Marriage Ordinance*, 1929.

OP 7/13/97, *Awgu-Rex versus Unaegbu and One Other Charged with Exposure of Twins and Committed to Trial to the Resident's Court*, 1926.

MINHEALTH 30/1/253, *Medical Development in Nigeria*, 1946.

NSUDIV 12/1/38, *Midwives General*, 1955–1960.

MISF 257, Box 161, F. A. M. Adewale-Abayomi, "African Traditional Healing through Ohun Ife," *Orunmila* 2 (1986): 25–26.

MISF 257, Box 161, Adeboye Oyesanya, "Ifa: The Do It Yourself for the Beginners," 8–9.

National Museum, Enugu Nigeria

"Ite Ola Okike."

National Archives, Ibadan

OYO PROF 662, *The Faith Healer-Babalola and the Faith Tabernacle Otherwise Known as the Aladura Religious Movement-Operation of in Oyo Province*, 1931–1947.

OYO PROF 1/28, *Aladura Movement (Apostolic Church)*, 1932.

OYO PROF 661, *Cherubim & Seraphim. Activities in Oyo Province*, 1930.

OYOPROF 105/1921, *Native Herbal Medicine Dealers: Practice and Sale of Herbal Preparations*, 1915–1933.

OYO PROF 1/1129, *Domestic Training for Girls-Suggestions as to*, 1933–1936.

J/1/a, *Medical Policy in the Colonial Empire*, 1943.

MH (Fed) 1/1/4075, *Infant Welfare Center Ondo Province*, 1942.

CSO 26/3, *Infant and Maternity Work in Nigeria II*, 133.

British National Archives, Kew

CO 583/248/6, *Training of Subordinate Staff in the Medical Department*, 1930.

CO 917/2, *Pan African Health Conference*, 1935.

CO 859/62/17, *Birth Control West Africa*, 1943.

CO 583/266/4, *Higher College of Yaba. Medical Training for Girls*, 1945.

CO 859/62/16, *Birth Control: West Indies*, 1941–1942.

CO 323/1463/5, *Medical Miscellaneous: Abortion in the Colonies*.

CO 583/296/4, *Resettlement of Africans in Overpopulated Areas*.

MH 55/269 *Maternal Mortality Departmental Committee Memorandum on Antenatal Clinics*, "Maternal Mortality in Childbirth."

Ministry of Health Annual Report 1957–1958, Vol. 1.

Ministry of Health Annual Report 1957–1958, Vol. 2.

DV 12/68, *Nigeria: Lagos Island Maternity Hospital*, 1959.

Wellcome Library London

Nigeria. Southern Provinces. Annual Medical and Sanitary Report for the Year Ended 31st December 1915.

Nigeria. Southern Provinces. Annual Medical and Sanitary Report for the Year Ended 31st December 1916.

Nigeria. Southern Provinces. Annual Medical and Sanitary Report for the Year Ended 31st December 1918.

ANN REP WA28 NH5 N68 1922–1925, *Annual Medical and Sanitary Report for the Year 1922.*

WA28 HN5 N68, *Nigeria. Annual Medical and Sanitary Report*, 1924.

WA28 HN5 N68, *Nigeria. Annual Medical and Sanitary Report*, 1925.

ANN REP WA28 NH5 N68 1926–1928, *Annual Medical and Sanitary Report for the Year 1926.*

Nigeria. Southern Provinces. Annual Medical and Sanitary Report for the Year Ended 31st December 1929.

Nigeria. Southern Provinces. Annual Medical and Sanitary Report for the Year Ended 31st December 1930.

Report on the Medical and Health Department for the Year 1931.

H1B 948, *Annual Report of the Federal Medical Service*, Nigeria, 1958.

7720600, *Choices. Lyrics.*

SA/ICM/7/1/1, *JSG 1970–1980*, "International Federation of Gynecology and Obstetrics. International Confederation of Midwives."

954574379, *Lagos Health and Baby Week*, April 22 to 29, 6.

MEDK22987, Robert Rene Kuczynski, *Demographic Survey of the British Colonial Empire, Vol. 1 (West Africa)*. London: Oxford University Press, 1948.

Cadbury Research Library, Birmingham

H7/B/42/101, CAC, "The Christ Apostolic Church, Its History, Beliefs and Organization," *Ecumenical Review* 28, no. 4 (1976): 423.

H7/B/42/124, *Africa Nigeria, Recent Developments in the Healing Concepts and Activities of Aladura Churches*.

H7/B/42/101, *Africa, Nigeria*, John Ferguson, "Christianity in Interaction with Yoruba Culture."

H7/B/51/3/21, *Nigeria*, "The Social Impacts of New Religious Movements on Yoruba Life," 41.

ACC 716 F8, *Church Missionary Outlook*, vol. LIX, 1931.

ACC 716 F8, *Church Missionary Outlook*, vol. LIX, 1932.

ACC 780/F1, Dorothy Ross, *The Pattern of a Life*, 19.

ACC/165/F27, *The Private Owned Maternity Home in Nigeria*.

E. O. A. Adejobi, *An Address Entitled "Facts about Faith, Psychic or Spiritual Healing" Delivered to the Teachers in Theological Colleges at the Emmanuel College, Ibadan*, May 1974.

Christ Apostolic Church, *The Constitution and the Order of Service* (Nigeria, n.d.).

C/2/1/8 1905–1909.

G/Y/A/2/2.

G/Y/A/9/2, *Northern Nigeria Mission*.

M/Y/A3/1 1916–1933.

M/Y/A2/1 1918–1945.

Medical Missions Quarterly, Nos IX to XVI, 1895–96. London: Church Missionary Society, Salisbury Square, E.C., 1897.

Mercy and Truth: A Record of CMS Medical Missions, vol. I. London: Church Missionary Society, 1897.

Mercy and Truth: A Record of CMS Medical Missions, vol. III. London: Church Missionary Society, 1899.

Mercy and Truth: A Record of CMS Medical Mission Work, vol. 9, 1903.

Mercy and Truth: A Record of CMS Medical Mission Work, vol. 12, 1908.

The Mission Hospital: A Record of Medical Missions of the CMS, vol. XXIX, 1925.

The Mission Hospital: A Record of Medical Missions of the CMS, vol. XXX, 1926.

The Mission Hospital: A Record of Medical Missions of the CMS, Vol. XXXI, 1927.

The Mission Hospital: A Record of Medical Missions of the C.M.S., vol. XXXII, 1928.

The Mission Hospital, A Record of Medical Missions of the C.M.S., vol. XXXII, 1929.

The Mission Hospital: A Record of C.M.S Medical Missions, vol. xxxiv, 1930.

M/C 2/1/7 (1898–1905).

M/FL1 N1/1.

G3/A3/0, *Henry Dobinson to R. Lang*, May 5, 1890.

G3/A3/0, *Annual Report of Onitsha Station for 1886*.

G/3/A/9/0, *Map of Northern Nigeria*.

Rockefeller Archives Center

JDR III 80/667/670, *Population Interests General*, 1952–1961, 8.

JDR III 85/718-719/FA108, 104.54.1, *Population Council Williamsburg Conference*, 1952.

Ford Foundation (RAC FF) FA571/3/7, *Family Planning Communications in Nigeria*.

Ford Foundation (FF) FA571/4/4, *A Report on a Visit to Nigeria to Consult on Communications Activities of the Family Planning Council of Nigeria*, 1973.

Population Council (PC) S 107/FA432, *Nigeria, Post-partum Program D&I-S*, 1967.

US National Archives, Maryland

R286/P792/4-7, *Nigeria-Reports, Correspondence*, 1965–1982.

R286/P811/3, *Nigeria 08 Birth Spacing Project*.

R286/P822/4, *Economic Assistance Task Force FY 61*, 1961–1972.

R286 P606, *AHEA Consultations, Field Visits, Workshops (Nigeria-Panama)*, 1972.

International Planned Parenthood Federation Archives (IPPFA), *IPPF Governing Body, 14th Meeting (Special Meeting) 5th–7th November*.

R286 P606, *AHEA International Family Planning Conference*.

R286/P646/11, *AHEA IPF Workshop London*, 1975.

University of Illinois

Colonial Annual Reports, No. 1030, Nigeria, "Reports for 1918."

Colonial Annual Reports, No. 1315, Nigeria, "Reports for 1925."

3064634, *Annual Report of the Social and Economic Progress of the People of Nigeria*, 1931.

Newspaper Publications

Nigerian Daily Times / Daily Times

W. H. S. Curryer, B.A., "Mothercraft in Southern Nigeria," *Nigerian Daily Times*, March 4, 1927.

"The Education of the African Woman (Final Article)," *Nigerian Daily Times*, November 2, 1928, 6.

"The Education of the African Woman," *Nigerian Daily Times*, October 31, 1928, 8.

"The Education of the African Woman," *Nigerian Daily Times*, November 1, 1928, 6.

"Appointment of Lady Medical Officer," *Nigerian Daily Times*, March 23, 1928, 4.

"The Education of the African Woman (Final Article)," *Nigerian Daily Times*, November 2, 1928, 6.

"Misunderstanding Cleared on Colonial Question," *Daily Times*, December 19, 1949, 3.

Daily Times Photo Interview, "Boys and Girls Must Be Given Equal Education," *Daily Times*, December 21, 1949, 6.

Mrs. Ibiyemi Bright, "Should Married Women Work," *Daily Times*, April 10, 1950, 5.

London Correspondent, "Training of Women Reviewed," *Daily Times*, August 15, 1949, 15.

"Lagos Clinic Critics Are Replied," *Daily Times*, April 28, 1950, 11.

Sunday Abukuru, "Hospitals without Doctors," *Daily Times*, April 14, 1978, 21.

Festus Ijilade, "Stories of Woe in State Hospitals," *Daily Times*, April 1978, 3.

Nekpen Ebohon and Pat Ibude, "Childless Marriage: Is the Woman to Blame," *Sunday Times*, October 18, 1992, 13.

"Baby Show at Abeokuta," *Daily Times*, January 14, 1938, 1.

"Developing Britain's Colonies," *Daily Times*, December 28, 1949, 3.

D. O. Dinyo, "Women Should Pay No Income Tax," *Daily Times*, April 17, 1950, 4.

"Give Traditional Medicine a Chance, NMA," *Daily Times*, April 2, 1981, 15.

Inatimi Spiff, "The Trials of Traditional Medicine," *Daily Times*, December 31, 1991, 36.

Layi Olajide, "Family Planning Is Very Necessary," *Daily Times*, January 20, 1973, 13.

G. B. Ajayi, "Birth Control Controversy. Extended Family: Core of African Society," *Daily Times*, January 8, 1973, 7.

"Training in Family Planning," *Daily Times*, December 2, 1972.

"Childlife in Nigeria," *The Nigerian Daily Times*, August 20, 1928, 4.

Bose Orishawo, "Times Woman," *Daily Times*, September 30, 1991, 32.

Pat Odedina, "Should Teenagers Use Contraceptives?" *Daily Times*, September 29, 1991, 13.

Clarkson de Majomi, "Africa Accepts Birth Control," *Daily Times*, January 8, 1973, 7.

Kenule Sarowiwa, "We Need More Babies Here," *Daily Times*, November 12, 1971.

Alexander Akinyele, "Pill Pedlars Are Welcome," *Daily Times*, December 11, 1971, 7.

Felix Adenaike, "We Want More Babies Here But . . ." *Daily Times*, December 11, 1971, 7.

I. B. Abodunrin, "Where Tsaro-Wiwa Is Wrong," *Daily Times*, December 11, 1971, 7.

Cofie Annan and Kehinde Opadeji, "75,000 Nigerian Women die Yearly from Pregnancy Problem," *Daily Times*, September 24, 1991, 2.

Bolaji Olaribigbe, "Surrogate Mom and the African Tradition," *Daily Times*, February 20, 1991, 16.

"Patients Ejected as Nurses Join Strike," *Daily Times*, December 28, 1991, 1.

"Doctors in Edo Continue Strike," *Daily Times*, December 27, 1991, 3.

"The Nurses' Strike," *Daily Times*, February 22, 1991, 14.

"Patients Now Wait for 3 Months before Getting Treatment . . . As Hospital Lacks Facilities," *Daily Times*, March 5, 1990, 4.

"New Deal for Doctor," *Daily Times*, October 31, 1990, 14.

Dr. Friday Njoku, "Overseas Medical Checkup Should Be Discouraged," *Daily Times*, April 4, 1981, 15.

Daily Times Opinion, "The Quality of Private Medicine," *Daily Times*, April 4, 1981, 16.

West African Pilot

Crab Ewulu, "Nursing and Midwifery," *West African Pilot*, December 20, 1963.

Nigerian Observer

Air Iyare, "Birth Control through Family Planning," *Nigerian Observer*, September 7, 1973, 10.

S. C. Onoguwe, "Family Planning and Our Social Problems," *Nigerian Observer*, October 8, 1973, 9.

Our Reporter, "Treatment of the Sick in Churches: Aladuras Warned," *Sunday Observer*, July 1, 1973, 1.

Lagos Weekend

"The Role of Family Planning in Nigeria," *Lagos Weekend*, September 30, 1977, 16.

"Family Planning Helps Families," *Lagos Weekend*, August 8, 1980, 10.

Sketch
O. A. Ojo (Jr.), "Population Growth and Its Problems," August 20, 1972, *Sunday Sketch*, 2.

Truth Weekly
"Dr. Adetoro on Family Planning," *Truth Weekly*, November 8–14, 1968, 1.
"Chief Awolowo on Family Planning," *Truth Weekly*, October 25–31, 1968, 8.
"Birth Control," *Truth Weekly*, November 8–14, 1968, 7.

Nigerian Tide
"Beware of the Pill," *Nigerian Tide*, September 2, 1981, 8.
Awusinba Iyalla, "Contraception and What It Does to Your Health," *Sunday Tide*,
    August 30, 1981, 13.

Nigerian Standard
Francis Agbo, "Family Planning Has Its Advantage," *Nigerian Standard*, June 20, 1977.

International Health News
K. Mazzocco, "Nigeria's New Population Policy," *International Health News*, March 9, 1988,
    1–12.

Deseret News
"Nigeria Chief Urges 4-Child Limit," *Deseret News*, April 16, 1989.

New York Times
Henry Kamm, "Pope to Nigerians: Defend the Family," *New York Times*, February 14, 1982, 4.

Newswatch
Soji Akinrinade, "The Snarl of Fortune: Structural Adjustment Program Brings Mixed
    Blessings to Industries, Others," *Newswatch*, August 29, 1988, 17–19.
Bala Dan Abu, "A Bog on the Path: Babangida's Well-Laid Social Programs Are Frustrated
    by Poor Execution," *Newswatch*, August 29, 1988, 20–22.

Vanguard
Adeyanju, "How Ondo Govt's Agbebiye Project Improves Maternal Healthcare," *Vanguard*,
    May 25, 2015.
Adeyanju, "How Ondo Govt's Agbebiye Project Improves Maternal Healthcare," *Vanguard*,
    May 25, 2015.

Books and Articles
Abugideiri, Hibba. *Gender and the Making of Modern Medicine in Colonial Egypt*. Burlington,
    VT: Ashgate Publishing, 2010.
Achebe, Nwando. *Farmers, Traders, Warriors, and Kings: Female Power and Authority in
    Northern Igboland, 1900–1960*. Westport, CT: Praeger, 2005.
Acobson-Widding, Anita, and David Westerlund. *Culture Experience and Pluralism: Essays
    on African Ideas of Illness and Healing*. Uppsala: Academiae Upsaliensis, 1989.

Adanikin, A. I., U. Onwudiegwu, and A. Akintayo. "Reshaping Maternal Services in Nigeria: Any Need for Spiritual Care?" *BMC Pregnancy Childbirth* 14, no. 196 (2014): 1–6. https://doi.org/10.1186/1471-2393-14-196.

Addae, Stephen. *History of Western Medicine in Ghana 1880–1960.* Edinburgh: Durham Academic Press, 1997.

Ade Ajayi, J. F. K. *Christian Missions in Nigeria: The Making of a New Elite, 1841–1891.* London: Longman, 1965.

Adekson, Olufunmilayo Mary. *The Yorùbá Traditional Healers of Nigeria.* New York: Routledge, 2003.

Adelakun, Abimbola. *Performing Power in Nigeria: Identity, Politics, and Pentecostalism.* New Brunswick, NJ: Rutgers University Press, 2022.

Aderinto, Saheed. *When Sex Threatened the State: Illicit Sexuality, Nationalism, and Politics in Colonial Nigeria, 1900–1958.* Champaign: University of Illinois Press, 2014.

Adeyemi, Gabriel, and Freeman Okosun, *The Great Woman of God Archbishop (Dr.) Dorcas Siyanbola. Olaniyi at 70.* Ibadan: Freeman Productions, 2004.

Agbasiere, Joseph. *Women in Igbo Life and Thought.* London: Routledge, 2000.

Agyei-Mensah, Samuel, and Johnson B. Castreline, eds. *Reproduction and Social Context in Sub-Saharan Africa: A Collection of Micro Demographic Studies.* Westport, CT: Greenwood Press, 2003.

Airhihenbuwa, Collins. *Health and Culture: Beyond the Western Paradigm.* Thousand Oaks, CA: Sage, 1995.

Allman, Jean. "Making Mothers: Missionaries, Medical Officers and Women's Work in Colonial Asante, 1924–1945." *History Workshop* 38 (1994): 23–24.

Allman, Jean Marie, Susan Geiger, and Nakanyike Musisi. *Women in African Colonial Histories.* Bloomington: Indiana University Press, 2002.

Alokan, Joshua. *Christ Apostolic Church @ 90, 1918–2008.* Ile-Ife: Timade Ventures, 2010.

Amadi, Lawrence. "Church-State Involvement in Educational Development in Nigeria, 1842–1948." *Journal of Church and State* 19, no. 3 (1977): 483–484.

Amadiume, Ifi. *Male Daughters, Female Husbands: Gender and Sex in an African Society.* London: Zed Books, 1987.

Amadiume, Ifi. *Re-inventing Africa: Matriarchy, Religion, and Culture.* London: Zed Books, 1997.

Amba, Mercy, and Musimbi Kanyoro. *The Will to Rise: Women, Tradition, and the Church in Africa.* New York: Orbis Books, 1992.

Amzat, J. *Medical Sociology in Africa.* Cham, Switzerland: Springer International Publishing, 2014.

Appiah-Kubi, Kofi. *Man Cures, God Heals: Religion and Medical Practice Among the Akans of Ghana.* Totowa, NJ: Allanheld, Osmun, 1981.

Arnold, David. *Imperial Medicine and Indigenous Societies.* Manchester: Manchester University Press, 1988.

Asare, M., and S. Danquah. "The African Belief System and the Patient's Choice of Treatment from Existing Health Models: The Case of Ghana." *Acta Psychopathology* 3, no. 4 (2017): 1–4.

Ayandele, E. A. *The Missionary Impact on Modern Nigeria 1842–1914: A Political and Social Analysis.* London: Longman, 1966.

Babalola, Joseph. *Joseph Ayo Babalola, Thoughts of an Apostle: His Collected Works and Teachings*, compiled and translated by Moses Idowu. Lagos: Artillery Christian Ministries, 2000.

Bankole, Akinrinola, et al. *Barriers to Safe Motherhood in Nigeria*. New York: Guttmacher Institute, 2009.

Baranov, David. *The African Transformation of Western Medicine and the Dynamics of Global Cultural Exchange*. Philadelphia: Temple University Press, 2008.

Barnes, Andrew. *Making Headway: The Introduction of Western Civilization in Colonial Northern Nigeria*. Rochester, NY: University of Rochester Press, 2009.

Bascom, William. *The Yoruba of Southwestern Nigeria*. New York: Holt, Reinhart, and Winston, 1969.

Basden, George. *Among the Ibos of Nigeria*. Gloucestershire: Nonsuch Publishing Limited, 2006.

Bastian, Misty. "The Naked and the Nude: Historically Multiple Meanings of Oto (Undress) in Southeastern Nigeria," in *Dirt, Undress, and Difference: Critical Perspectives on the Body's Surface*, edited by Adeline Masquelier. Bloomington: Indiana University Press, 2005.

Beidelman, T. O. *Colonial Evangelism*. Bloomington: Indiana University Press, 1981.

Berger, Iris. *Women in Twentieth Century Africa*. Cambridge, UK: Cambridge University Press, 2016.

Black, Edwin. *War against the Weak: Eugenics and America's Campaign to Create a Master Race-Expanded*. Cary, NC: Dialog Press, 2008.

Blakely, T. D., et al., eds. *Religion in Africa: Experience and Expressions*. London: James Currey, 1994.

Boahen, Abu. *African Perspectives on Colonialism*. Baltimore: John Hopkins University Press, 1987.

Boggs, Belle. *The Art of Waiting: On Fertility, Medicine, and Motherhood*. Minneapolis, MN: Graywolf Press, 2016.

Bourbonnais, Nicole. *Birth Control in the Decolonizing Caribbean: Reproductive Politics and Practice on Four Islands, 1930–1970*. Cambridge, UK: Cambridge University Press, 2016.

Bourbonnais, Nicole. *Reproductive Rights and Race Struggle in the Decolonizing Caribbean, Black Perspectives*, April 1, 2017. https://www.aaihs.org/reproductive-rights-and-race -struggle-in-the-decolonizing-caribbean/.

Bruce-Chwatt, L. J. "Obituary: Sir Samuel L.A. Manuwa." *Transactions of the Royal Society of Tropical Medicine and Hygiene* 70, no. 2 (1976): 173.

Bruinius, Harry. *Better for All the World: The Secret History of Forced Sterilization and America's Quest for Racial Purity*. New York: Vintage Press, 2007.

Buckley, Anthony. *Yoruba Medicine*. Oxford: Clarendon Press, 1985.

Bush, Barbara. "Gender and Empire: The Twentieth Century," in *Gender and Empire*, edited by Philippa Levine. London: Oxford University Press, 2007, 77–111.

Callaway, Barbara. *Muslim Hausa Women in Nigeria: Tradition and Change*. Syracuse, NY: Syracuse University Press, 1987.

Callaway, Helen. *Gender, Culture and Empire: European Women in Colonial Nigeria*. London: Oxford and Macmillan, 1987.

Campbell, Chloe. *Race and Empire: Eugenics in Colonial Kenya*. Manchester: Manchester University Press, 2007.

Chalmers, Beverley. *African Birth: Childbirth in Cultural Transition*. River Club, South Africa: Berev Publications CC, 1990.

Chesterman, Clement. *In the Service of the Suffering: Phases of Medical Missionary Enterprise*. London: Edinburgh House Press, 1940.

Chuku, Gloria. *Igbo Women and Economic Transformation in Southeastern Nigeria, 1900–1960*. New York: Routledge, 2005.

Chuku, Gloria. "Igbo Women and Political Participation in Nigeria, 1800s–2005." *The International Journal of African Historical Studies* 42, no. 1 (2009): 81–103.

Coles, Catherine, and Beverly Mack, eds. *Hausa Women in The Twentieth Century*. Madison: University of Wisconsin Press, 1991.

Comaroff, Jean. "Medicine and Culture: Some Anthropological Perspectives." *Social Science and Medicine* 12b (1978): 247–254.

Comaroff, John, and Jean Comaroff. *Ethnography and the Historical Imagination*. Boulder, CO: Westview Press, 1991.

Connelly, Matthew. *Fatal Misconception: The Struggle to Control World Population*. Cambridge, MA: Harvard University Press, 2008.

Cooke, Jennifer, and Farha Tahir. *Maternal Health in Nigeria: A Report of the CSIS Global Health Policy Center*. Washington, DC: Center for Strategic & International Studies, 2013.

Cooper, Barbara. *Countless Blessings: A History of Childbirth and Reproduction in the Sahel*. Bloomington: Indiana University Press, 2019.

Cooper, Frederick. *Tensions of Empire: Colonial Cultures in a Bourgeois World*. Berkeley: University of California Press, 1997.

Cooter, R. *Studies in the History of Alternative Medicine*. Houndsmill: Macmillan, 1988.

Coquery-Vidrovitch, Catherine. *African Women: A Modern History*. Boulder, CO: Westview Press, 1997.

Cosslet, Tess. *Women Writing Childbirth: Modern Discourses of Motherhood*. Manchester: Manchester University Press, 1994.

Critchlow, Donald. *Intended Consequences: Birth Control, Abortion and the Federal Government in Modern America*. London: Oxford University Press, 1999.

Crumbley, Deirdre. "Patriarchies, Prophets, and Procreation: Sources of Gender Practices in Three African Churches." *Africa* 73, no. 4 (2003): 586.

Crumbley, Deirdre. *Spirit, Structure, and Flesh: Gendered Experiences in African Instituted Churches among the Yoruba of Nigeria*. Madison: University of Wisconsin Press, 2008.

Davin, Anna. "Imperialism and Motherhood." *History Workshop* 5 (Spring 1978): 9–65.

de Barros, Juanita. *Reproducing the British Caribbean: Sex, Gender, and Population Politics after Slavery*. Chapel Hill: University of North Carolina Press, 2014.

Dekker, M., and Rijk van Dijk. *Markets of Well-Being: Navigating Health and Healing in Africa*. Leiden: Brill, 2010.

Denzer, L. "Domestic Science Training in Colonial Yorubaland, Nigeria," in *African Encounters with Domesticity*, edited by K. T. Hansen. New Brunswick, NJ: Rutgers University Press, 1992.

Dwork, Deborah. *War Is Good for Babies and Other Young Children: A History of the Infant and Child Welfare Movement in England 1898–1918*. London: Tavistock, 1987.

"Editorial." *British Journal of Nursing*, June 30, 1917, n.p.

Ehrenreich, John, ed. *The Cultural Crisis of Modern Medicine*. New York: Monthly Review Press, 1978.

Ekanem and A. Asira. "Religion and Medicine in the 21st Century Nigeria." *SOPHIA* 9, no. 1 (2006): 56–61.

Ekechi, F. K. "The Holy Ghost Fathers in Eastern Nigeria, 1885–1920: Observations on Missionary Strategy." *African Studies Review* 15, no. 2 (1972): 221–222.

Ekechi, F. K. "The Medical Factor in Christian Conversion in Africa: Observations from Southeastern Nigeria." *Missiology* 21, no. 3 (1993): 289–309.

Ekechi, F. K. *Missionary Enterprise and Rivalry in Igboland 1857–1914*. London: Frank Cass, 1971.

Ellen, Ross. *Love and Toil: Motherhood in Outcast London 1870–1918*. New York: Oxford University Press, 1993.

Elling, Ray H. *Cross-National Study of Health Systems: Political Economics and Health Care*. New Brunswick, NJ: Transaction Books, 1980.

Ene, Ebele. "Family Planning, Fertility Control and the Law in Nigeria—The Choices for a New Century." *African Journal of Reproductive Health* 2, no. 2 (1998): 90.

Erken, Arthur, ed. *My Body Is My Own: Claiming the Right to Autonomy and Self-Determination*. New York: UNFPA, 2021.

Ernst, Waltraud. *Plural Medicine Tradition and Modernity 1800–2000*. London: Routledge, 2002.

"Exodus," chapter 1, verse 19, *Holy Bible*, New International Version.

Falola, Toyin, and Nana Amponsah, eds. *Women, Gender, and Sexuality in Africa*. Durham, NC: Carolina Academic Press, 2012.

Falola, Toyin, and Matthew Heaton, eds. *Health Knowledge and Belief Systems in Africa*. Durham, NC: Carolina Academic Press, 2008.

Falola, Toyin, and Adam Paddock. *The Women's War of 1929: A History of Anti-Colonial Resistance in Eastern Nigeria*. Durham, NC: Carolina Academic Press, 2011.

Federal Republic of Nigeria. *Second National Development Plan 1970–74*. Lagos: Federal Ministry of Information, 1970.

Feierman, Steven, and John Janzen. *The Social Basis of Health and Healing in Africa*. Oakland: University of California Press, 1992.

Feldman-Savelsberg, Pamela. *Plundered Kitchens Empty Wombs: Threatened Reproduction and Identity in the Cameroon Grassfields*. Ann Arbor: University of Michigan Press, 1999.

Ferngren, Gary. *Religion and Society in Nigeria: Historical and Sociological Perspectives*. Baltimore: Johns Hopkins University Press, 2014.

Fieldes, Valerie, Lara Marks, and Hilary Marland, eds. *Women and Children First: International Maternal and Infant Welfare, 1870–1945*. London: Routledge, 1992.

Fisher, Humphrey J. "Slavery and Seclusion in Northern Nigeria: A Further Note." *Journal of African History* 32, no. 1 (1991): 123–135.

Fletcher, Jeannine. *Motherhood as Metaphor: Engendering Interreligious Dialogue*. New York: Fordham University Press, 2013.

Flint, Karen. *Healing Traditions: African Medicine, Cultural Exchange, and Competition in South Africa, 1820–1948*. Athens: Ohio University Press, 2008.

Gaitskell, Debby. "'Getting Close to the Hearts of Mothers': Medical Missionaries among African Women and Children in Johannesburg between the Wars," in *Women and Children First: International Maternal and Infant Welfare 1870–1945*, edited by Valerie Fildes, Lara Marks, and Hilary Marland. New York: Routledge Revivals, 1992.

Galadanci, Hadiza, and Suwaiba Sani. "Childbirth in Nigeria," in *Childbirth across Cultures: Ideas and Practices of Pregnancy, Childbirth, and Post-Partum*, edited by Helaine Selin and Pamela Stone. New York: Springer, 2009, 212–220.

Galletti, R., K. D. S. Baldwin, and I. O. Dina, *The Nigerian Cocoa Farmer*. London: Oxford University Press, 1956.

Gampiot, Aurelien Mokoko. "Kimbanguism: An African Initiated Church." *Scriptura: International Journal of Bible, Religion and Theology in Southern Africa* 113 (2014): 1–11.

Gelfand, Michael. *Midwifery in Tropical Africa: The Growth of Maternity Services in Rhodesia*. Salisbury: University of Rhodesia, 1978.

Geurts, Kathryn Linn. "Childbirth and Pragmatic Midwifery in Rural Ghana." *Medical Anthropology* 20, no. 4 (2001): 379–408.

Good, Charles. *Ethnomedical Systems in Africa: Patterns of Traditional Medicine in Rural and Urban Kenya*. New York: The Guilford Press, 1987.

Grayzel, Susan. *Women and the First World War*. Harlow: Longman, 2002.

Green, Monica. *Making Women's Medicine Masculine: The Rise of Male Authority in Pre-Modern Gynaecology*. New York: Oxford University Press, 2008.

Grimshaw, Anna. *The Ethnographer's Eye: Ways of Seeing in Anthropology*. Cambridge, UK: Cambridge University Press, 2001.

Handwerker, W. P., ed. *Birth and Power: Social Change and the Politics of Reproduction*. Boulder, CO: Westview Press, 1990.

Hardiman, James, ed. *Healing Bodies, Saving Souls: Medical Missions in Asia and Africa*. New York: Rodopi, 2006.

Harneit-Seivers, Axel. *Constructions of Belonging: Igbo Communities and the Nigerian State in the Twentieth Century*. New York: University of Rochester Press, 2006.

Harrison, Kelsey A. *Sowing the Seeds of Safe Motherhood in Sub-Saharan Africa*. London: Adonis & Abbey, 2010.

Hartmann, Betsy. *Reproductive Rights and Wrongs: The Global Politics of Population Control*. Boston: South End Press, 1995.

Hastings, Adrian. *Church and Mission in Colonial Africa*. London: Burns and Oates, 1967.

Holloway, Kris. *Monique and the Mango Rains: Two Years with a Midwife in Mali*. Long Grove, IL: Waveland Press, Inc., 2006.

Hunt, Nancy Rose. *A Colonial Lexicon of Birth Ritual, Medicalization, and Mobility in the Congo*. Durham, NC: Duke University Press, 1999.

Hunt, Nancy Rose. "Le Bebe en Brousse: European Women, African Birth Spacing and Colonial Intervention in Breast Feeding in the Belgian Congo." *International Journal of African Studies* 21 (1988): 401–432.

Isichie, Elizabeth. *A History of the Igbo People*. London: The Macmillan Press, 1976.

Isichie, Elizabeth. *The Ibo People and the Europeans*. London: Faber and Faber Limited, 1970.

Isichie, Elizabeth. *Igbo Worlds: An Anthology of Oral Histories and Historical Descriptions*. Philadelphia: Institute for the Study of Human Issues, 1978.

Imperato, Pascal. *African Folk Medicine*. Baltimore: York Press Inc., 1977.

Iwu, Chinedu, et al. "Empowering Traditional Birth Attendants as Agents of Maternal and Neonatal Immunization Uptake in Nigeria: A Repeated Measures Design." *BMC Public Health* 21, no. 287 (2021): 1–8. https://doi.org/10.1186/s12889-021-10311-z.

Izugbara, Chimaraoke, and Joseph Ukwayi, "The Hospital as a Birthing Site: Narratives of Local Women in Nigeria," in *Reproduction, Childbearing, and Motherhood: A Cross-Cultural Perspective*, edited by Pranee Liamputtong. New York: Nova Science, 2007.

Jacobson, Jodi. *Challenge of Survival: Safe Motherhood in the SADCC Region*. New York: Family Care International, 1991.

Janzen, John. *The Social Fabric of Health: An Introduction to Medical Anthropology*. Boston: McGraw Hill, 2002.

Jenkins, Philip. *The Next Christendom: The Coming of Global Christianity*. Oxford: Oxford University Press, 2002.

Jennings, Michael. "'A Matter of Vital Importance': The Place of the Medical Mission in Maternal and Child Healthcare in Tanganyika, 1919–39," in *Healing Bodies, Saving Souls: Medical Missions in Asia and Africa*, edited by David Hardiman, 227–250. New York: Rodopi B.V., 2006.

Jett, J. *The Role of Traditional Midwives in the Modern Health Sector in West and Central Africa*. Washington, DC: US Agency for International Development, 1977.

Johnson-Hank, Jennifer. *Uncertain Honor: Modern Motherhood in an African Crisis*. Chicago: University of Chicago Press, 2005.

Kaler, Amy. *Running After Pills: Politics, Gender, and Contraception in Colonial Zimbabwe*. Portsmouth: Heinemann, 2003.

Kalusa, Walima. "From an Agency of Cultural Destruction to an Agency of Public Health: Transformations in Catholic Missionary Medicine in Post-Colonial Eastern Zambia, 1964–1982." *Social Sciences and Missions* 27 (2014): 219–238.

Kirk, Dudley. "Population Changes and the Postwar World." *American Sociological Review* 9, no. 1 (1944): 148–157.

Klausen, Susanne. *Race, Maternity, and the Politics of Birth Control in South Africa, 1910–39*. London: Palgrave Macmillan, 2004.

Kleinman, Arthur. *Patients and Healers in the Context of Culture*. Berkeley: University of California Press, 1980.

Kline, Wendy. *Building a Better Race: Gender, Sexuality, and Eugenics from the Turn of the Century to the Baby Boom*. Berkeley: University of California Press, 2005.

Korieh, Chima, and Ralph Chijioke Njoku. *Missions, States, and European Expansions in Africa*. New York: Routledge, 2007.

Lado, L., C. Felicien, and J. Azetsop. "The Social Construction of the Legitimacy of Christian Healing in Abidjan." *Journal of Contemporary African Studies* 36, no. 3 (2018): 334–350.

Langwick, Stacey. *Bodies, Politics and African Healing: The Matter of Maladies in Tanzania*. Bloomington: Indiana University Press, 2011.

Last, Murray, et al. *The Professionalization of African Medicine*. Manchester: Manchester University Press, 1986.

Lesthaeghe, Ron J., ed. *Reproduction and Social Organization in Sub-Saharan Africa*. Berkeley: University of California Press, 1989.

Levine, Philippa, ed. *Gender and Empire*. Oxford: Oxford University Press, 2004.

Lewis, Jane. *The Politics of Motherhood: Child and Maternal Welfare in England 1900–1939*. London: Croom Helm, 1980.

Linden, Jane, and Ian Linden. "John Chilembwe and the New Jerusalem." *Journal of African History* 12, no. 4 (1971): 629–651.

Loustaunau, Martha, and Elisa J. Sobo. *The Cultural Context of Health, Illness, and Medicine*. Westport, CT: Bergin and Garvey, 1997.

Lovejoy, Paul. "Concubinage and the Status of Women Slaves in Early Colonial Northern Nigeria." *Journal of African History* 29, no. 2 (1988): 245–266.

Lovejoy, Paul, and Jan Hogendorn. *Slow Death of Slavery: The Course of Abolition in Northern Nigeria, 1897–1936*. Cambridge, UK: Cambridge University Press, 1993.

Lugard, Frederick, and John Dealtry. *The Dual Mandate in British Tropical Africa*. London: William Blackwood and Sons, 1922.

Maglacas, Mangay-Maglacas A., and John Simons. *The Potential of the Traditional Birth Attendant*. Geneva: World Health Organization, 1986.

Makinde, M. Akin. *African Philosophy, Culture, and Traditional Medicine*. Athens: Ohio University Center for International Studies, 1988.

Marc, M., Misty L. Bastian, and Susan Kingsley Kent. *The Women's War of 1929: Gender and Violence in Colonial Nigeria*. Basingstoke: Palgrave Macmillan, 2011.

Marks, Shula. *Divided Sisterhood: Race, Class and Gender in Southern African Nursing Profession*. Witwatersrand: Wits University Press, 1994.

Martin, Emily. *The Woman in the Body: A Cultural Analysis of Reproduction*. Boston: Beacon Press, 1989.

Mathews, Holly F. "Doctors and Root Doctors: Patients Who Use Both," in *Herbal and Magical Medicine: Traditional Healing Today*, edited by James Kirkland et al., 68–98. Durham, NC: Duke University Press, 1992.

Mbah, Ndubueze. *Emergent Masculinities: Gendered Power and Social Change in the Biafran Atlantic Age*. Athens: Ohio University Press, 2019.

McClintock, Anne. *Imperial Leather: Race, Gender, and Sexuality in the Colonial Conquest*. New York: Routledge, 1995.

Meek, C. K. *Law and Authority in a Nigerian Tribe*. London: Oxford University Press, 1937.

Merchant, Emily. *Building the Population Bomb*. Oxford: Oxford University Press, 2021.

Mimiko, Olusegun. "Experiences with Universal Health Coverage of Maternal Health Care in Ondo State, Nigeria, 2009–2017." *African Journal of Reproductive Health* 21, no. 3 (2017): 9–26.

Mohr, Adam. "Faith Tabernacle Congregation and the Emergence of Pentecostalism in Colonial Nigeria, 1910s–1941." *Journal of Religion in Africa* 43 (2013): 196–221.

Morgan, Robert. "Family Planning Acceptors in Lagos, Nigeria." *Studies in Family Planning* 3, no. 9 (1972): 221–222. https://doi.org/10.2307/1964834.

Mukonyora, I. *Wandering a Gendered Wilderness: Suffering and Healing in an African Initiated Church*. New York: Peter Lang, 2007.

Mume, J. O. *Tradomedicalism: What Is It?* Warri: Jom Nature Cure Center, 1980.

Nasah, B. T., J. K. G. Mati, and J. M. Kasonde. *Contemporary Issues in Maternal Health Care in Africa*. Luxembourg: Hardwood Academic Publishers, 1994.

National Population Commission. *Nigeria Demographic and Health Survey 2008*. Abuja: National Population Commission, Federal Republic of Nigeria and MEASURE DHS+ ORC Macro, 2009.

Nzegwu, Nkiru. *Family Matters: Feminist Concepts in African Philosophy of Culture*. Albany: State University of New York Press, 2006.

Oakley, Ann. *Essays on Women, Medicine, and Health*. Edinburgh: Edinburgh University Press, 1993.

Obermeyer, Carla Makhlouf, ed. *Cultural Perspectives on Reproductive Health*. New York: Oxford University Press, 2001.

Ochonu, Moses. "Conjoined to Empire: The Great Depression and Nigeria." *African Economic History* 34 (2006): 103–145.

Oduntan, O. "Culture and Colonial Medicine: Smallpox in Abeokuta, Western Nigeria." *Social History of Medicine* 30, no. 1 (2017): 48–70.

Ohadike, D. C. "The Influenza Pandemic of 1918–19 and the Spread of Cassava Cultivation on the Lower Niger: A Study in Historical Linkages." *Journal of African History* 22, no. 3 (1981): 379–386.

Ohaja, M., Jo Murphy-Lawless, and Margaret Dunlea, "Midwives Views of Traditional Birth Attendants within Formal Healthcare in Nigeria." *Women and Birth* 32, no. 2 (2020): 111.

Okeke, Edward, et al. *The Better Obstetrics in Rural Nigeria (Born) Study: An Impact Evaluation of the Nigerian Midwives Service Scheme*. Santa Monica, CA: Rand Corporation, 2015.

Olajubu, Aanuoluwapo, et al. "Mothers' Experiences with mHealth Intervention for Postnatal Care Utilisation in Nigeria: A Qualitative Study." *Bmc Pregnancy and Childbirth* 22 (2022): 1–11. https://doi.org/10.1186/s12884-022-05177-x.

Olsen, William, and Carolyn Sargent, eds. *African Medical Pluralism*. Bloomington: Indiana University Press, 2017.

Olupona, Jacob, and Toyin Falola. *Religion and Society in Nigeria: Historical and Sociological Perspectives*. Ibadan: Spectrum Books Ltd., 1991.

Olusanya, G. O. "The Freed Slaves' Homes—An Unknown Aspect of Northern Nigerian Social History." *Journal of the Historical Society of Nigeria* 3, no. 3 (1966): 523–538.

Onabamiro, Sanya. *Why Our Children Die: The Causes and Suggestions for Prevention of Infant Mortality in West Africa*. London: Methuen, 1949.

Orobator, A. E. *Religion and Faith in Africa: Confessions of an Animist*. Maryknoll, NY: Orbis Books, 2018.

Osseo-Asare, Abena. *Bitter Roots: The Search for Healing Plants in Africa*. Chicago: University of Chicago Press, 2014.

Osseo-Asare, Abena. "'Don't Use Herbs in Labor!': Plants, Pharmaceuticals, and the Unmaking of Traditional Birth Attendants in Ghana, 1970–2000." *Social Science and Medicine* 329 (2023): 1–10. https://doi.org/10.1016/j.socscimed.2023.115980.

Otsea, Karen, and Family Care International. *Progress and Prospects: The Safe Motherhood Initiative, 1987–1992*. Washington, DC: The World Bank, 1992.

Oyewumi, Oyeronke. *Gender Epistemologies in Africa: Gendering Traditions, Spaces, Social Institutions, and Identities*. New York: Palgrave Macmillan, 2010.

Oyewumi, Oyeronke. *The Invention of Women: Making an African Sense of Western Gender Discourses*. Minneapolis: University of Minnesota Press, 1997.

Oyewumi, Oyeronke. *What Gender Is Motherhood? Changing Yoruba Ideals of Power, Procreation, and Identity in the Age of Modernity*. London: Palgrave Macmillan, 2015.

Patton, Adell. *Physicians, Colonial Racism, and Diaspora in West Africa*. Gainesville: University Press of Florida, 1996.

Peek, Philip. *Twins in African and Diaspora Cultures: Double Trouble, Twice Blessed*. Bloomington: Indiana University Press, 2011.

Peel, J. D. Y. *Aladura: A Religious Movement among the Yoruba*. London: Oxford University Press, 1968.

Pierce, Tola Olu. "She Will Not Be Listened to in Public: Perceptions among the Yoruba of Infertility and Childlessness in Women." *Reproductive Health Matters* 7, no. 13 (1999): 69.

Pierce, Tola Olu. "Women's Reproductive Practices and Biomedicine: Cultural Conflicts and Transformations in Nigeria," in *Conceiving the New World Order: The Global Politics of Reproduction*, edited by Faye Ginsburgh and Rayna Rapp. Berkeley: University of California Press, 1995.

Practicing Midwifery in Nigeria (Ordinances and Laws) 1930–1992, compiled by P. N. Ndatsu. Abuja: Nursing and Midwifery Council of Nigeria, 1999.

Pretorius, H. L. *Historiography and Historical Sources Regarding African Indigenous Churches in South Africa: Writing Indigenous Church History*. Lewisten, ME: E. Mellen Press, 1995.

Quaye, Randolph. *Underdevelopment and Health Care in Africa: The Ghanaian Experience*. New York: Edwin Mellen Press, 1996.

Ranger, Terence. "The Invention of Tradition in Colonial Africa," in *The Invention of Tradition*, edited by Eric Hobsbawm and Terence Ranger. New York: Cambridge University Press, 1983.

Rasmussen, Susan J. *Those Who Touch: Tuareg Medicine Women in Anthropological Perspectives*. Dekalb: Northern Illinois University Press, 2006.

Riedmann, Agnes. *Science That Colonizes: A Critique of Fertility Studies in Africa*. Philadelphia: Temple University Press, 1993.

Roberts, Dorothy. *Killing the Black Body: Race, Reproduction, and the Meaning of Liberty*. New York: Pantheon Books, 1997.

Roberts, Jonathan. *Sharing the Burden of Sickness: A History of Healing and Medicine in Accra*. Bloomington: Indiana University Press, 2021.

Roseveare, Margaret. *High Spring: The Story of Iyi-Enu Hospital*. London: Church Missionary Society, 1946.

Sackey, B. *New Directions In Gender and Religion: The Changing Status of Women in African Independent Churches*. Lanham, MD: Rowman & Littlefield, 2006.

Sacks, K. "An Overview of Women and Power in Africa," in *Perspectives on Power: Women in Africa, Asia, and Latin America*, edited by J. O'Barr. Durham, NC: Duke University, Center for International Studies, 1982.

Sai, F. T. "The Safe Motherhood Initiative: A Call for Action." *IPPF Medical Bulletin* 21, no. 3 (1987): 1–2.

Sanneh, Lamin. *West African Christianity: The Religious Impact*. London: Allen and Unwin, 1983.

Sargent, C. *Maternity, Medicine, and Power: Reproductive Decisions in Urban Benin*. Berkeley: University of California Press, 1989.

Schram, Ralph. *A History of the Nigerian Health Services*. Ibadan: Ibadan University Press, 1973.

Selin, Helaine, and Pamela K. Stone. *Childbirth across Cultures: Ideas and Practices of Pregnancy, Childbirth and the Postpartum*. London: Springer, 2009.

Shiloh, Ailon. *Faith Healing: The Religious Experience as a Therapeutic Process*. Springfield, IL: Thomas, 1981.

Singer, Philip, ed. *Traditional Healing: New Science or New Colonialism?* New York: Conch Magazine Limited, 1977.

Stephens, Rhiannon. *A History of African Motherhood: The Case of Uganda, 700–1900*. Cambridge, UK: Cambridge University Press, 2013.

Stevenson, Robert. *Population and Political Systems in Tropical Africa*. New York: Columbia University Press, 1968.

Stirrett, A. P. *Medical Book for the Treatment of Diseases in West Africa*. Jos: The Niger Press, 1922.

Strobel, Margaret. *European Women and the Second British Empire*. Bloomington: Indiana University Press, 1991.

Summers, Carol. "Intimate Colonialism: The Imperial Production of Reproduction in Uganda, 1907–1925." *Signs* 16 (1991): 807.

Sundkler, Bengt, and Christopher Steed. *A History of the Church in Africa*. Cambridge, UK: Cambridge University Press, 2000.

Talbot, Amaury. *Some Nigerian Fertility Cults*. New York: Barnes and Nobles, 1927.

Talbot, Amaury. *Woman's Mysteries of a Primitive People, the Ibibios of Southern Nigeria*. London: Cassell and Company Limited, 1915.

Tasie, G. O. M. *Christian Missionary Enterprise in the Niger Delta, 1864–1918*. Leiden: E. J. Brill, 1978.

Thomas, Lynn. *Politics of the Womb: Women, Reproduction, and the State in Kenya*. Berkeley: University of California Press, 2003.

Turner, H. W. *History of an African Independent Church*. Oxford: Clarendon Press, 1967.

Turrittin, Jane. "Colonizing Midwives and Modernizing Childbirth in French West Africa," in *Women in African Colonial Histories*, edited by Susan Geiger, Jean Allman, and Nakanyike Musisi. Bloomington: Indiana University Press, 2002, 72–115.

Turshen, Meredith, ed. *Women and Health in Africa*. Trenton, NJ: Africa World Press Inc., 1991.

Ubah, C. N. "The Colonial Administration in Northern Nigeria and the Problem of Freed Slave Children." *Slavery and Abolition* 14, no. 3 (1993): 208–233.

Uchenna, Chinenye, and Banke-Thomas Aduragbemi. "There Is No Ideal Place but It Is Best to Deliver in a Hospital: Expectations and Experiences of Health Facility-Based Childbirth in Imo State Nigeria." *Pan African Medical Journal* 36, no. 317 (2020): 1–14. https://doi.org/10.11604/pamj.2020.36.317.22728.

Ulin, P. R., Good Rappaport, and Anita Spring. *Traditional Healers and Primary Health Care in Africa*. New York: Syracuse University, African Series 35, 1980.

Van Allen, Judith. "'Sitting on a Man': Colonialism and the Lost Political Institutions of Igbo Women." *Canadian Journal of African Studies/Revue Canadienne Des Études Africaines* 6, no. 2 (1972): 165–181.

Van Teijlingen, Edwin R., George W. Lowis, Peter McCaffery, and Maureen Porter, eds. *Midwifery and the Medicalization of Childbirth: Comparative Perspectives*. New York: Nova Publishers, 2004.

Van Tol, Deanne. "Mothers Babies and the Colonial State: The Introduction of Maternal and Infant Welfare Services in Nigeria 1925–1945." *Spontaneous Generations: A Journal for the History and Philosophy of Science* 1 (2007): 110–131. https://doi.org/10.4245/sponge.v1i1.1761.

Vaughan, Megan. *Curing Their Ills: Colonial Power and African Illness*. Stanford, CA: Stanford University Press, 1991.

Wall, Andrew. "Crowther, Samuel Adjai (or Ajayi)," in *Biographical Dictionary of Christian Missions*, edited by Gerald H. Anderson. New York: Macmillan Reference USA, 1998.

Wall, Andrew. "The Legacy of Samuel Ajayi Crowther." *International Bulletin of Missionary Research* 16, no. 1 (1992): 19–20.

Wall, L. Lewis. *Hausa Medicine: Illness and Well-Being in a West African Culture*. Durham, NC: Duke University Press, 1988.

Washington, Harriet. *Medical Apartheid: The Dark History of Medical Experimentation on Black Americans from the Colonial Times to the Present*. New York: Harlem Moon, 2008.

Wendland, Claire. *Partial Stories: Maternal Death from Six Angles*. Chicago: University of Chicago Press, 2022.

Williams, Ogechukwu. "A Blur between the Spiritual and the Physical: Birthing Practices among the Igbo of Nigeria in the Twentieth Century," in *Sacred Inception: Reclaiming the Spirituality of Birth in the Modern World*, edited by Marianne Delaporte and Morag Martins, 97–112. Lanham: Lexington Books, 2018.

Williams, Ogechukwu. "Medical Legitimacy: Childbirth, Pluralism, and Professionalization in Nigeria's Faith- Based Aladura Birthing Homes." *Journal of African History* 64, no. 1 (2023): 96–111.

Williams, Ogechukwu. "The Politics of Labels: Imperial Categorizations and the Marginalisation of Ethnomedicine in Nigeria during the 20th Century." *Social History of Medicine* 34, no. 1 (2021): 1297–1316.

World Health Organization. *World Health Day, Safe Motherhood 7 April 1998*. Geneva: Division of Reproductive Health, 1998.

Index

Figures and tables are indicated by "f" and "t" following page numbers.